Patient-Centered Medicine
Transforming the Clinical Method

THIRD EDITION

MOIRA STEWART, JUDITH BELLE BROWN,
W. WAYNE WESTON, IAN R MCWHINNEY,
CAROL L MCWILLIAM AND
THOMAS R FREEMAN

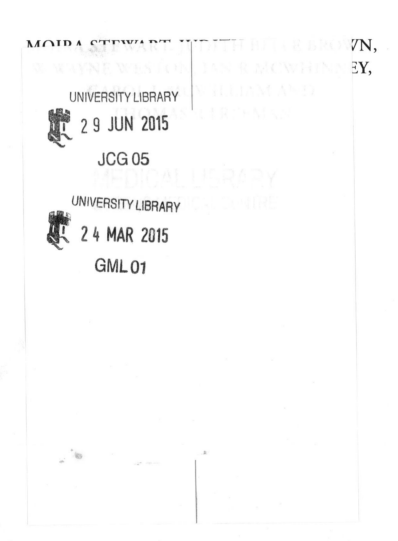

Radcliffe Publishing
London • New York

Radcliffe Publishing Ltd
St Mark's House
Shepherdess Walk
London N1 7LH
United Kingdom

www.radcliffehealth.com

First Edition 1995 (Sage)
Second Edition 2003

British Library Cataloguing in Publication Data

A catalogue record for this book is available from the British Library.

ISBN-13: 978 184619 566 2

The paper used for the text pages of this book is FSC® certified. FSC (The Forest Stewardship Council®) is an international network to promote responsible management of the world's forests.

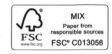

Typeset by Darkriver Design, Auckland, New Zealand
Printed and bound by TJI Digital, Padstow, Cornwall, UK

Contents

Preface to the Third Edition

The principles underpinning the patient-centered clinical method remain constant but the components have changed: there are now four components instead of six. "Being Realistic," one of the previous components, was considered not to be part of clinical care and so its material on time and teamwork was moved to other parts of the book. "Prevention and Health Promotion," the second of the previous components to be changed, was considered to be incorporated into each patient-clinician interaction and therefore has become part of the other components. Conceptual clarity has been achieved regarding where Health Promotion fits in patient-centered care and where Prevention fits (*see* Chapter 1). The teaching and learning chapters comprise an up-to-the-minute compendium of the relevant education literature and methods. The research chapters illuminate patient-centered concepts through stories of lived experiences, and they also provide clear, positive, and uplifting messages about the important impact of patient-centered clinical care.

This book is divided into five parts. Part One contains an introduction to the patient-centered clinical method, including its evolution and relationship to other models of care. In addition, common misconceptions about the meaning of patient-centeredness are elucidated. The second chapter in this part is a historic perspective written by Ian R McWhinney.

Part Two describes the four interactive components of the patient-centered clinical method. Chapters 3–7 elaborate in detail Components 1–4, respectively. The clinical reader will notice the cases illustrating each of the four components of the patient-centered approach that are embedded in Chapters 3–7. Those most interested in the application of patient-centeredness in everyday practice might enjoy reading the cases first. As McWhinney (2001: 88) has wisely noted, "An actual case brings things alive for us in a way that aggregated data cannot do." Taken together, the cases represent a typical series of patients in the practice of a busy doctor. All the cases are based on actual clinical encounters; however, the names, dates, and places have been altered to ensure the confidentiality of the participants.

Part Three, on teaching and learning, contains five chapters. Chapter 8 examines the experience of medical education. The parallel between the learner-centered method of medical education and patient-centered practice is described in Chapter 9. Practicing, learning, and teaching patient-centered medicine has many personal, professional, and systemic challenges, as Chapter 10 illustrates. Chapter 11 contains details on teaching strategies and practical tips for teaching the patient-centered clinical method. A particular teaching tool, the patient-centered case presentation, is described in Chapter 12.

Part Four of the book deals with two key health care contexts within which patient-centered clinical care is enacted. In Chapter 13 the context of teamwork is explored. In Chapter 14 the preoccupation with cost restraint in health care is dealt with by providing the news that patient-centered care saves money.

Part Five, on research, combines reviews of relevant literature with descriptions of important measures. Qualitative and quantitative methodologies are represented. Chapter 15 presents a description of qualitative findings that illuminate the patient-centered clinical method. Chapter 16 is a review of quantitative studies – in particular, a number of stunning systematic reviews. In Chapter 17 we present measures of patient perceptions of patient-centered care and their use in research and education. Chapter 18 describes a measure we have developed that uniquely assesses encounters according to the patient-centered clinical method.

In the final chapter, we summarize the key messages of this book and look to the future of challenge and reward in the practice, teaching, and research of the patient-centered clinical method.

Moira Stewart
Judith Belle Brown
W Wayne Weston
Ian R McWhinney
Carol L McWilliam
Thomas R Freeman
London, Ontario, Canada
October 2013

About the Authors

Judith Belle Brown, PhD in Social Work from Smith College, Northampton, Massachusetts, is a Professor in the Centre for Studies in Family Medicine, the Department of Family Medicine, Schulich School of Medicine & Dentistry at Western University, and in the School of Social Work at King's University College, London, Ontario, Canada. She is the Chair of the Masters in Clinical Science and PhD programs in Family Medicine at Western University, both of which are offered via distance education. She has been conducting research on the patient-centered clinical method for over 3 decades. Dr Brown has presented papers and conducted workshops both nationally (Canada and the United States) and internationally (the United Kingdom, Holland, Spain, Hong Kong, Sweden, New Zealand, Australia, Denmark, Argentina, Brazil, Japan) on the patient-centered method. She is the co-author of *Patient-Centered Medicine: transforming the clinical method* and is a series editor, along with Moira Stewart and Thomas R Freeman, of the following books all published by Radcliffe Publishing: *Substance Abuse: A Patient-Centered Approach* (2002), *Chronic Fatigue Syndrome: A Patient-Centered Approach* (2002), *Chronic Myofascial Pain: A Patient-Centered Approach* (2002), *Eating Disorders: A Patient-Centered Approach* (2002), *Patient-Centered Prescribing: Seeking Concordance in Practice* (2007), *Palliative Care: A Patient-Centered Approach* (2008), *Pregnancy and Childbirth: A Woman-Centered Approach* (2010), and *Serious Mental Illness: Person-Centered Approaches* (2011). She has also published papers dealing with patient-doctor communication in *Social Science and Medicine, Family Practice: An International Journal, Patient Education and Counseling, Canadian Family Physician*, and *Journal of Family Practice*. Dr Brown was a co-recipient of The American Academy on Physician and Patient Award for Outstanding Research in 1996. In the same year, Dr Brown was made an Honorary Member of the College of Family Physicians of Canada. She was a co-recipient of the College of Family Physicians of Canada Best Original Research Article Award (2009) and the Dean's Award of Excellence – Team Award for the Centre for Studies in Family Medicine, The Schulich School of Medicine & Dentistry, Western University (2010).

Thomas R Freeman, BSc, MD, MClSc, CCFP, FCFP, is a medical graduate of Western University, London, Ontario, Canada, completing his residency training in Family Medicine at Dalhousie University, Halifax, Nova Scotia, Canada. He practiced full service, comprehensive family medicine in a small town in Southwestern Ontario for 11 years, during which time he was involved with undergraduate education on a part-time basis and acquired a Masters of Clinical Science degree. He moved to a full-time academic practice at Western University in 1989. He is a Professor and Past Chair/Chief of Family Medicine at Western University and the London Health Sciences Centre and St. Joseph's Health Care London. Areas of research interest include vaccine adverse effects, risk perception and risk communication, health service delivery, health human resources, primary care renewal, and conflict of interest in academic medicine. He has published in the *Journal of Family Practice, Family Practice: An International Journal, Canadian Family Physician,* and the *Canadian Medical Association Journal* and he is a series editor, along with Moira Stewart and Judith Belle Brown, of the books *Substance Abuse: primary care challenges for patients providers and communities* (2002), *Patient-Centered Care of People with Chronic Fatigue Syndrome (CFS)* (2002), *Patient-Centered Approach to Chronic Myofascial Pain in Primary Care* (2002), *Eating Disorders: A Patient-Centered Approach* (2002), *Palliative Care: A Patient-Centered Approach* (2008), *Patient-Centered Prescribing: Seeking Concordance in Practice* (2007), *Challenges and Solutions: Narratives of Patient-Centered Care* (2012), *Women-Centered Care in Pregnancy and Childbirth* (2010), and *Serious Mental Illnesses: Person-Centered Approaches* (2011) all published by Radcliffe Publishing. He is co-author, with Dr Ian McWhinney, of the *Textbook of Family Medicine,* 3rd ed. (Oxford University Press, 2009).

Ian R McWhinney, OC, MD, FCFP, FRCP, is Professor Emeritus in the Department of Family Medicine at Western University, London, Ontario, Canada. He was born in Burnley, Lancashire, and educated at Cambridge University and St. Bartholomew's Hospital Medical School. For 14 years he was a general practitioner in Stratford-on-Avon. In 1968 he was appointed Foundation Professor of Family Medicine at Western University. He retired in 1992 and had a post-retirement appointment in the Centre for Studies in Family Medicine. His most recent books are a third edition of the *Textbook of Family Medicine* (2009) and *A Call to Heal* (Benchmark Press, 2012).

Carol L McWilliam, MScN, EdD, is a Professor in the Arthur Labatt Family School of Nursing, Faculty of Health Sciences, at Western University, London,

Ontario, Canada. She conducts research in the areas of health promotion, health services delivery, and relationship building, with a focus on patient-professional and interprofessional communication. She makes a unique contribution to the field as a qualitative research methodologist, with work published in *Social Science and Medicine*, *Family Medicine*, *Patient Education and Counseling*, *Journal of Advanced Nursing*, *International Journal of Quality in Health Care*, and *International Journal of Health Promotion*.

Moira Stewart, PhD, is a Distinguished University Professor at the Centre for Studies in Family Medicine at Western University, London, Ontario, Canada, and the Dr Brian W Gilbert Canada Research Chair in Primary Health Care Research. Dr Stewart has published widely on the topic of patient-centered care and has edited, with colleagues, an international series of books applying the patient-centered clinical method. The series now has eight books elaborating patient-centered principles on the topics of serious mental illness, pregnancy and childbirth, prescribing, palliative care, substance abuse, chronic fatigue, eating disorders, and chronic myofascial pain. She is Co-Principal Investigator of a National Team Grant on Patient-Centered Innovations for Persons with Multimorbidity. She trains young researchers as the Principal Investigator on a CIHR Strategic Training Grant on interdisciplinary primary health care research called TUTOR-PHC. Dr Stewart works with clinicians on a project creating a researchable database of the Electronic Medical Record data with approximately 50 family physicians in Southwestern Ontario. She works closely with policy-makers on collaborative programs of research such as the Primary Health Care Program funded by Ontario's Health System Research Fund. Dr Stewart received the James Mackenzie Medal of the Royal College of General Practitioners (2004), The College of Family Physicians of Canada Family Medicine Researcher of the Year Award (2007), and the Martin J Bass Recognition Award, Department of Family Medicine (2008), and she is co-recipient of the Dean's Award of Excellence – Team Award at the Schulich School of Medicine & Dentistry (2010) and The College of Family Physicians of Canada Lifetime Achievement Award in Family Medicine Research (2012).

W Wayne Weston, MD, CCFP, FCFP, is Professor Emeritus of Family Medicine at the Schulich School of Medicine & Dentistry, Western University, London, Ontario, Canada. After graduating from the University of Toronto in 1964, he practiced in the small village of Tavistock, Ontario, for 10 years before joining the faculty at Western University where he has a special interest in patient-physician communication and medical education. He taught a graduate course on teaching and learning for 30 years as part of the Master of Clinical Science in Family Medicine at Western. He has published over 190 articles in such journals as *Canadian Family Physician, Canadian Medical Association Journal, Academic Medicine, Medical Teacher,* and *Medical Education.* He has provided over 400 presentations and workshops for faculty on many topics – including patient-centered interviewing, problem-based learning, and clinical teaching – in Canada, New Zealand, Scotland, the United States, the United Arab Emirates, and Kazakhstan. He has received the Dean's Award of Excellence for Teaching from the Schulich School of Medicine & Dentistry, Western University (2001), the Douglas Bocking Award for Excellence in Medical Teaching from the Schulich School of Medicine & Dentistry, Western University (2005), and the prestigious 3M Award for Excellence in University Teaching in Canada (1992). He was the first recipient of the Ian McWhinney Family Medicine Education Award (1998) and the first family physician to receive the Canadian Association for Medical Education Award for Distinguished Contribution to Medical Education (2001). Now retired from practice, after almost 40 years, he continues to be active in educational consulting.

List of Contributors

Ms Christina Bodea
Former Research Assistant, Centre for Studies in Family Medicine
Schulich School of Medicine & Dentistry, Western University
London, Ontario

Ms Lynn Brown
Social Worker, WestBridge Associates Counselling and Consulting Services
London, Ontario

Dr Clarissa Burke
Family Physician, Middlesex Centre Regional Medical Clinic
Ilderton, Ontario
Assistant Professor, Department of Family Medicine
Schulich School of Medicine & Dentistry, Western University
London, Ontario

Dr Sonny Cejic
Family Physician
Associate Professor, Department of Family Medicine
Schulich School of Medicine & Dentistry, Western University
London, Ontario

Dr Sara Hahn
Family Physician Resident, Department of Family Medicine
Schulich School of Medicine & Dentistry, Western University
London, Ontario

Ms Vera Henderson
Family Practice Nurse, Middlesex Centre Regional Medical Clinic
Ilderton, Ontario

Dr Gina Higgins
Family Physician, Killick Health Services
Grand Falls, Newfoundland

Dr Gerald Choon-Huat Koh
Associate Professor and Director of Undergraduate Medical Education
Saw Swee Hock School of Public Health
Joint Associate Professor, Dean's Office, Yong Loo Lin School of Medicine
National University of Singapore/National University Health System
Singapore

Dr Barry Lavallee
Acting Director, University of Manitoba's Centre for Aboriginal Health
Education
Centre for Human Rights Research
University of Manitoba
Winnipeg, Manitoba

Ms Leslie Meredith
Research Associate, Centre for Studies in Family Medicine
Schulich School of Medicine & Dentistry, Western University
London, Ontario

Ms Joan Mitchell
Nurse Practitioner, Byron Family Medical Centre
London, Ontario

Dr Christine Rivet
Associate Professor, Department of Family Medicine
University of Ottawa
Ottawa, Ontario

Dr Bridget L Ryan
Postdoctoral Fellow, Centre for Studies in Family Medicine
Schulich School of Medicine & Dentistry, Western University
London, Ontario

Dr Lynn Shaw
Occupational Therapist, Associate Professor, Field Chair, Occupational Science
School of Occupational Therapy
Faculty of Health Sciences, Western University
London, Ontario

Dr Darren Van Dam
Family Physician, Middlesex Centre Regional Medical Clinic
Ilderton, Ontario
Assistant Professor, Department of Family Medicine
Schulich School of Medicine & Dentistry, Western University
London, Ontario

Dr Jamie Wickett
Family Physician, Victoria Family Medical Centre
London, Ontario
Assistant Professor, Department of Family Medicine
Schulich School of Medicine & Dentistry, Western University
London, Ontario

Acknowledgments

We thank the Department of Family Medicine at Western University, Canada, for providing a supportive environment in which to write this book. In particular, we want to express our gratitude to Dr Brian KE Hennen, Chair of the Department of Family Medicine (from 1987 to 1999), and Chair Dr Thomas R Freeman (from 1999 to 2011) for their encouragement of scholarly activities.

We are indebted to our patients and research participants who generously shared their stories of suffering and coping with suffering; our colleagues who shared their stories of caring for patients, exposing both their failures and their triumphs; and our students who stimulated our thinking on patient-centered care and encouraged us to clarify the concepts.

Andrea Burt's combination of coordination skills and perpetual aura of calm has been indispensable. Her attention to detail and organizational abilities are extraordinary. Evelyn Levy has been stellar in completing the multiple drafts of the manuscript. Leslie Meredith created the excellent diagrams. Magda Catani and Michele VanderSpank assisted with the preparation of the chapters.

We would like to extend our sincere thanks to Gillian Nineham and her incredible team at Radcliffe Publishing. Again they have all been fabulous to work with.

Finally, we would like to express our heartfelt appreciation for all the support and encouragement provided by our families – in particular, Murray Brown, Kate and Amy Freeman, and Sharon Weston.

The Dr Brian W Gilbert Canada Research Chair in Primary Health Care Research funds Dr Moira Stewart.

This book is dedicated to Joseph H Levenstein, MD, for his inspiration to us and his outstanding contribution to the practice of medicine. We are grateful to Dr Levenstein for introducing us to the patient-centered clinical method during his time as a visiting professor in our department in 1981–1982.

We also dedicate this book to the late Ian R McWhinney, MD, who invited Joseph to come to Western University as a visiting professor and provided him and all of us with an intellectually stimulating and nurturing environment in which to co-create the ideas in this book.

PART ONE

Overview

1 Introduction

Moira Stewart, Judith Belle Brown, W Wayne Weston,
Thomas R Freeman, and Carol L McWilliam

In the 1980s, when the patient-centered clinical method was first being conceptualized and used in research and education, it was at the periphery of medicine (Brown *et al.*, 1986, 1989; Levenstein *et al.*, 1986; Stewart *et al.*, 1986, 1989; Weston *et al.*, 1989). Indeed, many educators and researchers viewed patient-centered medicine as a "soft science" – caring and compassion were acknowledged to be important aspects of humanitarian care but few people were aware of the pivotal role of patient-centered communication in modern scientific medicine. In the first edition of this book, we described the full patient-centered clinical method, with the goal of placing it at the epicenter of clinical practice and medical education (Stewart *et al.*, 1995).

Since that time we have learned much by presenting the patient-centered clinical method to many groups of medical students, residents, graduate fellows, community physicians, and medical school faculties across North America, Europe, Turkey, the United Arab Emirates, Argentina, Brazil, Australia, New Zealand, Japan, and Southeast Asia. The patient-centered clinical method now forms the basis of many educational curricula internationally, at both the undergraduate and the graduate level (Stewart & Ryan, 2012). Furthermore, the patient-centered clinical method serves as the guide for the summative evaluation of postgraduate training in several countries (Brown *et al.*, 1996; Tate *et al.*, 1999). Research, focusing on the patient-centered clinical method, has exploded in the past decade. International studies reinforce not only the patients' desire for, and satisfaction with, patient-centered care but also the positive impact of such care on patient outcomes, health care utilization, and costs of care (Dwamena *et al.*, 2012; Epstein, 2005b; Stewart *et al.*, 2011). These studies support an emerging international definition of patient-centered care.

There is still much work to be done! The current context of health care sometimes discourages patient-centered practice. For example, a recent study by Neumann *et al.* (2011) has found that empathy declines over the years of medical education. Those of us who had hoped that such findings were a thing of the past have had a wake-up call. Further, Cassell (2013: xii) says we "still do not know how to do it nor how to teach it." It has been 10 years since the second edition of this book. Our hope, in launching this third edition, is that it will aid those engaged in improving care through the patient-centered clinical method, by providing constructive information and encouragement.

THE PATIENT-CENTERED CLINICAL METHOD

The Department of Family Medicine at Western University, Ontario, Canada, began work on the patient-doctor relationship at its inception with the arrival in 1968 of the inaugural Chairperson, Dr Ian R McWhinney. His work elucidating the "real reason" the patient presented to the doctor (McWhinney, 1972) set the stage for explorations of the breadth of all patient problems, whether physical, social, or psychological, and depth, the meaning of the patient's presentation. The research of his PhD student Moira Stewart was guided by these interests and began to focus on the patient-physician relationship (Stewart *et al.*, 1975, 1979; Stewart & Buck, 1977). In 1982, Dr Joseph Levenstein, a visiting professor of family medicine from South Africa, shared with us his attempts to develop a model of practice and stimulated the department. The patient-centered clinical method evolved further through the work of the Patient-Doctor Communication Group at Western University.

In this book the patient-centered model and method is described and explained. A program of conceptual development, education, and research, which has been underway for the last 3 decades, provides the material. Although the program took place in the context of family medicine, its messages are relevant to all disciplines of medicine and to other health care professions, such as nursing, social work, physiotherapy, and occupational therapy. The overarching framework is the *model*. The way of implementing the framework reflects the clinical *method*. This book presents both a framework and its implementation, the patient-centered clinical method.

Patient-centered care presupposes several changes in the mindset of the clinician. First, the hierarchical notion of the professional being in charge and the patient being passive does not hold here. To be patient-centered, the practitioner must be able to empower the patient and share the power in the relationship, and this means renouncing control that traditionally has been in the hands of the professional. This is the moral imperative of patient-centered practice. In making this shift in values, the practitioner will experience the new direction the relationship can take when power is shared. Second, maintaining an exclusively objective stance in relation to patients produces an unacceptable insensitivity to human suffering. To be patient-centered requires a balance between the subjective and the objective, a bringing together of the mind and the body.

We have changed the conceptual framework and hence the diagram in significant ways since the first edition of this book. First, there are now four components, not six. The previous component "Being Realistic" was thought to be not so much a component as a comment on the context within which the patient-centered clinical method is enacted. The issues considered as part of "Being Realistic" – time and teamwork – are handled in other, later chapters. As well, the previous component "Incorporating Prevention and Health Promotion" was always conceived as occurring as part of the processes within the other components. Therefore, we have incorporated prevention and health

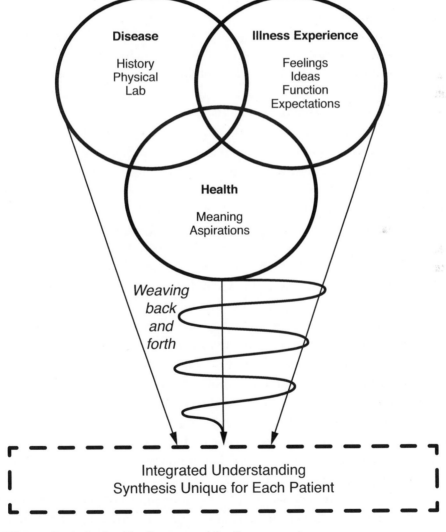

FIGURE 1.1 Exploring health, disease, and the illness experience

promotion as a portion within the chapters on each of the four remaining components.

We incorporated health promotion within Component 1. Health promotion conducted in interactions between patients and clinicians includes exploring the patient's perceptions and experience of health. Its incorporation into Component 1 has the added advantage of making explicit that part of the dialogue between patient and clinician that focuses on the patient's health and strengths. In addition to the explicit focus on a patient's function, which has always been an integral part of the patient's illness experience (in the patient-centered conceptual framework, the four dimensions of the illness experience are feelings, ideas, function, and expectations), the new attention to health (strengths and resilience) strengthens care designed for persons over a lifetime. It aligns with literature in nursing on health promotion and resilience; with literature in occupational and physical therapy highlighting functional strengths, not only functional deficits; and, finally, with new literature on the nature of healing that balances and integrates a patient's function, strengths, and disease into one vision of healing (Cassell, 2013).

Reflecting these considerations, Component 1 is now called "Exploring Health, Disease, and the Illness Experience." As well, the diagram depicting Component 1 has changed (*see* Figure 1.1), now having three intersecting circles (one for health, one for disease, and one for the patient's illness experience). Most important of all is the bottom of the new diagram, which stresses the integration of the relevant aspects of health, disease, and illness experience into a synthesis completely unique for each patient. This integration has always been part of our diagram but it has not always been stressed as much as it will be in the chapters of this current book. We have increased this emphasis here in order to underline that health care does not have two or three goals (such as treating diseases, assisting in mobilizing strengths, or caring for the patient) but, rather, one overarching goal, the holistic health of the patient.

Returning for a moment to the way we have incorporated prevention and health promotion into the remaining four components of the patient-centered clinical method, we included the one-on-one health promotion in Component 1 because it focused on exploring the dimensions of health with the patient. The activities of health education and disease prevention, being actions not explorations, are included in Component 3, "Finding Common Ground."

In this book, therefore, we describe the four interacting components of the patient-centered clinical method, summarized in Box 1.1 and illustrated in Figure 1.2.

Box 1.1 The Four Interactive Components of the Patient-Centered Clinical Method

1. Exploring Health, Disease, and the Illness Experience:
   - unique perceptions and experience of health (meaning and aspirations)
   - history, physical, lab
   - dimensions of the illness experience (feelings, ideas, effects on function and expectations).
2. Understanding the Whole Person:
   - the person (e.g., life history, personal and developmental issues)
   - the proximal context (e.g., family, employment, social support)
   - the distal context (e.g., culture, community, ecosystem).
3. Finding Common Ground:
   - problems and priorities
   - goals of treatment and/or management
   - roles of patient and doctor.
4. Enhancing the Patient-Clinician Relationship:
   - compassion and empathy
   - power
   - healing and hope
   - self-awareness and practical wisdom
   - transference and countertransference.

The first three interactive components encompass the interactions between patient and doctor. The fourth component focuses on the ongoing relationship that forms the foundation on which the interactions occur. Although components are used for ease in teaching and research, patient-centered clinical practice is a holistic concept in which components interact and unite in a unique way in each patient-clinician encounter.

The goal of the *first* component of the patient-centered clinical method is to explore disease and patients' perceptions of health and illness. In addition to assessing the disease process by history and physical examination, the clinician actively seeks to enter into the patient's world to understand both the perceptions of health (its meaning to the patient and his or her aspirations or life goals) and the unique experience of illness (the patient's feelings about being ill, his or her ideas about the illness, how the illness is affecting his or her functioning, and, lastly, what he or she expects from the clinician).

The *second* component is the integration of these concepts (health, disease,

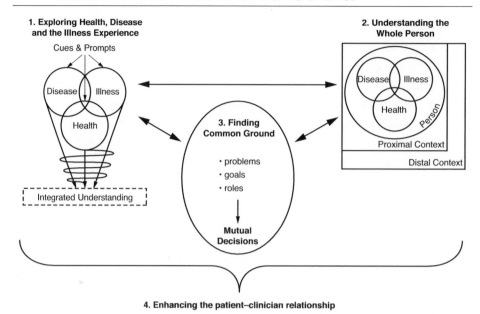

FIGURE 1.2 The patient-centered clinical method: four interactive components

and illness) with an understanding of the whole person. This includes an awareness of the multiple aspects of the patient's life, such as personality, developmental history, life cycle issues, and the multiple contexts in which he or she lives.

The mutual task of finding common ground between patient and clinician is the *third* component of the method and focuses on three key areas: defining the problem, establishing the goals of treatment, and identifying the roles to be assumed by patient and clinician.

The *fourth* component emphasizes that each contact with the patient should be used to build on the patient-clinician relationship by including compassion, empathy, a sharing of power, healing, and hope. To enact these skills requires both mindfulness and practical wisdom, as well as an appreciation of unconscious aspects of the relationship such as transference and countertransference.

THE PATIENT-CENTERED CLINICAL METHOD IN RELATION TO OTHER MODELS OF PRACTICE

Models of practice are valuable in several ways: first, they guide our perceptions by drawing our attention to specific features of practice; second, they provide a framework for understanding what is going on; and third, they guide our actions by defining what is important. A productive model will not only simplify the complexity of reality but also focus our attention on those aspects of a situation that are most important for understanding and effective action. The dominant model in medical practice has been labeled "the conventional medical model." No one would question the widespread influence of the conventional medical model, but it has often been challenged for oversimplifying the problems of sickness (Reiser, 2009; Schleifer & Vannatta, 2013). Engel (1977: 130) describes the problems with the conventional medical model this way:

> It assumes disease to be fully accounted for by deviations from the norm of measurable biological (somatic) variables. It leaves no room within its framework for the social, psychological, and behavioral dimensions of illness. The biomedical model not only requires that disease be dealt with as an entity independent of social behavior, it also demands that behavioral aberrations be explained on the basis of disordered somatic (biochemical or neurophysiological) processes.

Balint and colleagues (Balint *et al.*, 1970; Hopkins & Balint Society, 1972) introduced the term "patient-centered medicine" and contrasted it with "illness-centered medicine." An understanding of the patient's complaints, based on patient-centered thinking, was called "overall diagnosis," and an understanding based on disease-centered thinking was called "traditional diagnosis." Stevens (1974) and Tait (1979) elaborated the clinical method. Byrne and Long (1984) developed a method for categorizing a consultation as doctor-centered or patient-centered, their concept of a doctor-centered consultation being close to other writers' "illness"- or "disease"-centered methods. Wright and MacAdam (1979) also described a doctor- and patient-centered approach to care.

The patient-centered clinical method we describe joins the work of Rogers (1951) on client-centered counseling, Balint (1957) on person-centered medicine, Newman and Young (1972) on the total person approach to patient problems in nursing, and the "Two-Body Practice" in occupational therapy (Mattingly & Fleming, 1994). In addition, there are strong similarities between our work and that of Pendleton *et al.* (2003), who defined, independently, a similar model of practice. Their approach of defining their model as a set of tasks for the physician to perform in the consultation appealed to us and we incorporated this idea into our own model. We refer to the elements of our method as components, rather than tasks, to avoid the misconception that the method is a rigid, linear technique. The practice of medicine cannot be reduced to technique but rather is embedded in a way of thinking about the clinical tasks of medicine that need to be explained clearly and pragmatically (White, 1988).

Epstein *et al.* (1993) have described, compared, and contrasted a number of approaches to patient-doctor communication, including the biopsychosocial model (Engel, 1977; Frankel *et al.*, 2003), the three-function model (Cole & Bird, 2009), the family systems approach to patient care (Doherty & Baird, 1987; McDaniel *et al.*, 2005), physician self-awareness (Balint, 1957), and the patient-centered clinical method presented in this book. Epstein *et al.* (1993: 386) conclude that "on a theoretical level, the complementarity of the approaches is more powerful than their difference." In our view, where they are similar is in their attempt to broaden the conventional medical approach to include psychosocial issues, the family, and the clinician him- or herself.

Two other frameworks for improving care and education have become prominent in the past decade and can be compared and contrasted with the patient-centered clinical method: shared decision making and narrative medicine.

The central tenet of the shared decision-making framework is that power must be more equally shared between patient and practitioner, and we agree (Légaré *et al.*, 2003, 2010; Elwyn *et al.*, 2012; Stiggelbout *et al.*, 2012). Shared decision making and the patient-centered clinical method are most aligned in Component 3, "Finding Common Ground." The approaches are most different in the following three aspects. First. the patient-centered clinical method stresses an emotional engagement with the patient that goes beyond sharing information about experiences, beliefs, and values. Second, the patient-centered clinical method stresses the need for a unique approach to each patient, and even each visit with each patient, using the structure as a guide only, with the main injunction being to follow the patient's lead. The shared decision-making approach, while similar in its attempt to balance the formulaic and the idiosyncratic, has chosen a more standardized approach. Further, its goal is to increase shared decision making. Third, the patient-centered clinical method seeks to integrate its approach into clinical practice, hence its name as a clinical method.

Narrative medicine, in common with the patient-centered clinical method, stresses the patient's particular story (Components 1 and 2 of the patient-centered clinical method) revealed in the context of an ongoing patient-practitioner relationship (Charon, 2006; Launer, 2002). The two approaches also seek to enhance the clinician's comfort in engaging patients at an emotional level. Narrative medicine in Component 3, "Finding Common Ground," is a process of the patient and clinician co-constructing the patient's story to promote both understanding and change. One difference is that narrative medicine separates itself from the tasks of conventional medicine, in contrast to the patient-centered clinical method, which attempts to integrate its work with the medical tasks.

These models in general, and the patient-centered clinical method in particular, set out to make the implicit in patient care explicit. While models help clarify the basics, they never completely capture what happens in reality. The tacit knowledge of the doctor and patient are not captured in the models, which are, by definition, oversimplifications. Stewart (2001: 445) stated that while models do help in teaching and research they "fail to capture the indivisible whole of a healing relationship."

VALUE OF THE PATIENT-CENTERED CLINICAL METHOD

In order to convince colleagues, education committees, and policy-makers of the value of transitioning to a patient-centered approach, one needs to be able to answer the essential questions: Does it work? Do patients want it, and why? Is it more costly?

The series of studies by Little *et al.* (2001a) in the United Kingdom indicate that, whereas only a minority of patients want an X-ray or medication, more than 75% of patients want the elements of a patient-centered approach. Furthermore, the patients wanted all components of patient-centeredness.

We do not find this surprising, given the following data. Recent studies show that adult patients come for medical care with not one condition but multiple conditions at the same time. A focus on one disease will not satisfy these patients. Twenty-three percent of all adult patients have two or more chronic conditions, and of the 65-year-old patients more than 65% have two or more chronic conditions (Barnett *et al.*, 2012). Furthermore, this is only part of the picture – one must add acute conditions. Also, until recently we have not known how frequently patients express their illness experience in their medical visits; such expressions are remarkably common. Figure 1.3 shows that 89% of adult patients expressed ideas about their problems; 72% expressed an expectation about their care; 57% expressed problems with functioning; 55% expressed family, life cycle, or context issues; and 42% expressed concerns, fears, or anger (data from the study called Patient-Centered Care and Outcomes). With this complex of issues being present at each visit with a health professional, a single disease focus will not likely meet the patients' needs.

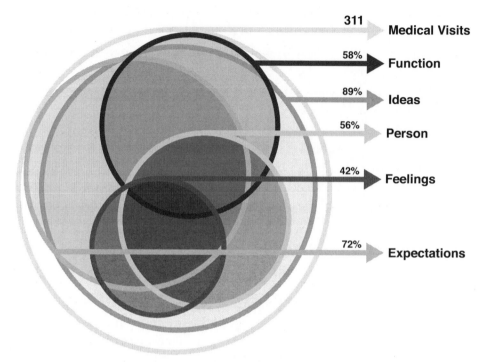

311 → **Medical Visits**

58% → **Function**

89% → **Ideas**

56% → **Person**

42% → **Feelings**

72% → **Expectations**

EXPECTATIONS: patients expressing expectations; **FUNCTION:** patients expressing effects on function; **PERSON:** patients expressing issues regarding the whole person; **IDEAS:** patients expressing ideas; **FEELINGS:** patients expressing feelings during the consultations.
71% of patients expressed 3 or more of the 5 issues depicted in this figure.

FIGURE 1.3 Patients' issues expressed during visits with their family physician

Does patient-centered medicine work? What evidence is there that it positively affects important outcomes? In our view, this is one of the great strides that has been made over the last decade. Chapter 16 shows that the results of several key systematic reviews are very positive. Education interventions to improve patient-centered practice are effective in changing physician behavior. Such interventions are also having more of an impact on patient health outcomes than was the case with previous systematic reviews.

In the context of severe economic restraint, health care costs are an overriding concern for health care managers and policy-makers. Chapter 14 provides Canadian data on patient-centered care in relation to health care costs; as well, there are US data to demonstrate that patient-centered care results in lower costs for diagnostic tests and subsequent use of services (Epstein *et al.*, 2005b).

CHALLENGES TO THE PATIENT-CENTERED CLINICAL METHOD IN THE TWENTY-FIRST CENTURY: THE NEW CONTEXT OF CARE

There are a remarkable number of changes in our society that challenge the practice of patient-centered care. However, some changes can improve the interaction between patients and doctors – for example, emphasis on patient autonomy, interest in ethnic diversity, and increased attention by the public on prevention and health promotion activities. These changes enhance the abilities of patients to become more involved in their own health care.

Paradoxically, being patient-centered actually saves costs to the system, as is shown in Chapter 15; however, this news is not widely known and may not feel like good news for a clinician feeling conflicted between the patient's expressed expectations and his or her need to contain costs.

An emerging trend of decreasing continuity of care, because of pressure either from overworked clinicians or from policy-makers, is likely to be deleterious to the future of patient-centered care. The positive outcomes of continuity of care are well known (Freeman, 2012) and it is a key prerequisite to patient-centered care.

Two aspects of the pervasiveness of information technology may have varied effects on patient-centered care. One is the empowering of patients to learn, in advance of coming to a health professional, about their symptom or condition. Practitioners can consider this a distraction and a time-consuming issue, but it can be reframed as a positive experience. The patient is certainly engaged and ready to learn. The Internet information brought by patients to their practitioners is a new kind of cue that sheds light on the level of the patients' concerns and expectations. Using this information can be a mutual learning experience.

The second aspect of information technology is the use of electronic medical records (EMRs), which has been shown to have some negative effects on the interaction of patients with their health care professionals (Margalit *et al.*, 2006; Noordman *et al.*, 2010). Lown and Rodriguez (2012: 392) suggest that EMRs

> introduce a "third party" into exam room interactions that competes with the patient for clinicians' attention, affects clinicians' capacity to be fully present, and alters the nature of communication, relationships, and physicians' sense of professional role. Screen-driven communication inhibits patients' narratives and diminishes clinicians' responses to patients' cues about psychosocial issues and emotional concerns.

On the other hand, other authors have pointed out improvements in screening for health risks using EMRs (Adams *et al.*, 2003) and better information exchange by being able to show the patient graphs or test results (Shachak & Reis, 2009).

Doctors are being directed to follow a plethora of clinical practice guidelines, with more being produced every day. This can be overwhelming, and particularly daunting, when the guidelines are unclear because of insufficient evidence, and at worst conflicting when two or more respected organizations produce differing guidelines. However, guidelines are *just* guidelines and their application must be geared to the individual needs and context of each particular patient. This is where being patient-centered can be extremely useful (Tudiver *et al.*, 2001). The balance between patient-centered medicine and evidence-based medicine is also explored in the next section.

EVIDENCE-BASED MEDICINE AND THE PATIENT-CENTERED CLINICAL METHOD: THE CONFLUENCE OF TWO WORLDVIEWS

On superficial examination of the current literature of evidence-based medicine and the approach described in this book as the patient-centered clinical method, some could conclude that the two are in conflict with each other. This view is sometimes further simplified by saying that evidence-based medicine represents the "hard science" of medicine and the patient-centered clinical method is the "soft" side of it. This is to misrepresent both evidence-based medicine and the patient-centered clinical method, which, in truth, have significant areas of confluence.

The early writings describing evidence-based medicine make clear that it is not intended to replace clinical judgment. Clinical decision making is described as taking into account three elements: the evidence, patient particulars, and patient preference (Haynes *et al.*, 2002; Sackett *et al.*, 2000). Evidence-based medicine has made tremendous strides in describing and putting into practice a method for acquiring the best available evidence about an issue in health care. The concurrent improvements in electronic databases and retrieval systems make it possible to access this information at the site of care and to integrate with the EMR. Evidence-based medicine is, in essence, a robust and extremely useful method for framing questions and evaluating evidence. It is not itself a clinical method, although it does inform the clinician.

Research on the patient-centered clinical method has made clear that finding common ground between both the physician's and the patient's perspective is key to a successful clinical outcome. Evidence-based medicine assists the physician in determining what elements might be appropriate for a part of the physician's perspective. It is not a substitute for clinical judgment or clinical intuition, which arises out of a specific interaction between a particular patient and a particular clinician. The patient-centered clinical method describes a method for ensuring that the patient's particulars and preferences are taken into account and an agreed plan arrived at. From this vantage point, the patient-centered clinical method incorporates or subsumes evidence-based medicine.

One could look at this in another way, however. It is increasingly apparent that the patient-centered clinical method is itself evidence-based. Taking into account the illness experience, the person and the context and arriving at common ground have together been demonstrated to improve patient health outcomes, patient satisfaction, and physician satisfaction. This burgeoning literature detailing the evidence to support this clinical method is covered in Chapter 16.

In summary, evidence-based medicine and the patient-centered clinical method are not ideas in conflict; rather, they are synergistic. The field of action between them is best understood as one of creative tension. Complexity science (Plsek & Greenhalgh, 2001: 627) calls the "edge of chaos" those circumstances in which there is "insufficient agreement and certainty to make the next choice obvious, but not so much disagreement and uncertainty that the system is thrown into chaos." This calls for complex adaptive behavior. Such areas of human interaction are the genesis of humane moral action from which arises true value. The patient-centered clinical method explicitly addresses this domain.

COMMON MISCONCEPTIONS ABOUT THE PATIENT-CENTERED CLINICAL METHOD

Over the last 30 years, as the patient-centered clinical method has been disseminated to students, clinicians, educators, and researchers, we have observed many misconceptions about the model. These misconceptions have concluded that being patient-centered takes more time; it focuses primarily on the patients' psychosocial issues versus their diseases; it requires acquiescing to patients' demands; it means being rigid and following a standard approach; it expects sharing all information and all decisions with patients; and, finally, that the patient-centered clinical method is a set of tasks that do not need to be applied during each visit but, rather, that can be cherry-picked – that is, some used or some discarded.

In addition, the acronym FIFE (feelings, ideas, function, and expectations) can be very useful for students as they are learning to inquire about the patient's illness experience. However, it can also be dangerous if it becomes an appendage to the conventional review of systems: "Any visual problems – blurred vision . . .?" "What do you feel about this?" "How are your bowels – any constipation; diarrhea . . .?" "Any ideas about what is causing this?" Thus "FIFEing" the patient, as we have heard students remark, becomes just another interviewing technique or an additional step in their review of systems and does not reflect a genuine interest in and concern about the patient's unique illness experience and does not encourage attentive listening.

Having said that, sometimes patients' expectations are very clear and straightforward. They want treatment for their athlete's foot or completion of a medical form for insurance purposes. Thus it is not always essential to explore, in depth, the patient's perceptions of health or his or her illness experience. What is essential is that doctors listen to patients' cues and prompts in order to make appropriate and sensitive inquiries. In a similar vein, being patient-centered means taking into account the patient's desire for information and for sharing decision making and responding appropriately.

The notion that patient-centeredness recommends a single style of practice is worrisome (Lussier & Richard, 2008). We find it difficult to present a diagram and an approach and, at the same time, avoid giving the impression that a standard approach is recommended. Nonetheless, a standard approach is *not* recommended; rather, the diagrams are a guide and the goal is different conversations with different patients.

The argument that a physician does not need to be patient-centered in all visits – for example, when a patient presents a straightforward problem – is supported by the description of visits as falling into types: routines, rituals, or dramas (Miller, 1992). Arguing in favor of the view that doctors are not patient-centered all the time is our own result that doctors with low average scores on patient-centeredness show small standard deviations for these scores, perhaps revealing a more rigid and inflexible approach. However high-scoring doctors show wide standard deviations, suggesting a flexibility in their clinical approach. Nonetheless, our contention is that physicians do not know whether the visit ought to be routine, a ritual, or a drama, unless they are patient-centered and ask brief and appropriate questions at the beginning of the visit. A brief patient-doctor dialog about a minor sore throat serves as an example.

Doctor: *(While reaching for a tongue depressor)* Is there anything unusually worrying about this sore throat?

Patient: No. *(Pause)*
Doctor: Do you think this is anything out of the ordinary?
Patient: No . . . I don't think so.
Doctor: Anything else going on in your life that you want to tell me about today?
Patient: No. Things are great!

Only after such a 5-second interchange can a doctor be sure that this visit is going to be routine as opposed to a drama.

CONCLUSION

In this introductory chapter we have provided a historical perspective of the evolution of the patient-centered model, and of the clinical method that serves to implement the theoretical framework. The place of the patient-centered model and clinical method was examined in relation to other models of practice and current trends in health care. This chapter has briefly provided empirical evidence supporting the adoption of the patient-centered clinical method. In the final sections, challenges in practicing the patient-centered clinical method in the current context were explored, with attention given to some common misconceptions about the patient-centered clinical method.

2   The Evolution of Clinical Method

Ian R McWhinney

The clinical method practiced by physicians is always the practical expression of a theory of medicine, even though it is not made explicit. The theory embraces such concepts as the nature of health and disease, the relation of mind and body, the meaning of diagnosis, the role of the physician, and the conduct of the patient-doctor relationship. The theory and practice of medicine is strongly influenced in any era by the dominant theory of knowledge and by societal values. Medicine is always a child of its time.

In recent times, medicine has not paid much attention to philosophy. When our efforts have been crowned with such great successes as they have in the past century, why be concerned if someone questions our assumptions? Indeed, we often behave as if they are not assumptions but simply the way things are. Crookshank (1926) marks the end of the nineteenth century as the time when medicine and philosophy became completely dissociated. Physicians began to see themselves as practitioners of a science solidly based on observed facts, without a need for inquiry into how the facts are obtained and, indeed, what a fact is (Fleck, 1979). We believe ourselves to be at last freed from metaphysics, while at the same time maintaining a belief in the theory of knowledge known as physical realism.

Although continuous with the Hippocratic tradition of Greek medicine, the clinical method that has dominated Western medicine for nearly 200 years had its main origins in the European Enlightenment of the seventeenth century. Whitehead (1975) called this the century of genius, on whose capital of ideas we have lived ever since. It was the century of Galileo and Newton, of Descartes, Locke, and Bacon. Bacon urged mankind to dominate and control nature, thus lightening the miseries of existence. In *The Advancement of Learning* (1605) he provided, as his agenda for medical science, a revival of the Hippocratic method of recording case descriptions, with their course toward recovery or death; and the study of the pathological changes in organs – the "footsteps of disease" – with a comparison between these and the manifestations of illness during life. Clinical medicine at this time was dominated by untested theory ungrounded in bedside observation. The new scientific ideas had recently been applied to medicine by men such as Vesalius and Harvey, but their discoveries had been in anatomy and physiology, not in pathology and clinical science. Medicine was still practiced in ignorance of these discoveries. If Bacon set the agenda for science, it was Descartes who provided the method: the separation of mind and matter, with value residing only in mind; the separation of subject and object; and the reduction of complex phenomena to their simplest components.

Of all seventeenth-century figures, none has had more influence on science and medicine than René Descartes. In his *Traité de l'homme*, published in 1634, he wrote: "The body is a machine, so built up and composed of nerves, muscles, veins, blood and skin, that even though there were no mind in it at all, would not cease to have the same functions" (Foss, 2002: 37). Descartes' concept of the body as machine had enormous consequences for medicine. It replaced the vitalist concept of premodern medicine and made possible the basic sciences of medicine and all the benefits they have conferred on us. Descartes' reductionist approach to inquiry, and his separation of *res extensa* from *res cogitans* enabled biology to make great progress. However, the problems left unresolved by Descartes have been gnawing away at the conceptual foundations of medicine and science. The questions include how can a non-material mind act on a material substance, and what is the relationship between the mind of the observer and the world of phenomena? The philosopher Burtt (1954: 324) wrote: "An adequate cosmology will only begin to be written when an adequate philosophy of mind has appeared."

It was in the century of genius that reason was enthroned and modern science was born. However, it was a reason defined as formal logic, divorced from human experience and seeking for universal laws to explain natural phenomena. Mathematics was the model and Newton's *Principia* was the great exemplar. The idea of nature as a vast machine – including the human body – seemed eminently plausible. The aim was to attain knowledge that was universal and certain. Toulmin (1992: 34–5) describes this as a radical shift in the paradigm of knowledge:

> From 1630 on, the focus of philosophical inquiries has ignored the particular, concrete, timely and local details of everyday human affairs: instead it has shifted to a higher, stratospheric place on which nature and ethics conform to abstract, timeless, general and universal theories.

In his book *Return to Reason* (1991) Toulmin reminds us that a "universal" was for the Greeks a concept that was true "on the whole" or "generally," but not invariably applicable in every case. "In real-life situations, many universals hold generally rather than invariably" (1991: 11). This applies especially in biology and the human sciences.

Since the seventeenth century, physics has been the model for all sciences. However, physics, writes the biologist Yates (1993: 189), is "characterized by uniformity and generality":

> Biology, in contrast, presents diversity and specialness of form and function and sometimes a striking localness of distribution of its objects. Biological systems are *complex*. Physics is a strongly reductionist science and has prospered in that style; [the metaphor of organisms as machines] is false and destructive of conceptual advances in the understanding of complex living systems that self-organize, grow, develop, adapt, reproduce, repair and maintain form and function, age and die. (italics in the original)

Our patients do all these things. They are complex systems – organisms – and our clinical method should enable us to deal with complexity.

THOMAS SYDENHAM

It was in the intellectual climate of the 1600s that there arose the first modern physician to use systematic bedside observation: Thomas Sydenham. Sydenham described the symptoms and course of disease, setting aside all speculative hypotheses based on unsupported theories. He classified diseases into categories – a novel idea at the time – believing that they could be classified by description in the same way as botanical specimens. Finally, he sought a remedy for each "species" of disease, exemplified by the newly introduced Peruvian bark (quinine). His great innovation, however, was to correlate his disease categories with their course and outcome, thus giving them predictive value. His method bore fruit in the distinction, for the first time, of syndromes such as acute gout and chorea. Sydenham was a close friend of John Locke, who took a great interest in his observations, sometimes accompanying him on his visits to patients.

FROM SYDENHAM TO LAENNEC

After Sydenham, the work of classifying diseases was taken up by others, notably Sauvages of Montpellier, a physician and botanist, who sought to group diseases into classes, orders, and genera in the same way that biologists were classifying plants and animals. Biology and medicine were at this time predominantly descriptive sciences. Sauvages was a strong influence on Carl von Linné, the Swedish physician and botanist who was responsible for the

Linnaean system of botanical classification – another instance of the connection between medicine and the ideas of the Enlightenment. The groupings of Sydenham's successors, however, were of little practical value because they were not correlated with the course and outcome of disease and represented only random combinations of symptoms with no basis in the natural order.

Sydenham died in 1689 and for the next hundred years no system for classifying diseases proved to be of lasting value. The next great step, and the one that laid the foundations for the modern clinical method, was taken by the French clinician-pathologists in the years after the French Revolution. The political turmoil engendered by Enlightenment ideas was associated with a further application of these ideas to medicine. Laennec, the greatest genius of the French school, described the method:

> The constant goal of my studies and research has been the solution of the following three problems:
> 1. To describe disease in the cadaver according to the altered states of the organs.
> 2. To recognize in the living body definite physical signs, as much as possible independent of the symptoms . . ..
> 3. To fight the disease by means which experience has shown to be effective: to place, through the process of diagnosis, internal organic lesions on the same basis as surgical disease. (Faber, 1923: 35)

For the first time, clinicians examined their patients, using new instruments such as the Laennec stethoscope. Then they linked together two sets of data: (1) signs and symptoms from the clinical inquiry and (2) the descriptive data of morbid anatomy. At last medicine had a classification system based on the natural order of things: the correlation between symptoms, signs, and the appearance of the organs and tissues after death. The system proved to have great predictive value, and it was further vindicated when Pasteur and Koch showed that some of these entities had specific causal agents. The clinical method based on this system developed gradually during the nineteenth century, until by the 1870s it had taken the form familiar to us today.

As is always the case, this development in clinical method was associated with a change in the perception of disease. Since classical times, Western medicine has used two different explanatory models of illness (Crookshank, 1926; Dubos, 1980). According to the ontological model, a disease is an entity located in the body and conceptually separable from the sick person. According to the physiological or ecological model, disease results from an imbalance within the organism, and between organism and environment; individual diseases have no real existence, the names being simply clusters of observations used by physicians as a guide to prognosis and therapy. According to the latter view, it becomes difficult to separate the disease from the person and the person from the environment.

Each model is identified with a clinical method, the ontological with a conventional or academic, and the physiological with a natural or descriptive method. The natural, concerned with the organism and disease, attempts to describe the illness in all its dimensions, including its individual and personal features. The conventional, concerned with organs and diseases, attempts to classify and name the disease as an entity independent of the patient.

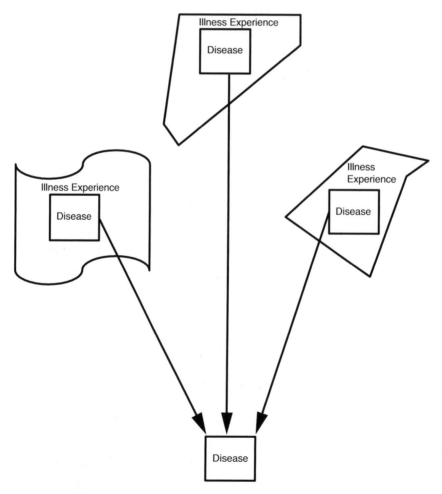

FIGURE 2.1 The process of abstraction (adapted from McWhinney [2000: 135]; reprinted with permission of the publisher, Mediselect GV.)

Crookshank (1926), who introduced these terms, also observed that the best physicians in all ages have used a balance of the two methods. The patient-centered clinical method can be seen as the restoration of balance to a clinical method that has gone too far in the ontological direction.

The success of the new clinical method in the late 1800s soon resulted in a dominance of the ontological model, a dominance it has retained ever since. Whereas in former times the word diagnosis often meant the diagnosis of a patient, the aim of diagnosis was now to identify the disease. Disease was located in the body. As in all taxonomies, the disease categories were abstractions that, in the interest of generalization, left out many features of illness, including the subjective experience of the patient.

Figure 2.1 illustrates the process of abstraction. The three irregular shapes represent patients with similar illnesses. They are all different because no two illnesses are exactly the same. The four squares represent what the patients have in common. In the process of abstraction we take the common factors and form a disease category – multiple sclerosis, carcinoma of the lung, and so on. Abstraction gives us great predictive power and provides us with our taxonomic language. It enables us to apply our therapeutic technologies with precision, but it comes at a price. The power of generalization is gained by distancing ourselves from individual patients and all the particulars of their illness. "A large acquaintance with particulars," said William James (1958: ix), "often makes us wiser than the possession of abstract formulas, however deep." If we look closely, every patient is different in some way. It is in the care of patients that the particulars become crucial. If we are to be healers, we need to know our patients as individuals; they may have their diseases in common, but in their responses to disease they are unique.

TABLE 2.1 Levels of Abstraction in a Patient with Multiple, Fluctuating Neurological Symptoms and Signs

Level 1	Level 2	Level 3	Level 4
Patient's sensations and emotions	Patient's expressed complaints, feelings, interpretations	Doctor's analysis of illness: clinical assessment	MRI scan
Preverbal	Second-order abstraction	Third-order abstraction	Fourth-order abstraction
Illness	"Illness" (doctor's understanding)	"Disease" (clinical diagnosis: multiple sclerosis)	"Disease" (definitive diagnosis: multiple sclerosis)

Source: McWhinney IR (1997a: 77); reprinted with permission of Oxford University Press, New York.

With its predictive and inferential power, the new clinical method was highly successful. Indeed, the application of new technologies to medicine depended on it. It had other strengths: it gave the clinician a clear injunction, "identify the patient's disease or rule out organic pathology"; it broke down a complex process into a series of easily remembered steps; and it provided canons of verification – the pathologist was able to tell the clinician whether he or she was right or wrong.

So successful was the method that its weaknesses only became apparent much later, as its abstractions became further and further removed from the experience of the patient. No abstraction is ever a complete picture of what it represents: it becomes less and less complete as levels of abstraction and power of generalization increase. Table 2.1 illustrates degrees of abstraction in a patient with multiple, fluctuating neurological symptoms. The first and lowest level is the patient's experience before it has been verbalized: his or her raw experience that something is not right. Level 2 is the patient's expressed sensations, feelings, and interpretations, and his or her understanding by the doctor. Level 3 is the doctor's clinical assessment and analysis of the illness: the clinical diagnosis of multiple sclerosis. Level 4 is the definitive diagnosis after an MRI scan. As we increase the levels of abstraction, individual differences are ironed out in the interest of generalization. The lower levels of abstraction are closest to the patient's lifeworld. As we increase the level of abstraction, the danger is that we forget that our abstraction is not synonymous with the real world. The diagnosis of multiple sclerosis and the MRI scan are not the patient's experience. To forget this, in Alfred Korzybski's (1958) aphorism, is mistaking the map for the territory. Many of the recently published illness narratives have drawn our attention to this weakness.

ILLNESS NARRATIVES

In the past 3 decades there has been a remarkable increase in the number of books and articles describing personal experiences of illness. These writings, by patients themselves or by their relatives, are often bitterly critical of clinicians and, by implication, of the modern clinical method. Hawkins (1993) sees this literature as a possible reaction to a medicine "so dominated by a biophysical understanding of illness that its experiential aspects are virtually ignored." Two themes recur in these stories:

> the tendency in contemporary medical practice to focus primarily not on the needs of the individual who is sick but on the nomothetic condition we call

the disease, and the sense that our medical technology has advanced beyond our capacity to use it wisely. (Hawkins, 1993)

Some illness narratives are written by patients who have a professional perspective as physicians, philosophers, sociologists, or poets. Sacks (1984) viewed his experience of a body image disorder from the perspective of an existential neurologist and medical theorist. Stetten (1981) found that his fellow physicians were interested in his vision, but not in his blindness. Toombs (1992), a phenomenologist who has multiple sclerosis, noted that the attention of physicians is directed to their patients' bodies rather than their patients' problems of living. The patient feels "reduced to a malfunctioning biological organism" (1992: 106). Toombs (1992: 106) writes:

> no physician has ever inquired of me what it is like to live with multiple sclerosis or to experience one of the disabilities that have accrued . . . no neurologist has ever asked me if I am afraid, or . . . even whether I am concerned about the future.

Writing of his experience with testicular cancer, Frank (1991), a sociologist, observed that the more critical his illness became, the more his physicians withdrew.

True to its origins in the age of reason, this clinical method was analytical and impersonal. Feelings and the life experience of the patient did not figure in the process. The meaning of the illness was established on one level only – that of physical pathology. The focus was on diagnosis, with much less attention to the detailed care of the patient. In keeping also with its Cartesian origins, it divided mental from physical disorder, bringing the two together in dubious terms such as "functional illness," "psychosomatic disease," and "somatization" (McWhinney *et al.*, 1997b).

The central idea on which the modern clinical method was based came into being at a time when Enlightenment ideas had become the dominant worldview of the West. Man had become the measure of all things, metaphysics devalued, tradition weakened, progress proclaimed, and knowledge put to practical use for the benefit of mankind. The fruits born by these ideas in our own time include this clinical method and all the benefits and problems of modern medicine.

Modern medicine continues to make great advances, many of them based on the mechanical metaphor. Training these technologies on their target has required diagnostic precision and the modern clinical method has rightly attached great importance to the linear logic of differential diagnosis. However, the promise of new technologies often falls short of expectations when they are applied in the real world of practice. It is here that linear logic meets the logic of complexity. Whether they are preventive, therapeutic, or rehabilitative, the technologies require acceptance by the patient, motivation, cooperation, and often determination. They may require a different way of life and the giving up of lifelong habits or cherished pleasures. The changes must be timely, and consistent with lifetime goals and priorities. The patient must be convinced that his or her efforts are justified.

Many illnesses are themselves complex and multifactorial, requiring an approach different from the linear logic and targeted technology that can work so well in diseases with a specific etiology. Illnesses such as chronic pain, eating disorders, depression, and addiction have an existential dimension that must be addressed if they are to be understood. Attention must be paid to patients' sufferings, to their emotions, beliefs, and relationships, not only for humanitarian reasons but also because they have an important bearing on the origins of illness (Foss, 2002).

The patient-centered clinical method is designed to deal with complexity. While using linear logic where appropriate, its essence is the understanding of the patient as a whole, a knowledge of his or her illness experience, and an attempt to attain common ground. Common ground is the key to therapeutic success, but it is often difficult to obtain. It tests the doctor's ability to motivate the patient by resolving objections, laying doubts to rest, allaying fears, and clearing up misconceptions (Botelho, 2002). The art of persuasion has ancient roots in medicine. The Greeks spoke of a "therapy of the word" (Entralgo, 1961). Before the Enlightenment, rhetoric – the art of persuasion – was a respected field of study. Its purpose was to take general fundamental principles and apply them in practical situations such as clinical medicine, taking into account all the local circumstances of time and place. The fact that rhetoric is now a derogatory term is a reflection on the limits of our knowledge. The search for common ground should be an exchange and synthesis of meanings. The physician interprets the patient's illness in terms of physical pathology, the name of the disease, causal inferences, and therapeutic choices. The patient interprets it in terms of experience: what it is *like* for him or her to suffer from the illness, beliefs about its nature, and expectations of therapy. Ideally, the exchange results in a synthesis of perspectives: they are, after all, different perspectives – concrete or abstract – of the same reality. However, there are some reasons why synthesis may not be achieved – at least initially. For the patient, the encounter with the physician is often emotionally charged. The physician's interpretation or management of the illness may be rejected. The physician may not believe the patient – a disbelief not necessarily conveyed in words. There are a hundred ways of saying, "I don't believe you."

Attaining empathetic understanding requires attention to the patient's emotions. This is something that the modern clinical method does not do in any systematic way. True to Descartes' supposed separation of mind from body,* the method of most clinical disciplines does not include attention to the emotions. Internal medicine attends to the body; psychiatry attends to the emotions. Family practice is one of the few clinical fields that transcend this deep fault line. As long ago as 1926, Crookshank, writing on the theory of diagnosis, noted that the handbooks of clinical diagnosis, which appeared in the early 1900s, "give excellent schemes for the physical examination of the patient while strangely ignoring, almost completely, the psychical [sic]" (1926: 941). The price we have paid for the benefits of abstraction is a distancing of doctor from patient. We have justified this to ourselves as objectivity, but to our patients it is often seen as indifference to their suffering.

The teaching with regard to the patient-doctor relationship was "don't get involved." In one respect, fear of the emotions was well founded – to be involved at the level of one's unexamined emotions is potentially harmful. However, what the teaching did not say was that involvement is necessary if one is going to be a healer as well as a competent technician. There are right and wrong ways of being involved and the teaching gave no guidance about finding the right way. The teaching was also profoundly mistaken in suggesting that one can encounter suffering and not in some way be affected. Our emotional response may be repressed, but this exacts a heavy price, for repressed emotion may be acted out in ways that are destructive of relationships. There is no such thing as noninvolvement and only self-knowledge can protect us from the pitfalls of involvement at the level of our egocentric emotions. Without self-knowledge, moral growth is likely to have shallow roots. This is why the patient-centered clinical method includes attention to the patient-doctor relationship, and, by implication, to the physician's self-awareness. The daily encounter with suffering can evoke strong emotions: helplessness in the face of incurable illness, fear of discussing questions that frighten us, guilt at our failures, anger at our patient's demands, and sadness at the suffering of someone who has become a friend. If we fail to acknowledge and deal with our disturbing emotions, they may be acted out in avoidance of the patient,

---

* Contrary to modern assumptions, Descartes did not deny mind-body interactions but maintained that most aspects of affective states are primarily somatic.

emotional distancing, exclusive concentration on the technical aspects of care, and even cruelty. Lack of emotional insight can disturb or destroy the relationship between patient and doctor, adding to the patient's sufferings and often leaving the doctor with a sense of failure. It is not easy to look suffering in the face without flinching.

All this implies that we see ourselves no longer as detached observers and dispassionate dispensers of therapy. To be patient-centered means to be open to a patient's feelings. It means becoming involved in a way that was made difficult by the old method. This has the potential for making medicine a much richer experience for us, as well as more effective for our patients. However, there are pitfalls. There are right and wrong ways of becoming involved. There are ways of dealing with some of the disturbing things our new openness will expose us to. Hence the importance of the knowledge and insight I have referred to. It is through such experiences that students can develop emotionally as well as intellectually.

If we are to recapture our capacity to heal, we will have to transcend the literal-mindedness that seems to follow when we become prisoners of our abstractions. A new clinical method should find room for the exercise of imagination and for restoring the balance between thinking and feeling.

KURT GOLDSTEIN'S HOLISTIC APPROACH TO MEDICINE

Any serious illness or injury sends reverberations throughout the organism. Total attention to the main symptom can miss any attention to a problem brought on by the illness or injury, a problem that turns out to be a change that assists the patient's recovery.

Goldstein (1995: 18) describes the holistic approach:

> *The Organism* consists mainly of a detailed description of the new method, the so-called holistic, organismic approach. Certainly, isolated data acquired by the dissecting method of natural science could not be neglected if we were to maintain a scientific basis. But we had to discover how to evaluate our observations in their significance for the total organism's functioning and thereby to understand the structure and existence of the individual person. We were confronted then with a difficult problem of epistemology. The primary aim of my book is to describe this methodological procedure in detail, by means of numerous observations.
>
> The great number of examples from various fields in which the usefulness of the method was to be demonstrated may make the reading of the book at

times difficult. But it seemed to me relevant to include such diverse observations since in this way I could exemplify the characteristic feature of the new method, namely, that by using this principle much of what we observe in living beings can be understood in the same manner. This created another advantage. Such diverse material, from the fields of anatomy, physiology, psychology, and philosophy, that is, from those disciplines concerned with the nature of man, were correlated for the reader. In this way he could observe that the method may be useful for the solution of various problems that may, superficially, seem to be divergent and that have, until now, been treated as unrelated.

A DIFFERENT WAY OF THINKING ABOUT HEALTH AND DISEASE

Most difficult of all, perhaps, will be the transition from linear, causal thinking to cybernetic thinking. Linear thinking is deeply ingrained in our culture. The notion of a cause is based on the Newtonian model of a force acting on a passive object, as when a moving billiard ball collides with a stationary one. The action is in one direction only. In medicine, this notion is exemplified by the doctrine of specific etiology – of an environmental agent acting on a person to produce a diseased state.

The notion of cybernetic causation is based on the model of self-organising systems. The human organism can be viewed as a self-organising system, maintaining itself by interaction with its environment and by a system of feedback loops from the environment and from its own output. Self-organizing systems have the ability both to renew and to transcend themselves. Healing is an example of self-renewal in which constituent parts are renewed while the integrity of the organization is maintained. Organisms transcend themselves by learning, developing, and growing. Self-organizing systems require energy, but as organizations they are maintained and changed by information. The notion of cause in self-organizing systems is based on the model of information that triggers a process that is already a potential of the system. The response is not the direct result of the original stimulus but the result of rule-governed behavior that is a property of the system. If the process is long term, destabilizing, and self-perpetuating, then the question of cause becomes much more complex than that of identifying the trigger. The trigger that initiated the process may be quite different from the processes perpetuating it. We have to consider the processes in the organism that are perpetuating the disturbance. The key to enhancing healing may be in strengthening the organism's defenses, changing the information flow, or encouraging self-transcendence, rather than neutralizing an agent.

Nonlinear logic is "both-and" rather than "either-or." Perspectives that we regard as opposites can be seen as complementary polarities – different aspects of the same reality. The pitfalls of either-or thinking are exemplified by a leading neurologist's perspective on migraine: "Practitioners should realize that migraine is a neurobiologic, not a psychogenic disorder" (Olesen, 1994: 1714). Nonlinear logic would say: "Why can it not be both?"

It is self-knowledge that enables us to know where we are on the scale of these complementary polarities: between involvement and detachment, between concrete and abstract, between the particular and the general, or between uncertainty and precision.

THE REFORM OF CLINICAL METHOD

It is not surprising that criticism of the modern clinical method from within the profession has come mainly from fields of medicine that most experience the ambiguities of abstraction and the importance of the patient's life story, notably general practice and psychiatry. In the 1950s Michael Balint (1964), a medical psychoanalyst, began to work with a group of general practitioners, exploring difficult cases and the doctors' affective responses to them. Balint distinguished between "overall" diagnosis and traditional diagnosis; he emphasized the importance of listening and of the personal change required in the doctor; and he introduced new terms such as "patient-centered medicine"; "the patient's offers" and the doctor's "responses"; the doctor's belief in his "apostolic function"; and the "drug doctor" – the powerful influence for good or harm of the patient-doctor relationship. The idea that physicians should attend to their own emotional development as well as the emotions of the patient was revolutionary in its day. In other ways, Balint's method conformed to the dualistic approach of the period. The method was intended to apply only to certain patients with "neurotic illnesses," not to those with straightforward clinical problems.

In the 1970s Engel (1977, 1980), an internist and psychiatrist with a psychoanalytic orientation, used systems theory as a model for integrating biologic, psychologic, and social data in the clinical process. Engel's critique of the modern clinical method focused on the unscientific nature of the physician's judgments on interpersonal and social aspects of patients' lives, based on "tradition, custom, prescribed rules, compassion, intuition, common sense, and sometimes highly personal self-reference" (1980: 543).

Any successor to the modern clinical method must propose another method with the same strengths: a theoretical foundation, a clear set of injunctions about what the clinician must do, and canons of verification by which it may be judged. Laín Entralgo (1956) attributes the failure of Western medicine to integrate the patient's inner life with the disease to the lack, among other things, of a method – "a technique [for] laying bare, to clinical investigation and to subsequent pathological consideration the inner life of the patient . . . an exploration method – the dialogue with the patient." Balint and Engel both provided a theory, but they were less clear about what the clinician must do and how the process is to be validated. Although Engel emphasized that the verification must be scientific, validation of both models was bound to depend on qualitative methods that were barely accepted as scientific. A model is an abstraction; a method is its practical application; and medicine had to wait longer for the transition to occur. The patient-centered clinical method is an answer to Laín Entralgo's challenge.

Clinical medicine, it seems, took a long time to fall under the domination of the Enlightenment paradigm of knowledge. Although the modern clinical method was concerned with abstractions, until our own time the individual case or series of cases remained the focus of attention for study and for teaching. Our abstractions have been low level, not far removed from experience of patients. In more recent times, however, the development of clinical method can be seen as moving toward increasing levels of abstraction, and an increasing distance from the experience of illness. The fact that a ward round can now be done around the charts rather than around the beds is an indication of how far we have gone.

THE DIFFICULTIES OF CHANGE

It is important not to underestimate the magnitude of the changes implied by the transformation of our clinical method. It is not simply a matter of learning some new techniques, although that is part of it. Nor is it only a question of adding courses in interviewing and behavioral science to the curriculum. The change goes much deeper than that. It requires nothing less than a change in what it means to be a physician, a different way of thinking about health and disease, and a redefinition of medical knowledge.

A glance at any medical school curriculum is usually sufficient to show that it is dominated by the modern paradigm of knowledge. Of course, this kind of knowledge is important, but restoring the balance in medicine requires that it be balanced by other kinds of knowledge: an understanding of human experience and human relationships, moral insight, and that most difficult of accomplishments, self-knowledge. Whitehead (1975) criticized professional education for being too full of abstractions, a condition he described as "the celibacy of the intellect" (1975: 223), the modern equivalent of the celibacy of the medieval learned class. Wisdom, he believed, is the fruit of a balanced development. What we need is not more abstractions but, rather, an education in which the necessary abstractions are balanced by concrete experiences, an education that feeds both the intellect and the imagination. Much of this is not the kind of knowledge that can be learned in the classroom or from books, although some of it can. There is now, for example, a rich literature describing personal experiences of illness. If we are to give as much attention to care as we give to diagnosis we will need to feed our imagination with accounts of what it is like to go blind, have multiple sclerosis, suffer bereavement, bring up a handicapped child, and the many other experiences our patients live with. We will need also to know the many practical ways in which life for them can be enriched or made more tolerable.

Human relationships and moral insight, again, are not principally classroom subjects, except insofar as students learn moral lessons from the way they are treated by their teachers. However, once its importance is acknowledged, and time allowed for it, understanding of relationships can be deepened with the help of teachers who are sensitive, reflective, and prepared to expose their own vulnerability. Self-knowledge, by definition, cannot be taught. However, its growth can be fostered by teachers who are themselves embarked on this difficult journey – a journey that is never complete. The patient-centered clinical method is the most recent version of the historic struggle to reconcile two often competing notions of the nature of disease and the role of the physician. The past century has seen the increasing dominance of abstraction and the devaluation of experience. The patient-centered clinical method can be viewed as a move to bring medical practice and teaching back to the center, to reconcile clinical with existential medicine (Sacks, 1982). It may seem paradoxical that the modern clinical method does not have a name. It is simply the way clinical medicine has been taught in the medical schools in modern times. Giving the successor method a name has its dangers – notably, that of conveying different meanings to different people. In this transition period, however, it does seem necessary to have a name for the new method, but when the transition is complete, perhaps it can simply become "clinical method."

The new method should not only restore the Hippocratic ideal of friendship between doctor and patient but also make possible a medicine that can see illness as an expression of a person with a moral nature, an inner life, and a unique life story: a medicine that can heal by a therapy of the word and a therapy of the body.

PART TWO

The Four Components of the Patient-Centered Clinical Method

Introduction

Judith Belle Brown and Moira Stewart

In this section of the book, the four interactive components of the patient-centered clinical method are described in detail, with each component being illustrated by several case examples. Of note, the "Whole Person" component, because of its magnitude, is examined in two separate but interconnected chapters. While each component is, for the most part, described as a discrete entity, the expert clinician weaves among the components throughout the process in response to the patient's expressed needs and concerns. There is both an art and a science to this process that comes together with time, training, and experience.

3 The First Component: Exploring Health, Disease, and the Illness Experience

Moira Stewart, Judith Belle Brown, Carol L McWilliam, Thomas R Freeman, and W Wayne Weston

HEALTH, DISEASE, AND ILLNESS

There is a long history documenting the failure of conventional medical practice in meeting patients' perceived needs and expectations. Component 1 of the patient-centered clinical method addresses this failure by proposing that clinicians cast a wider gaze beyond disease, to include an exploration of health and the illness experience of their patients. In the earlier editions of this book we have elaborated on a conceptual distinction between disease and illness; in this edition, we add a third distinction: health.

This chapter is organized as follows. First, the terms used in this chapter are broadly defined: health, disease, and the illness experience. Then, their interconnectedness is described in a diagram. Next the clinical method, to help clinicians explore these issues with patients, is presented. Finally, the literature and powerful quotations justifying and elaborating the dimensions are provided – especially useful for the academic audience.

Effective patient care requires attending as much to patients' perceptions of health and personal experiences of illness as to their diseases. Health, for the purposes of this chapter, is defined in a way that is akin to the most recent World Health Organization definition of a "resource for living," which is among the several important concepts presented later in this chapter under the heading "Dimensions of Health: Relevance to Health Promotion and Disease Prevention." We define health as encompassing the patients' perception of health and what health means to them, and their ability to pursue the aspirations and purposes important to their lives.

Disease is diagnosed by using the conventional medical model by analysis of the patient's medical history and objective examination of his or her body by physical examination and laboratory investigation. It is a category, the "thing" that is wrong with the body-as-machine or the mind-as-computer. Disease is a theoretical construct, or abstraction, by which physicians attempt to explain patients' problems in terms of abnormalities of structure and/or function of body organs and systems and which includes both physical and mental disorders. Illness, for its part, is the patient's personal and subjective experience of sickness: the feelings, thoughts, and altered function of someone who feels sick.

In the biomedical model, sickness is explained in terms of pathophysiology – abnormal structure and function of tissues and organs. "The medical model is materialist and assumes that the mechanisms of the body can be revealed and understood in the same way that the working of the solar system can be understood through gazing at the night sky" (Wainwright, 2008: 77). This model is a conceptual framework for understanding the biological dimensions of sickness by reducing sickness to disease. The focus is on the body, not the person. A particular disease is what everyone with that disease has in common, but the health perceptions and illness experiences of each person are unique. Disease and illness do not always coexist; health and disease are not always mutually exclusive. Patients with undiagnosed asymptomatic disease perceive themselves to be healthy and do not feel ill; people who are grieving or worried may feel ill but have no disease. Patients and practitioners who recognize these distinctions and who realize how common it is to perceive a loss of health or feel ill and yet have no disease are less likely to search needlessly for pathology. However, even when disease is present, it may not adequately explain the patient's suffering, since the amount of distress a patient experiences refers not only to the amount of tissue damage but also to the personal meaning of health and illness.

Several authors have described similar distinctions among health, disease, and illness from different perspectives and these are presented in detail later in this chapter under the heading "Distinctions among Health, Disease, and the Illness Experience."

Research has long supported the contention that disease and illness do not always present simultaneously. For some illnesses patients do not even seek medical advice (Green *et al.*, 2001; Frostholm *et al.*, 2005).

> Many people present with medically unexplained symptoms. For example, more than a quarter of primary care patients in England have unexplained chronic pain, irritable bowel syndrome, or chronic fatigue, and in secondary and tertiary care, around a third of new neurological outpatients have symptoms thought by neurologists to be 'not at all' or only 'somewhat' explained by disease. (Hatcher & Arroll, 2008: 1124)

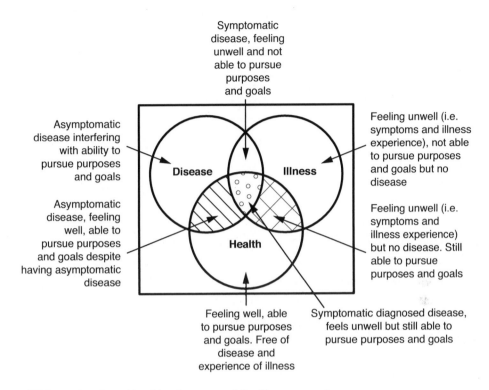

Symptomatic disease, feeling unwell and not able to pursue purposes and goals

Asymptomatic disease interfering with ability to pursue purposes and goals

Asymptomatic disease, feeling well, able to pursue purposes and goals despite having asymptomatic disease

Disease   Illness

Health

Feeling unwell (i.e. symptoms and illness experience), not able to pursue purposes and goals but no disease

Feeling unwell (i.e. symptoms and illness experience) but no disease. Still able to pursue purposes and goals

Feeling well, able to pursue purposes and goals. Free of disease and experience of illness

Symptomatic diagnosed disease, feels unwell but still able to pursue purposes and goals

FIGURE 3.1 Overlap of health, disease, and the illness experience

In Figure 3.1, the patient with a sensation of being ill but having no disease is in the upper right-hand part of the Venn diagram or in the cross-hatched portion on the right. There are a variety of reasons for feeling ill but having no disease: the problem may be transient; it may be managed so early that it never reaches a diagnosis (e.g., impending pneumonia); it may be a borderline condition that is difficult to classify; the problem may remain undifferentiated; and/ or the problem may have its source in factors such as an unhappy marriage, job dissatisfaction, guilt, or lack of purpose in life (McWhinney & Freeman, 2009). Patients falling into the group at the center of Figure 3.1, represented by the dots, where disease, illness, and health overlap, would have experiences of ill-health (sensory, cognitive, and emotional), a diagnosed disease and perceptions of their health, and what health means to them. For example, it is known that people with chronic disease may rate their health as good or very good despite having the disease. People in the center of the diagram have potential for health-enhancing attitudes and activities. The patient in the portion of Figure 3.1 with the diagonal lines in the left-hand overlap would have no feelings of ill-health but would have a diagnosed disease as well as perceptions of his or her health and what health means to him or her. Patients in the upper left-hand part of Figure 3.1 have a disease that is asymptomatic and also feel their disease interferes with their aspirations and life purposes. Examples of such patients may be those sometimes called partial patients, with high cholesterol, high blood pressure, high blood sugars (pre-diabetes or early diabetes).

THE CLINICAL METHOD TO EXPLORE THE DIMENSIONS OF HEALTH

We propose that clinicians keep in mind the definition of health as being unique to each patient and encompassing not only absence of disease but also the *meaning* of health to the patient and the patients' ability to realize *aspirations* and purpose in their lives. For one person health may mean being able to run in the next marathon; for another, health is when the back pain is brought under control.

Assuming the importance of the role of health promotion in all of health care, we recommend that clinicians ask persons coming to the clinic for periodic health examinations or minor ailments: "What does the term 'health' mean to you in your life?" Such questions adapted to the culture and individuality of each patient will serve two purposes clinically: first, the questions will reveal to the clinician previously unknown dimensions in the patient's life; second, the questions will "develop the patients' knowledge," as Cassell (2013) says, a health-promoting act in itself. Some of the dimensions that the clinician may learn about (all are important as identified by the literature in this chapter under the heading "Dimensions of Health: Relevance to Health Promotion and Disease Prevention") are the patient's perceived susceptibility; his or her perceived health status and sense of well-being; his or her attitudes toward health consciousness and health behaviors; his or her perceptions of the benefits and barriers to health in his or her life; and the degree to which the patient feels he or she can create his or her own health, often called "self-efficacy."

When patients are very sick, perhaps with chronic multimorbidities and experiencing hospitalizations, the clinician can explore the aspirations and purposes using the following types of questions taken from Cassell (2013: 89): "What is really bothering you about all this? . . . Are there things that you feel are very important that you want to do now . . . things that, if you got those done or started . . . you would have a better sense of well-being?"

THE CLINICAL METHOD TO EXPLORE THE FOUR DIMENSIONS OF THE ILLNESS EXPERIENCE: FIFE

We propose four key dimensions of illness experience that practitioners should explore: (1) patients' feelings, especially their fears, about their problems; (2) their ideas about what is wrong; (3) the effect of the illness on their functioning; and (4) their expectations of their clinician (*see* Figure 3.2).

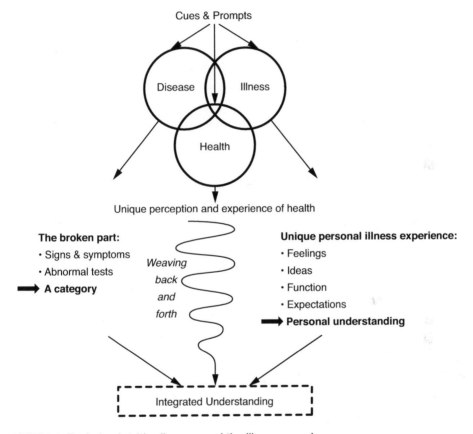

FIGURE 3.2 Exploring health, disease, and the illness experience

What are the patient's *feelings*? Does the patient fear that the symptoms he or she presents may be the precursor of a more serious problem such as cancer? Some patients may feel a sense of relief and view the illness as a reprieve from demands or responsibilities. Patients often feel irritated or culpable about being ill.

What are the patient's *ideas* about his or her illness? On one level the patient's ideas may be straightforward – for example, "I wonder if these headaches could be migraine headaches." However, at a deeper level, patients may struggle to make sense of their illness experience. Many persons face illness as an irreparable loss; others may view it as an opportunity to gain valuable insight into their life experience. Is the illness seen as a form of punishment, or, perhaps, as an opportunity for dependency? Whatever the illness, knowing the patients' explanation is significant for understanding the patient.

What are the effects of the illness on *function*? Does it limit the patient's daily activities? Does it impair his or her family relationships? Does it require a change in lifestyle? Does it compromise the patient's quality of life by preventing him or her from achieving important goals or purposes?

What are the patient's *expectations* of the clinician? Does the presentation of a sore throat carry with it an expectation of an antibiotic? Does the patient want the clinician to do something or just listen? In a review and synthesis of the literature on patient expectations of the consultation, Thorsen *et al.* (2001) provide a further conceptualization of patients' expectations of the visit. They suggest that patients may come to a visit with their practitioner with "a priori wishes and hopes for specific process and outcome" (2001: 638). At times these expectations may not be explicit and, in fact, patients may modify or change their expectations during the course of the consultation.

The following examples of patient-practitioner dialogue contain specific questions that clinicians might ask to elicit the four dimensions of the patient's illness experience.

- To the clinician's question, "What brings you in today?" a patient responds, "I've had these severe headaches for the last few weeks. I'm wondering if there is something that I can do about them."
- The patient's *feelings* about the headaches can be elicited by questions such as: "What concerns you most about the headache? You seem anxious about these headaches; do you think that something sinister is causing them? Is there something particularly worrisome for you about the headaches?"
- To explore the patient's *ideas* about the headaches, the clinician might ask questions such as: "What do you think is causing the headaches? Have you any ideas or theories about why you might be having them? Do you think there is any relationship between the headaches and current events in your life? Do you see any connection between your headaches and the guilty feelings you have been struggling with?"
- To determine how the headaches may be impeding the patient's *function*, the clinician might ask: "How are your headaches affecting your day-to-day living? Are they stopping you from participating in any activities? Is there any connection between the headaches and the way your life is going?"
- Finally, to identify the patient's *expectations* of the practitioner at this visit,

the clinician might ask: "What do you think would help you to deal with these headaches? Is there some specific management that you want for your headaches? In what way may I help you? Have you a particular test in mind? What do you think would reassure you about these headaches?"

As the following case illustrates, listening to the patient's story and exploring the disease and illness experience are essential aspects of patient-centered care.

Case Example

At 3 a.m. Jenna Jamieson was awakened by a sharp pain in her right lower quadrant. She dismissed it as bothersome menstrual pain and tried to get back to sleep. However, sleep was not an option, as the pain became unremitting.

Jenna was a 31-year-old single woman who lived alone. A committed teacher of special needs children she had just begun working at a new school. She was also an accomplished rower who had led her team to several national victories. At 3:30 a.m. Jenna, feeling feverish and nauseated, staggered to the bathroom. In her stupor of pain she was thankful on two counts: it was Saturday – at least she would have a couple of days to recover from whatever this was before returning to school – and being winter there was no rowing practice.

By 6 a.m. the pain had reached the point that Jenna could hardly get her breath. She felt weak, sweaty, and nauseated. In desperation Jenna called a close friend to take her to the hospital.

Three hours later, after undergoing numerous tests and examinations, the surgeon on call diagnosed acute appendicitis. Jenna was promptly taken to the operating room for surgery. While medication had alleviated Jenna's pain, her anxiety and fear had intensified. In a few brief hours she had gone from feeling healthy and vital to someone who was very ill.

In the recovery room Jenna felt groggy and disoriented. She sighed and then blinked to see her surgeon standing over her. "Well, Jenna" he said "It was not your appendix after all. In fact it was a bit more serious." Jenna had had a Meckel's diverticulitis requiring a partial bowel resection. Because it had ruptured and she developed peritonitis, she would be in hospital for several days for intravenous antibiotics. Her recovery would require at least 4–6 weeks. The diagnosis was a shock and the surgery had been intrusive. Jenna found it hard to comprehend how all this had transpired and to some extent she denied her current reality.

Daily, her surgeon came to see her and offer support. On one occasion, sensing her irritability, he asked Jenna if she was angry. While initially surprised by his question, upon reflection Jenna realized that she was angry and also felt as if her once healthy body had betrayed her. She was struggling to make sense of why this had happened. Her life had been turned upside down and the things that were important to her were now even more precious. She missed her students and her work and wondered if she would have the physical stamina to return to work. She was also fearful that her other passion, rowing, would have to be forsaken – at the pinnacle of her career. Her team was so close to an international victory – an event she might now miss.

Jenna's surgeon listened and understood her anger and fears. He did not dismiss them or render them superfluous. Rather, he validated Jenna's concerns and reassured her that she would be able to enjoy all her activities and zest for living. These actions on the part of the doctor were central to Jenna's recovery. The doctor's acknowledgment of her present anger and future fears assisted in Jenna's own self-knowledge and belief in becoming well again. Had the surgeon only focused on her disease, her emotional recovery could have been delayed. Exploring Jenna's unique illness experience and supporting her through the recovery period to regain her health was as essential to her care as the surgical intervention.

Certain illnesses or events in the lives of individuals may cause them embarrassment or emotional discomfort. As a result, patients may not always feel at ease with themselves or their clinician and may cloak their primary concerns in multiple symptoms. The doctor must, on occasion, respond to each of these symptoms to create an environment in which patients may feel more trusting and comfortable about exposing their concerns. Often, the doctor will provide them with an avenue to express their feelings by commenting: "I sense that there is something troubling you or something more going on. How can I help you with that?"

Identifying how to ask key questions ought not to be taken lightly. Malterud (1994) has described a method for clinicians to formulate and evaluate the most effective wording of key questions. By trying out different wording, the physician was able to discover key questions with wording that facilitated patients answering questions that they had previously avoided. For example:

By including . . . 'let me hear' . . . or . . . 'I would like to know' . . ., I heard myself signalling an explicit interest towards the patient's thoughts . . . When asking the women directly about their expectations, they often responded – somewhat embarrassed: . . . 'I thought that was up to the doctor to decide . . .' The response became more abundant when I hinted that she surely had been imagining what might happen (. . . '*of course* you have *imagined*' . . .)." (Malterud, 1994: 12)

Key questions were usually open-ended, signalled the doctor's interest, invited the patient to use her imagination and conveyed that the doctor would not withdraw from medical responsibility.

The following case provides another illustration of the patient-centered clinical method and explicitly describes dimensions of health, disease, and the illness experience.

Case Example

Mr Rex Kelly was a 58-year-old man who had been a patient in the practice for 10 years. He had been a healthy man with few problems until 8 months ago, when he had a massive myocardial infarction and required triple coronary artery bypass surgery. He was married, with grown children, and he worked as a plumber. He had come to the office for diet counseling about his elevated cholesterol.

The following excerpt from the visit demonstrates the doctor's use of the patient-centered approach. The interaction began with Dr Wason stating, "Hi Rex, I'm glad to see you again. I understand you are back to check on your progress since your heart attack. Is there anything else you would like to discuss today?"

"That's right, doc, I'm sticking to our plan. I'm feeling pretty good about my weight. I'm down 5 more pounds and almost at my goal. I'm wondering how my last cholesterol turned out."

"Congratulations, Rex, you have done really well with the diet and that has helped bring down your cholesterol – it's now almost at the target level, too."

The interview then shifted to Rex's exercise program, and he stated that he had been regularly following his exercise regimen throughout the summer months and was walking up to 4 miles a day. Dr Wason asked, "Will you be able to continue your walking during the winter?"

"I think so," indicated Rex. "I don't mind walking in the winter as long as it's not too cold."

"Yes, you do need to be cautious during the severe weather," replied Dr Wason. Rex looked away and appeared sad. The doctor paused and asked,

"Is there something concerning you, Rex?"

"Oh well ... no," stated Rex quickly. "No, not really."

"Not really?" reflected Dr Wason.

"Well," replied Rex, "I was just thinking about the winter and ... well ... no, I guess I'll be able to snowmobile if I just keep warm."

"Why are you concerned that you won't be able to do that, Rex?" asked the doctor.

"Well, I don't know. I'd just miss it if I couldn't participate."

"It sounds as if that activity is important to you," responded Dr Wason.

"Well, yes, it has been a very important family activity. We have some land and a little cabin up north of here, and it's really how we spend our winter weekends – the whole family together."

"It sounds as if not being able to participate in something that's been an important family activity would be very difficult for you," reflected the doctor.

"Yes, it would be. I just feel that so many things have been taken away from me that I really would miss not being able to do that."

The doctor responded, "Rex, during the last several months you have experienced a lot of changes and a lot of losses. I sense it has been very difficult for you."

Rex solemnly replied: "Yes, doc, it has. It's been tough. I've gone from being a man who is really healthy and has no problems to having a bad heart attack and a big operation and being a real weight watcher. And I still don't have the energy I used to have and sometimes I worry about having another heart attack. And my wife is worried too – she is always reminding me to be careful and we are both anxious about resuming our lovemaking. It has been a big change, and it has had its tough moments, but I'm alive and I guess that is what matters."

"It seems that you – and your wife too – still have a lot of feelings surrounding your heart attack and the surgery and the changes that have occurred," observed Dr Wason.

"Yes, we have," Rex noted soberly, "... we have."

"I'm glad I can tell you that you have passed the most dangerous period after your heart attack and now your risk is quite low. In some ways, because of your better diet and regular exercise, you are healthier than you were before your heart attack. That's good news, but I am concerned about your sadness and wonder if it would be helpful at your next appointment for us to talk about that more, to set aside some time just to look at that?" inquired Dr Wason.

"Yes it would. It's hard to talk about, but it would be helpful," Rex answered emphatically.

"Are you encountering any problems with sleep or appetite Rex?" asked the doctor.

"No, none at all," stated Rex.

The doctor asked a few more questions exploring possible symptoms of depression. Finding none, he again offered to talk further with Rex at their next visit and suggested it might be helpful to invite his wife to an upcoming appointment. The patient answered affirmatively.

In this example the patient's situation can be summarized by using the health, illness, and disease framework, which is part of the patient-centered model illustrated in Figure 3.3.

The doctor already knew the patient's medical conditions before the interview began. He picked up on the patient's sadness and his initial hesitancy in exploring how the heart attack had made him fearful. At the same time, the doctor ruled out serious depression by asking a few diagnostic questions and offered the patient an opportunity to explore further his feelings about his health and illness experience. Also the doctor and patient explored the patient's aspirations for a healthy life, in his case including snowmobiling with his family and resuming lovemaking. The reader will notice that the interview effortlessly weaved among the disease, health, and the illness experience.

By considering the patient's health and illness experience as a legitimate focus of enquiry and management, the physician has avoided two potential errors. First, if only the conventional biomedical model had been used, by seeking a disease to explain the patient's distress, the doctor might have labeled the patient depressed and given him unnecessary and potentially hazardous medication. A second error would have been simply to conclude that the patient was not depressed and move on to the next part of the interview. Had the physician decided that the patient's distress was not worthy of attention, he might have delayed the patient's emotional and physical recovery and the patient's adjustment to living with a chronic disease.

This case also illustrates that, although medical management after a myocardial infarction has improved considerably in recent years, it is not enough to limit treatment to the biological dimensions of the problem. This patient was following all of the guidelines but he still did not feel healthy or secure in his body. Also, his fears were shared by his wife, thus compounding his anxiety. Dealing with this patient's experience of health and illness, and including his wife in the discussions, may be helpful in promoting health, alleviating fears,

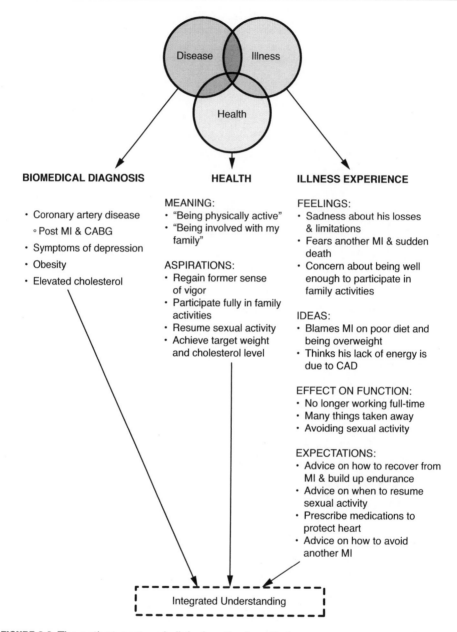

FIGURE 3.3 The patient-centered clinical method applied

correcting misconceptions, encouraging him to discuss his discouragement, or simply "being there" and caring what happens to him. At the very least, this compassionate concern is a testimony to the fundamental worth and dignity of the patient; it might help prevent him from becoming truly depressed; it might even help him to live more fully.

DISTINCTIONS AMONG HEALTH, DISEASE, AND THE ILLNESS EXPERIENCE

In analyzing medical interviews, Mishler (1984) identifies contrasting voices: the voice of medicine and the voice of the lifeworld. The voice of medicine promotes a scientific, detached attitude and uses questions such as: Where does it hurt? When did it start? How long does it last? What makes it better or worse? The voice of the lifeworld, on the other hand, reflects a "commonsense" view of the world. It centers on the individual's particular social context, the meaning of health and illness, and how they may affect the achievement of personal health goals. Typical questions to explore the lifeworld include: How would you describe your health? What are you most concerned about? How does your loss of health disrupt your life? What do you think it is? How do you think I can help you?

Mishler (1984) argues that typical interactions between doctors and patients are doctor-centered – they are dominated by a technocratic perspective. The physician's primary task is to make a diagnosis; thus, in the interview, the doctor selectively attends to the voice of medicine, often not even hearing the patient's attempts to make sense of his or her suffering. What is needed, he maintains, is a different approach, in which doctors give priority to "patients' lifeworld contexts of meaning as the basis for understanding, diagnosing and treating their problems" (Mishler, 1984: 192).

In a qualitative study, Barry *et al.* (2001) applied Mishler's concepts in the analysis of 35 case studies of patient-doctor interactions. Their findings revealed an expansion of Mishler's ideas, adding two communication patterns: "lifeworld ignored," where patients' use of the voice of the lifeworld was ignored, and "lifeworld blocked," where doctors' use of the voice of medicine blocked patients' expressions of the lifeworld. These two communication patterns were found to have the poorest outcomes. When both the patient and the doctor used the voice of medicine exclusively, Barry *et al.* (2001) called this "strictly medicine," as the emphasis was on simple, acute physical complaints. "Mutual lifeworld" was the term applied to interactions where both the patient and the doctor used the voice of the lifeworld, thus highlighting the uniqueness of the patient's life and experience. Of note, Barry *et al.* (2001) found that the best outcomes were in patient-doctor encounters categorized as either "mutual lifeworld" or "strictly medicine." They offer four possible interpretations of the latter finding: (1) the patient has come to view his or her problems from the perspective of the voice of medicine; (2) the patient has learned from experience that the voice of the lifeworld has no value in medical encounters; (3) the patient is goal oriented in these encounters and wants a quick, efficient encounter; and, finally, (4) the structure of these encounters is such that the patient has no opportunity to use the voice of the lifeworld. Because the encounters incorporating "mutual lifeworld" reflected excellent outcomes, too, Barry *et al.* (2001) conclude that doctors need to be sensitized to the importance of attending to patients' concerns of the lifeworld.

Typically, when patients become seriously ill, they find some way to make sense of it – they may blame their own bad habits (eating too much, not exercising enough); they may blame fate or bad luck; or they may attribute it to "bad genes" or environmental toxins; some may even believe they have been cursed. Patients' "explanatory models" are their own personal conceptualizations of the etiology, course, and sequelae of their problem (Green *et al.*, 2002). Medical anthropologists such as Kleinman have described ways to elicit the patients' "explanatory models" of their illness and offer a series of questions to ask patients – a "cultural status exam." The physician might ask, for example: "How would you describe the problem that has brought you to me? Does anyone else that you know have these problems? What do you think is causing the problem? Why do you think this problem has happened to you and why now? What do you think will clear up this problem? Apart from me, who else do you think can help you get better? What do you think you could do to feel healthy?" (Kleinman *et al.*, 1978; Galazka & Eckert, 1986; Katon & Kleinman, 1981; Good & Good, 1981; Helman, 2007).

The following views on the importance of distinguishing between health, disease, and illness are offered from the perspective of the patient and the doctor. The patient is Anatole Broyard, who taught fiction writing at Columbia University, New York University, and Fairfield University. An editor, literary critic, and essayist for the *New York Times*, he died from prostate cancer in October 1990.

> I wouldn't demand a lot of my doctor's time. I just wish he would brood on my situation for perhaps five minutes, that he would give me his whole mind just once, be bonded with me for a brief space, survey my soul as well as my flesh to get at my illness, for each man is ill in his own way . . . Just as he orders blood tests and bone scans for my body, I'd like my doctor to scan me, to grope for my spirit as well as my prostate. Without some such recognition, I am nothing but my illness. (Broyard, 1992: 44–5)

The doctor is Loreen A Herwaldt, an internist and epidemiologist in Iowa.

> The big lesson for me was learning the difference between treating the disease and treating the human being. It's not always the same thing. There are times

you can kill the person – in a sense, killing their spirit – by insisting that some-thing be done a certain way. (Herwaldt, 2001: 21)

Eric Cassell (2013) challenges physicians to broaden their concept of their role to include a careful assessment of how disease impairs the patient's function:

> The focus is wider. Knowing the disease, the healer is concerned with establish-ing the functional status of the patient – what the patient can and cannot do. What is interfering with the accomplishment of the patient's goals? How does the patient attempt to surmount these impairments? (2013: 126)

He suggests expanding the scope of questions:

> "Fatigue (or dyspnea, heartburn, or abdominal pain)?" "Does that get in your way?" or "Does that interfere in your life?" "How?" "Tell me about it." (2013: 128)

> We are trying to uncover anything in any dimension of the patient's existence that is interfering with the patient's ability to achieve his or her goals or pur-poses. In what sphere do we find these purposes? Those in which people strive to make life worth living. For example, love and human connections – does the patient feel left out, isolated, wanted, or loved . . . Of a belief that there are things larger and more enduring than the self – fulfilling purposes in work (e.g., medicine, art, machine shop, or finance), social existence, or family. This is expressed in the ability to communicate, be creative, or fulfill expectations of the self or others and in doing things that the patient has identified as impor-tant, or other things that are central to particular individuals. (2013: 129)

COMMON RESPONSES TO ILLNESS

The reasons patients present themselves to their practitioners when they do are often more important than the diagnosis. Frequently the diagnosis is obvious or it is already known from previous contacts; often there is no biomedical label to explain the patient's problem. Thus, it is often more helpful to answer the question "Why now?" than the question "What's the diagnosis?" In chronic illness, for example, a change in a social situation, or a change in the internal sense of health agency/control, are more common reasons for presenting than a change in the disease or the symptoms.

Illness is often a painful crisis that will overwhelm the coping abili-ties of some patients and challenge others to increased personal growth

(Sidell, 2001; Wainwright, 2008; Marini & Stebnicki, 2012; Lubkin & Larsen, 2013). Livneh and Antonak (2005) describe common negative psychological responses to chronic illness and disability.

> Increased stress is experienced because of the need to cope with daily threats to (a) one's life and well-being; (b) body integrity; (c) independence and autonomy; (d) fulfillment of familial, social, and vocational roles; (e) future goals and plans; and (f) economic stability. (2005: 12)

A sudden disability or life-threatening diagnosis creates a crisis that upsets the patient's equilibrium and may be long-lasting. This triggers a mourning process over the loss of body part or function that serves as a constant reminder of the impairment. Unsuccessful adaptation to the loss may lead to chronic anxiety, depression, social withdrawal, and distortion of the body image. Self-concept and identity may be damaged. Patients with chronic disease may be stigmatized, resulting in social withdrawal and reduced self-esteem. Many medical conditions are unpredictable and lead to a life of uncertainty. Quality of life is often diminished.

It is helpful to understand these reactions as part of a predictable process described by Strauss and colleagues as a "trajectory framework" or "biography" (Glaser & Strauss, 1968; Strauss & Glaser, 1970). "The trajectory is defined as the course of an illness over time, plus the actions of clients, families, and healthcare professionals to manage that course" (Corbin & Strauss, 1992: 3). Even for persons with the same disease, the illness trajectory will be unique for each individual based on the strategies that the individual uses to manage his or her symptoms, illness beliefs, and personal situation.

> During the trajectory phase, signs and symptoms of the disease appear and a diagnostic workup may begin. The individual begins to cope with implications of a diagnosis. In the stable phase, the illness symptoms are under control and management of the disease occurs primarily at home. A period of inability to keep symptoms under control occurs in the unstable phase. The acute phase brings severe and unrelieved symptoms or disease complications. Critical or life-threatening situations that require emergency treatment occur in the crisis phase. The comeback phase signals a gradual return to an acceptable way of life within the symptoms that the disease imposes. The downward phase is characterized by progressive deterioration and an increase in disability or symptoms. The trajectory model ends with the dying phase, characterized by gradual or rapid shutting down of body processes. (Corbin, 2001: 4–5)

Reiser and Schroder (1980) describe a similar model of illness that has three stages: awareness, disorganization, and reorganization. The first stage, awareness, is characterized by ambivalence about knowing: on the one hand, wanting to know the truth and to understand the illness; on the other hand, not wanting to admit that anything could be wrong. At the same time patients are often struggling with conflicting wishes to remain independent and longing to be taken care of. Eventually, if the symptoms do not go away, the fact of the illness hits home and the patient's sense of being in control of his or her own life is shattered.

This disrupts the universal defense – the magical belief that somehow we are immune from disease, injury, and death. The patient who has struggled to forestall his awareness of serious illness and then has finally recognized the truth is one of the most fragile, defenseless, and exquisitely vulnerable people one can ever find. This is a time of terror and depression and reflects the second stage, disorganization (Reiser & Schroder, 1980).

At this stage, patients typically become emotional and may react to their caretakers as parents rather than as equals. They often become self-centered and demanding, and although they may be aware of this reaction and embarrassed by it, they cannot seem to stop it. They may withdraw from the external world and become preoccupied with each little change in their bodies. Their sense of time becomes constricted and the future seems uncertain; they may lose a sense of continuity of self. They can no longer trust their bodies, and they feel diminished and out of control. Their whole sense of their personal identities may be severely threatened. One reaction to this state of mind in some patients is rebellion, a desperate attempt to have at least some small measure of control over their lives even if it is self-destructive in the end.

The third stage is reorganization. In this stage patients call upon all of their inner strengths to find new meaning in the face of illness and, if possible, to transcend their plight. Their degree of mastery and sense of health and capability, in spite of a disease, will be affected by the nature and severity of the disease. However, in addition, the outcome is profoundly influenced by the patients' social supports, especially loving relationships within their families, and by the type of support their physician can provide.

These stages of illness are part of a normal human response to disaster and not another set of disease categories or psychopathology. This description emphasizes how the humanity of the ill person is compromised and points to an added obligation of physicians to their wounded patients.

So great is the assault of illness upon our being that

it is almost as if our natures themselves were ill, as if the strands or parts of us were being forced apart and we verged on the loss of our own humanness. A phenomenon so great in its effects that it can threaten us with the loss of our fundamental humanness clearly requires more than technical competence from those who would 'treat' illness. (Kestenbaum, 1982: viii–ix)

Stein (2007) describes four common feelings that accompany serious illness: terror, loss, loneliness, and betrayal. Understanding these predictable responses to illness can help prepare both patients and physicians for the struggles that patients may experience in attempting to come to terms with the impact of disease on their bodies and their lives. "Terror is the beginning of the end of the illusion that illness isn't that bad" (2007: 95). Losses associated with illness come one after another and sometimes feel endless. "Disfigurement offers the most literal understanding of loss, of change, of the fragility and vulnerability of the body" (2007: 165). Stein refers to the unbearable loneliness of serious illness, how patients conceal their struggles with pain or chemotherapy without revealing the fears and many inconveniences illness brings. Betrayal refers to the feeling that the body has let the patient down – it can no longer be trusted or counted on to let the patient do what matters to him or her. Stein describes betrayal this way:

> Health is familiar, predictable, reliable, and, we hope enduring. It provides a sense of orientation. Illness is a break in the established, continuous sameness and comfort of health. Betrayal arrives without arrangement, unpredictably, spontaneously, carrying danger. It is a threat, and we are vulnerable. It has revealed a secret about us. Personal worth and value are undermined. All of us idealize our own bodies (even if not every piece of them) so we are deeply disappointed by illness. We are strong and vigorous one moment, helpless the next; we have power one moment and are without it the next. We take account of our assets and resources, but when betrayed, we feel useless. (2007: 61)

Case Example

It all happened in a flash, or so Brenna thought. One day Brenna felt well, in her sailboat flying over the waves at the end of summer, and the next she was not. Fall had ascended – in so many ways.

Brenna had suffered an aneurism at the age of 47. She had been fit, healthy, and fully employed in the health care field. Now she was a patient, hospitalized and helpless. While headaches were not foreign to her, the headache she awoke with "at the onset of the episode" did feel unusual. However, she quickly passed it off. Brenna was not one to succumb to such inconveniences – or to appear weak and vulnerable.

With the holiday weekend coming to a close, Brenna had diligently secured the sailboat, pushing the pain in her head aside, and began the trip back to the city. "Perhaps a coffee would help," she reflected. It did not. An hour later, just as Brenna was turning off the highway, she lost control of her car and ripped through 13 guardrails on the exit ramp. The car was demolished but she was alive. Her next memory, although vague, was being in a white, sterile room in the hospital. Her head felt like it was about to explode.

Brenna had limited memories of the car accident or the events that followed. She struggled to make sense of the time line that expired over this short but very significant period in her life. While others, family and friends, said "Don't fret about it – that's the past, move on," she could not. Her past was connected to her future. Brenna could not ignore it or dismiss it as meaningless. It had meaning to her – meaning that radically informed who she was – today and what her future held. Because, at that moment, her future was uncertain.

From the outset, Brenna's neurologist, Dr Menin, had been kind and informative. The surgical team who repaired her aneurism were superlative in their handiwork. The neuropsychologist was efficient and also supportive. Brenna's health care team provided her with "optimal medical care." She recognized the initial denial she experienced regarding both the life-threatening diagnosis and the serious nature of the surgical procedure to repair her aneurism. However, she survived and was now on a journey to understand the neurological deficits she experienced and how they would change her life.

Months have now passed and, as the memories of that horrific assault on her brain and her personhood are slowly and painfully receding, she still struggles to understand what has happened. Brenna wonders, not "Why did this happened to me?" but rather, "Who have I become?" "Am I a sick person?" "Am I now disabled?" "What do these labels really mean – do they actually now define me as a person?"

PATIENTS' CUES AND PROMPTS

Patients often provide physicians with cues and prompts about the reason they are coming to the physician that day. These may be verbal or nonverbal signals. The patients may look tearful, sigh deeply, or be breathless. They may say directly, "I feel awful, Doctor. I think this flu is going to kill me." Or, indirectly, they may present a variety of vague symptoms that are masking a more serious problem such as depression. Other authors have described patients' cues and prompts using different terminology, such as clues (Levinson *et al.*, 2000; Lang *et al.*, 2000) or offers (Balint, 1964), but regardless of the name assigned, the patient behaviors are the same. Lang *et al.* (2000) describe a useful taxonomy of clues revealed in patients' utterances and behaviors reflecting their underlying ideas, concerns, and/or expectations:

- expression of feelings (especially concern, fear, or worry)
- attempts to understand or explain symptoms
- speech clues that underscore particular concerns of the patient
- personal stories that link the patient with medical conditions or risks
- behaviors suggestive of unresolved concerns or expectations (e.g., reluctance to accept recommendations, seeking a second opinion, early return visit).

Levinson *et al.* (2000) define

> a clue as a direct or indirect comment that provides information about any aspect of a patient's life circumstances or feelings. These clues offer a glimpse into the inner world of patients and create an opportunity for empathy and personal connection. . . . [thus] physicians can deepen the therapeutic relationship. (2000: 1021)

In order to assess how primary care physicians and surgeons respond to patient clues they assessed 116 patient-doctor encounters (54 of primary care physicians and 62 of surgeons). Through their qualitative analysis, Levinson and colleagues found that patients initiated the majority of clues and most were emotional in nature. The physicians frequently missed opportunities to adequately acknowledge patients' feelings, and as a result some patients repeatedly brought up the clue only to have it ignored again and again.

Thus as doctors sit down with patients and ask them, "What brings you in today?" they must ask themselves, "What has precipitated this visit?" They need to listen attentively to patients' cues not only of their diseases but also of their experience of illness and their perceptions of their health. Of equal importance to hearing patients' cues and prompts are empathic responses that help patients feel understood and recognized.

NARRATIVES OF HEALTH AND THE ILLNESS EXPERIENCE

A growing number of publications illustrate the importance of patients' narratives – in particular, their recounting of their story of illness (Greenhalgh & Hurwitz, 1998; Launer, 2002; Sakalys, 2003; Charon, 2004, 2006, 2007; Nettleton *et al.*, 2005; Haidet *et al.*, 2006; Greenhalgh, 2006; Brown *et al.*, 2012a; Herbert, 2013). As Arthur Kleinman (1999) observes, narratives of illness, the patients' stories of being unwell, open up untold vistas of experience and knowing.

> Stories open up new paths, sometimes send us back to old ones, and close off still others. Telling (and listening to) stories we too imaginatively walk down those paths – paths of longing, paths of hope, paths of desperation. We are, actually, all of us, physicians and patients and family members too, storied folk: stories are what we are; telling and listening to stories is what we do. (Kleinman, 1999: x)

Hunter's (1991) vision of the narrative expands this view, in that the story is not one-sided but involves two (and we suggest multiple) protagonists or story-tellers. "Understanding medicine as a narrative activity enables us – both physicians and patients – to shift the focus of medicine to the care of what ails the patient and away from the relatively simpler matter of the diagnosis of disease" (Hunter 1991, p. xxi). Expanding the focus of inquiry from simply the disease to include the patient's health and illness experience can provide a richer, more meaningful, and more productive outcome for all participants.

Yet research spanning almost 30 years (Beckman & Frankel, 1984; Marvel *et al.*, 1999; Rhoades *et al.*, 2001) indicates that physicians interrupt patients' accounts of their symptoms early in the consultation and hence their stories of health and illness are often untold. This reflects a failure on the physicians' part to weave back and forth between exploring the disease and illness experience, following the patients' cues. The patients' story of a troublesome sore throat may cloak their fear that this is a precursor to cancer, or patients may minimize their severe shortness of breath, explaining it as allergies, which, from the doctor's perspective, may indicate a more severe medical problem such as chronic obstructive pulmonary disease.

However, when clinicians assist patients to tell their story of health and illness, they are helped to gain meaning, and ultimately mastery, of their health and illness experience (Stensland & Malterud, 2001). When patients do not have a voice in the consultation, important dimensions of their health and illness experience, such as their feelings and ideas, will not be expressed (Barry *et al.*, 2000). Of equal concern is the potential for problematic outcomes such as nonuse of prescriptions and nonadherence to treatment (Barry *et al.*, 2000; Dowell *et al.*, 2007). Thus patient-centered practice requires attending to the patient's unique experience of health and illness as an important part of practicing good medical care.

DIMENSIONS OF HEALTH: RELEVANCE TO HEALTH PROMOTION AND DISEASE PREVENTION

Rex Kelly, the patient who was recovering from a previous myocardial infarction in the case study presented earlier in this chapter, saw himself as "no longer a healthy man." In general, patients' definitions of health undoubtedly influence their life and their care. Also, the providers' definition of health, and their role in promoting health, inevitably permeates the care offered. Just as understanding the illness experience requires inquiry into feelings, ideas, effect on function, and expectations, so too understanding the unique perceptions and experience of health requires an exploration of health meanings and aspirations as well as the individual's self-perceived health, susceptibility and seriousness of disease, ideas about health promotion, and the perceived benefits and barriers to health promotion and prevention.

To practice patient-centered care clinicians must think about the different conceptualizations of health as well as understand the patient's understanding (way of defining) health for him- or herself. Historically there have been three conceptualizations of health: (1) health has been understood to mean the absence of disease, and this meaning holds true within the biomedical model of clinical practice today; (2) in 1940, the World Health Organization (WHO, 1983) defined health as "a state of complete mental, social and physical well-being, not merely the absence of disease and infirmity"; and (3) in 1986, the World Health Organization (WHO, 1986a) redefined health as "a resource for everyday life, not the objective of living," a concept of health that emphasizes the individual's aspirations, social and personal resources, and physical capacities. Thus, the notion of health has been shifted from its former abstract focus on physical, and then physical, mental, and social, status toward "an ecological understanding of the interaction between individuals and their social and physical environment" (de Leeuw, 1989; Hurowitz, 1993; Stachtchenko & Jenicek, 1990; McQueen & Jones, 2010). While the earlier definitions direct attention to objective factual data, the most recent definition directs attention to the subjective and intersubjective experience and enactment of health. How patients and practitioners think about and, therefore, experience health continues to evolve. In fact, all partners in health care have unique and often differing understandings of health and, in turn, they all have different understandings of health promotion and disease prevention to contribute to these aspects of health care.

It might be said that Rex Kelly sees his "not healthy" state as the losing end of an all-or-nothing continuum. Engaging Rex Kelly in considering his health, as his ability to pursue his own aspirations, could be described as health-promoting patient-centered care.

HEALTH PROMOTION AND DISEASE PREVENTION WITH THE INDIVIDUAL PATIENT

Health promotion and disease prevention are important pillars in the "New Public Health Movement," as described in the Ottawa Charter (Epp, 1986). Much of the energy directed toward these thrusts has been devoted to developing public policy, screening, and other methods, and to addressing related ethical issues (Hoffmaster, 1992; Doxiadis, 1987). The population-based approach to health promotion continues to be of high priority. Less attention has been paid to implementing ideas of health promotion and disease prevention at the level of the individual practitioner and patient. Frequently, this effort has been related to chronic disease management (Barlow *et al.*, 2000; Bodenheimer *et al.*, 2002; Farrell *et al.*, 2004; Lorig *et al.*, 2001b; McWilliam *et al.*, 1997, 1999; Squire & Hill, 2006; Steverink *et al.*, 2005; Wagner *et al.*, 2001). As primary health care reform proceeds, achieving new directions clearly hinges on the efforts of both individual practitioners and interprofessional teams. Viewing a primary health care practice as serving both individual patients and a population at risk (McWhinney & Freeman, 2009) necessitates both an individualized and a population health approach.

Undoubtedly, the original concept of health as the absence of disease continues to dominate medical practice, creating a focus on health as a product of the physician's clinical work. The prevalence of chronic disease, multimorbidity, and the accompanying emphasis on self-care management also demand individualized attention to disease prevention as an ongoing part of medical care.

Additionally, however, as societal expectations for health as a state of complete physical, mental, and social well-being (WHO, 1986a) increase, both solo and interprofessional practice also have increasingly attended to the individual's and the community's holistic potential for health. Health as a resource for everyday living – specifically, the ability to realize aspirations, satisfy needs, and respond positively to the environment (WHO, 1986b) – has come to the fore. Thus, primary health care teams have begun to consider and address the involvement of individuals and communities in health promotion. Attention to efforts to promote health and prevent disease has become an essential part of primary health care reform, complementing the population health approach. The patient-centered clinical method provides a clear framework for the practitioner to apply health promotion and disease prevention efforts, using the patient's or the community's world as the starting point.

The Patient's Experience of Health and Illness

To understand the perspective of the patient, the practitioner needs to explore the patient's experiential learning about health and illness, consequential personal knowledge and beliefs in relation to health and illness, and what each means to that person. The practitioner needs to discover the patient's worldview of health and corresponding health-related values and priorities as one of many competing values in order to assess the patient's commitment to its pursuit. These are inherently very individualistic, reflecting a diversity of personal values, beliefs, and aspirations that are experienced uniquely, contextualized by ethnicity (Papadopoulos et al., 2003; Lai et al., 2007), and the many other social determinants of health, and hence they require exploration with each patient. In fact, research suggests important considerations in promoting health. One consideration is a person's perceived susceptibility to a particular health problem or to health problems generally. For example, perceived susceptibility has been found to be positively associated with screening and vaccination for hepatitis B virus among Vietnamese adults of lower socioeconomic and education levels (Ma et al., 2007) and is an important dimension in Becker's Health Belief Model (Janz & Becker, 1984). A second consideration is self-reported perceived health status, which has been correlated with a health-promoting lifestyle (Gillis, 1993).

A third element requiring exploration is health-valuing attitudes (or an image of being health-conscious), which may buffer socio-environmental risks (Reifman et al., 2001). Health-valuing attitudes have been found to be strong motivators for health-promoting activity (Gillis, 1993; Reifman et al., 2001; Wanek et al., 1999). An individual's perceptions of the benefits and barriers to health and a health-promoting lifestyle are important in determining whether or not a health-promoting strategy is adopted. Furthermore, individuals, who conceive health as the presence of wellness, rather than merely the absence of disease, have a significantly stronger engagement in health-promoting lifestyles (Gillis, 1993). Consistent with current notions of health as a process of mobilizing resources for everyday living, patients with chronic illness often experience health, and do much to create their own health (McWilliam *et al.*, 1996), with positive outcomes for themselves and the health care system (McWilliam *et al.*, 1999, 2004, 2007). Thus, it is important both to assess the patient's own perception of experienced health and illness and to assess what health really means in daily life.

The Patient's Potential for Health

The patient's potential for health is determined by his or her exposure to broader determinants of health throughout the life course, age, sex, genetic potential for disease, socioeconomic status, and personal goals and values. However, perhaps the most challenging aspect of assessing a patient's potential for health lies in identifying personal goals, values, and self-efficacy for health.

Personal aspirations and values are readily explored. However, self-efficacy – the power to produce one's own desired ends – is not. Yet self-efficacy is also fundamental to the patient's potential for health. Bandura (1986) suggests that self-efficacy behavior, which includes choice, effort, and persistence in activities related to desired goals or outcomes, is a function of (a) the individual's self-perceptions of ability to perform a behavior and (b) the individual's beliefs that the behavior in question will lead to the specific outcomes desired. Numerous studies document the positive correlation between these two factors and actual decision making and/or action regarding health behavior (Anderson *et al.*, 2001; Martinelli, 1999; Piazza *et al.*, 2001; Rimal, 2000; Shannon *et al.*, 1997; Sherwood & Jeffery, 2000). While research related to the influence of locus of control is contradictory, researchers have demonstrated that self-efficacy and health status are the most powerful predictors of a health-promoting lifestyle (Gillis, 1993; Stuifbergen *et al.*, 2000). Approaches that focus on increasing self-efficacy for health behaviors would improve health-promoting effort and quality of life (Burke *et al.*, 1999).

In summary, the more favorable the patient's potential for health, particularly as it relates to self-efficacy and health status, the more appropriate is the practitioner's role as facilitator of health enhancement.

CONCLUSION

In this chapter we have articulated the first component of the patient-centered clinical method, exploring health, disease, and the patient's illness experience. Prior research has demonstrated how physicians have failed to acknowledge the patient's personal and unique experiences of health and illness. Caring for patients in a way that promotes health and attends to the illness experience requires a broad definition of the goals of practice. The importance of exploring the dimensions of health (through thoughtful questions) and illness experience (particularly the four dimensions of the patient's illness experience: feelings, ideas, function, and expectations [FIFE]) has been described and demonstrated through case examples. The bridge between health promotion and patient-centered care has been elucidated; a person's perception of health and the practitioner's openness to that person's perceptions create opportunities for enhanced patient-centered healing.

The final two cases that follow bring to life the integrated approach, weaving among health, disease, and illness, leading to the clinician and the patient achieving a healing integrated understanding.

"I Don't Want to Die!": Case Illustrating Component 1
Judith Belle Brown, W Wayne Weston, and Moira Stewart

With shock and disbelief Hanna felt the lump in her breast. She felt it again and with mounting fear realized her cancer may have returned. Hanna had been diagnosed with localized cancer in her left breast 4 years ago. Treatment included lumpectomy and adjuvant radiotherapy. Axillary dissection showed no cancer in the axillary lymph nodes. She was given tamoxifen at that time, which she had taken faithfully. Since her surgery and treatments Hanna had been healthy with no symptoms. With vigor and determination she had resumed her active and busy life as a wife, mother, daughter, and worker.

Now, recognizing the need to seek medical advice immediately, Hanna contacted Dr Maskova, her surgeon, who performed a biopsy. A few days later, Hanna was called into the doctor's office, at which time Dr Maskova broke the news that the biopsy results indicated a new cancer in the right breast. During the appointment, Hanna, a normally strong and independent woman, became distraught and wanted to leave immediately after her physical examination. Dr Maskova, surprised by Hanna's response, suggested they meet again in a week to discuss the next steps. Hanna agreed.

Up until that fateful appointment with her surgeon Hanna had kept her fear of recurrence a secret. Hanna, age 48, had not wanted to alarm her 50-year-old husband, Arnold, who had been recently diagnosed with hypertension. A manager at a local food store, Arnold had been under extreme stress because of a possible strike action by the cashiers at the store. The last thing Hanna wanted to do was to add more stress to her already overburdened partner. Nor did Hanna wish to frighten her two children, Rachel (aged 14) and Jonah (aged 16). They had been very anxious and afraid of losing their mother when she was first diagnosed 4 years ago. Their worries had subsided and they were both currently excelling in their individual academic and social circles. Finally, Hanna wished to protect her 70-year-old mother from the fear and angst it would evoke to learn that her daughter might have cancer again. Her mother had endured enough losses in life; the loss of an infant son from sudden infant death syndrome and then the death of her husband 6 years ago of a myocardial infarction at age 64, just as he was about to retire. And now to possibly lose her daughter would be too much to bear. Hanna resolved to keep the diagnosis a secret – just a little longer.

Hence, in the intervening week until her next visit with her surgeon, Hanna searched the Internet. She also spoke with several friends regarding breast cancer recurrence and treatment. Since Hanna worked as a copywriter for a medical journal, she was comfortable with medical terminology and tests. She was also the type of patient who needed as much information as possible in order to make any decisions about her health. In addition, she had talked at length with her friend Adelle, also a breast cancer survivor. Unlike Hanna, Adelle had tried several different kinds of alternative therapies. Her cancer had not recurred in over 7 years and Hanna began to question if she should also have tried these alternative treatments. She had begun to question her faith in conventional treatments and, although normally quite decisive, she now felt confused and uncertain about how to proceed.

A week later Hanna returned to Dr Maskova's office.

Dr Maskova: Hello Hanna – I am glad to see you back today. How are you doing?

Hanna: Hi Dr Maskova. It has been a hard week since I last saw you.

Dr Maskova: How so?

Hanna: Oh Doctor, I'm really scared, I wasn't expecting anything like this. I haven't slept in a week. I can't eat, and my stomach is in knots . . .

Dr Maskova: It does sound like it's been an awful week for you.

Hanna: Yes it has been awful. I have so many questions, and I am so confused. Will I have to stop working? I'm already finding it hard to work . . . I DON'T WANT TO DIE. I'm not ready to die; my children are just teenagers – they still need me.

Dr Maskova: There is a lot going on Hanna – a lot to consider. Tell me more about what is happening.

Hanna: Yes, and I have been on the Internet and I've been talking to friends. I need to know if I should have done things differently. Should I have restricted fat from my diet? Should I have taken shark's cartilage or Essiac? My friend has done these things and her breast cancer has not come back in over 7 years. Could it be that they prevented a recurrence for Adelle? Why did I get a new cancer? Isn't that very rare? What am I doing wrong?

Dr Maskova: *(Feeling overwhelmed by the multitude and rapidity of his patient's concerns, the doctor decides to try to gain a better understanding of Hanna's life and context.)* You're asking a lot of important questions, Hanna. I feel I need more information before I can answer them properly. Can you tell me, Hanna, what's happening at home? – with you and the family?

Hanna explained that she had not told her family because her husband was under tremendous strain at work and had high blood pressure. She described her children's fear that they would lose their mother. Most important, Hanna did not want to upset her mother; she had already had enough losses in one lifetime. Hanna perceived that the well-being of all these people was basically on her shoulders and she clearly felt overwhelmed.

Hanna's confusion and anxiety dissipated as Dr Maskova took time to listen to her story. He was honest, caring, and understanding. Dr Maskova validated her concerns and worries about the effect of her diagnosis on her family and explored ways to address how best to involve them. He listened to her growing doubts about conventional treatments and allayed her fears that she could have, or should have, done more to stop her cancer from recurring. With respect, he explored her inquiries about alternative therapies and discussed how they could examine the efficacy of such treatments together. The doctor also provided Hanna with sufficient information at the appropriate moments and provided guidance in making informed decisions. Dr Maskova supported Hanna's decision to seek information about alternative medicine, offered advice on authoritative websites, and provided contact information for a local support group. Dr Maskova made it clear to Hanna that she would be given opportunities to choose between treatment options and be involved as much as she wanted in all the decisions throughout the course of her treatment.

At the conclusion of the consultation, Hanna felt more informed, more certain, more in control, and less overwhelmed. The doctor had achieved this by exploring Hanna's feelings and expectations and by building on his relationship with Hanna, resisting his temptation to take over and provide all the answers. Dr Maskova indicated that he would be there for her through her treatment and recovery.

Hanna's interactions with her surgeon consequently became pivotal in regaining control. She needed information from him that would assist her in the multiple treatment decisions before her. She needed a surgeon who would listen to and respect her concerns and wishes. For Hanna, a relationship with her surgeon, built on honesty and reciprocity, was paramount. Hanna also needed a surgeon who expressed an interest in both her and her family – taking into consideration their needs and anxieties. By developing a trusting and respectful relationship with her surgeon, Hanna was able to regain some semblance of control over the chaos she was experiencing. Dr Maskova did not dismiss Hanna's questions or negate her worries; rather, he took the time necessary to explore her fears and that in itself helped to alleviate her concerns.

As Hanna progressed from the shattering realization of the recurrence of cancer to the treatment phase, she and her physician engaged in a process of establishing a mutual understanding of what should and would transpire. At each point in her treatment they discussed the current situation, her various options and what would be the most appropriate plan. Hanna, by choice, became an active and informed partner in her care, thereby regaining the courage to live with cancer.

"I Should Write a Letter to the Editor!": Case Illustrating Component 1
Carol L McWilliam

Mrs Samm was an 80-year-old widow with chronic obstructive pulmonary disease and hypertension. Both the physiological incapacitation and the accompanying need for oxygen by nasal cannula severely limited her mobility, leaving her largely confined to her eleventh-floor apartment, where she lived alone. Mrs Samm managed from day to day with the assistance of her only daughter, 60-year-old Gloria, who lived on a farm 40 minutes outside of town but dutifully visited every Wednesday afternoon to clean her mother's apartment, to grocery shop, to assist with managing the household finances, and to organize meals, which she froze in individual meals for easy preparation by microwave. Additionally, Gloria visited every Sunday afternoon along with her farmer husband. Both were reluctantly pursuing this family routine despite the

24-hours-a-day, 7-days-a-week demands that the farm placed on them as an aging, childless, self-sustaining couple. Every week they listened to Mrs Samm's incessant complaining about everything from the weather to her lot in life.

Dr Aronson, Mrs Samm's aging family physician, had cared for her for many years, supporting her through a life-threatening diagnosis of meningitis that Gloria had contracted as a teenager, through her husband's 2-year battle with terminal lung cancer, and through her own struggle to quit smoking at the age of 75, as her own chronic obstructive pulmonary disease worsened. Now, Dr Aronson made a house visit to Mrs Samm once a month to monitor her condition and treatment.

In the past, Mrs Samm had managed to amuse herself by watching television, reading, and talking on the telephone. However, Mrs Samm's condition had begun to deteriorate in recent months. Increased difficultly breathing, loss of appetite, and anxiety related to a fear of developing lung cancer had begun to take its toll. Mrs Samm had become preoccupied with the fear of having to go to a nursing home, or worse, the possibility of death. As her preoccupation intensified, Mrs Samm had begun to make regular visits to the hospital emergency room, seeking urgent medical attention for chronic symptoms that were clearly being adequately managed at home under her family physician's care. In response, emergency department physicians were urging Dr Aronson to consider admitting Mrs Samm to a nursing home.

Familiar with Mrs Samm's larger life context and her personal goal of avoiding admission to a nursing home, Dr Aronson decided to explore the broader notions of health with Mrs Samm. He knew from his routinely provided care that her condition had not really deteriorated. Dr Aronson needed to know more about how Mrs Samm viewed health, and what personal resources she might have to optimize her health, despite her chronic illness. Also, he needed to learn what her commitment to the pursuit of optimizing her health, despite the chronic illness, might be. He recognized that there might be broader determinants of health entering into Mrs Samm's current inability to maintain the level of wellness and quality of life that she had managed to have for the last several years. He decided to see if he might promote health by engaging her as a partner in its enhancement.

Accordingly, during his next visit, the following conversation transpired.

Dr Aronson: While I see no change in your physical condition over the past year, you seem to be experiencing more illness in recent months. Can you tell me about your experience of health right now?

Mrs Samm: I've lost my confidence. I'm afraid I will end up in a nursing home. Now, every time I feel a little down, I think I've just got to get help! I go to the hospital's emergency department and they check me out and just send me home. That makes me angry and upset, and I begin to worry even more and get very frightened that I will end up in a nursing home. It's a vicious circle, and I don't know what to do, don't know what will happen, don't know where I'll end up.

Dr Aronson: You are afraid because you don't know what to do, don't know what will happen, and don't know where you'll end up.

Mrs Samm: Yes, that's it.

Dr Aronson: So it's fear of the unknown, isn't it.

Mrs Samm: Yes, that's it. And it's affecting my health.

Dr Aronson: So is there anything that can be done about this fear of the unknown in order to help your health?

Mrs Samm: I don't know, I just want to be able to do the things I want to do.

Dr Aronson: Yes. And what might some of those things be?

Mrs Samm: I don't know. I guess I'll have to think about it.

Following this lead, Dr Aronson agreed and suggested he would come again to monitor her condition next week. At the next visit, following his routine examination, Dr Aronson resumed his effort to engage Mrs Samm in health enhancement.

Dr Aronson: So have you come up with a list of things you'd like to do?

Mrs Samm: Well, for one thing, I'd like to able to be more actively involved in the community like I used to be, but that's out with this bad breathing problem!

Dr Aronson: Maybe, maybe not. I wonder if there is anything in particular you think you might like to do?

Mrs Samm: Well, I'd sure like to do something about the mess City Hall has made of our water bills! The latest billings are outrageous, and it's all because they've increased the rates to offset the cost of new housing developments!

Dr.Aronson: I wonder what you might be able to do about it from here?

Mrs Samm: Well, I should write a letter to the editor. Someone should tell them what this means to people like me on a fixed income!

Dr Aronson: Yes, that's a great idea. I think you should do that.

Dr Aronson made a commitment to check up on Mrs Samm in 2 weeks, and followed up accordingly.

Dr Aronson: How is your health today, Mrs Samm?

Mrs Samm: Well, I'll tell you, my blood pressure must be back to normal because I did write that letter to the editor, and I've since had telephone calls from many seniors who happen to agree with me, and from my city council member, who has agreed to address it at the next council meeting. I'm glad you helped me to get onto this. When the counselor called, I also told him what I thought he should do about the problem of vandalism in our parks, and I've written a letter to the editor about that too!

Dr Aronson: Sounds like you've found a new niche in the world.

Mrs Samm: (Chuckling) Well, perhaps I have. I certainly am going to keep on to these problems. Somebody has to!

Dr Aronson agreed, and proceeded to check Mrs Samm's vital signs, review her medication adherence, and make his usual assessment. Dr Aronson observed that Mrs Samm had not been making her usual trips to the emergency department and he and Mrs Samm agreed that she was well enough for him to go back to the routine of visiting once a month.

This case illustrates how patient-centered practice can facilitate the promotion of health as a resource for everyday living. Dr Aronson sought a broader understanding of Mrs Samm, and her experience of health, illness, and disease. He determined that health to her meant being able to do the things she wanted to do. He helped her explore her commitment to and options for achieving her notion of health. He also facilitated her determination of what and how much she might do to experience health more positively, despite her debilitating chronic medical problems, and within the broader parameters of her larger life context. He used a patient-centered approach and built on the continuity of his relationship with her to enable her to use her full resources for everyday living, thereby optimizing her ability to realize her aspirations, giving her a renewed sense of purpose in life, to satisfy her needs for social cohesion within her community, and to respond positively to the environment, despite her chronic medical problems.

4 The Second Component: Understanding The Whole Person, Section 1 – Individual and Family

Judith Belle Brown and W Wayne Weston

> It is impossible to practice effective primary medical care without attention to the range of psychological and social issues embedded in the lives of all human beings. (Pincus, 2004: 243)

We all face the many challenges and demands presented at each stage of human development. The ascendancy to independence in adolescence, the creation of intimate partnerships in adulthood, and the realignment of roles and tasks that transpire in the senior years are all examples of expected life cycle changes. How we traverse each stage will be influenced by prior life experience. For many individuals, the successful achievement of the tasks and expectations of each developmental phase steers them through life relatively unscathed. However, for others, each ensuing life phase may be marred by past failures and previous losses; for them, life's challenges are experienced as overwhelming and often unachievable.

The second component of the patient-centered clinical method is the integration of the concepts of health, disease, and illness with an understanding of the whole person, including an awareness of the patient's position in the life cycle and his or her life context. The patient's position in the life cycle takes into consideration the individual's own personality development, whereas the patient's context includes both his or her proximal (e.g., familial) and his or her distal (e.g., cultural) contexts. Distal context will be addressed in Chapter 5.

THE PERSON: INDIVIDUAL DEVELOPMENT

There are multiple theoretical frameworks that can help clinicians understand patients' individual development and provide both explanation and prediction about patient behavior and responses to illness. For example, they include psychoanalytic theory (i.e., ego psychology, object relations, and self-psychology);

feminist theory; and cognitive theory. A comprehensive overview of these various theoretical frameworks has been provided by numerous authors (e.g., Piaget, 1950; Erikson, 1950, 1982; Kohut, 1971, 1977; Bowlby, 1973, 1982; Gilligan, 1982; Berzoff *et al.*, 1996; Schriver, 2004; Guest, 2007; Santrock, 2007; Broderick & Blewitt, 2010; Harris, 2011). The intent of this section of the chapter is to highlight understanding individual development and to demonstrate how its exploration can be achieved in the practice of patient-centered care.

Healthy individual development is reflected by a solid sense of self, positive self-esteem, a position of independence, and autonomy, coupled with the capacity for connectedness and intimacy. The motives, attachments, ideals, and expectations that shape each individual's personality evolve as they traverse each developmental phase. Each person's life is profoundly influenced by each stage of development, which may be isolated and lonely for an elderly widow or vast and complex for a middle-aged woman with multiple responsibilities as wife, mother, daughter, and worker. Thus their position in the life cycle, the tasks they assume, and the roles they ascribe to will influence the care that patients seek. As an illustration of the impact of illness on human development, consider the teenager grappling with the demands of peer acceptance who is ostracized because of his or her acne, or the middle-aged woman coping with the "empty-nest syndrome" who is reminded of her loss of fertility by the symptoms of menopause.

Understanding the patient's current stage of development and the relevant developmental tasks that need to be accomplished assists clinicians in several ways. First, knowledge of expected life cycle crises that occur in individual development helps the clinician recognize the patient's problems as more than isolated, episodic phenomena. Second, it can increase the clinician's sensitivity to the multiple factors that influence the patient's problems and broaden awareness of the impact of the patient's life history. For example, the onset of a chronic illness at an early age may interfere with negotiation of age-specific tasks. Such is the case with juvenile-onset diabetes, which may create difficulty for an adolescent attempting to negotiate the turbulent process of becoming independent. Third, understanding the whole person may also expand the clinician's level of comfort with caring as well as curing.

In the following two case examples we witness the loss of independence and its devastating impact on two patients in their later years. The stories depict how disease not only affects organs and organ systems of the body but also diminishes patients' ability to achieve goals and aspirations that give meaning to their lives. Often the patients presenting before us bear no resemblance to their former selves. We view them in their present context and fail to understand their past.

Case Example

As the nurse cleaned up another soiled diaper of her patient in bed C, room 557, all she saw was a frail old man, eyes at half-mast, bent over in his wheelchair, unable to speak. What she failed to capture was Allen, the Renaissance man.

Allen had been diagnosed with Parkinson's disease at the age of 68 – shortly after the death of his wife, Maria, a year before after a protracted course of breast cancer. While her death had been devastating, Allen had adapted stoically. Together they had raised three children who had gone on to lead successful and happy lives – of this he was proud and content. Initially the diagnosis of Parkinson's had not fazed him, but as the symptoms of the disease rapidly progressed he was suddenly projected into a place he had never imagined. The family home was sold and Allen was placed in a long-term facility. At a frightening rate, Allen experienced a loss of multiple functions – he could no longer walk and was now confined to a wheelchair, and he was unable to dress or feed himself without some catastrophic incident such as a serious fall. Ultimately, he lost the ability to communicate – while his internal voice remained strong and his cognition intact, Allen's ability to speak was gone. Allen the Renaissance man had vanished, with only his children remembering the history of this amazing man.

In particular, his one daughter, Jordan, tried vehemently to retain her father's spirit and zest for life. She reminisced with him about his passion for classical music and their times together at the opera. Allen had been an avid sailor, and with care and devotion he had refitted an ancient teak sailboat that was the envy of his yacht club. Jordan and her father could now see the humor in his disastrous finish in the Boston Marathon when he was aged 60 – Allen had come in as the 300th runner, but at least he had finished! As a successful entrepreneur in the sale of "used but not abused" clothing he had done well, but more important was the commitment Allen had made to the betterment of his community – not just financially but also through active participation in campaigns to make it safer, cleaner, and viable for all who lived there.

Allen was a remarkable man in his time, but as his time began to diminish and slip away Jordan took note. She reflected on his life and grieved the inevitable loss of her beloved father, the Renaissance man – but at the same time she took hold of the moment to be with him as he, with her care and love, moved toward the end of his life.

Imagine how the health care professional's care of Allen may have changed if she had shown interest and taken the time to know the man he had been.

Case Example

At the age of 88, Thompson felt very satisfied with his life as he reflected on his loving marriage of 58 years with Victoria, his two successful children, Belle and Gibson, and a very fulfilling career in the technology industry. After being a widower for 3 years, Thompson had made the decision to sell the family home with the blessing of his children and he now resided in a retirement home. Thompson had gradually adjusted to this new lifestyle at the retirement home – although with some reluctance. He was still very independent and in fact still remained, although peripherally, engaged with the technology industry.

Thompson's health had been remarkable for his age – high blood pressure controlled by medications, and some intermittent arthritis. He viewed the latter as part of aging. But in the winter of his eighty-eighth year his health status and quality of life was dramatically altered. After an episode of shortness of breath, ankle edema, and general malaise, the nursing staff at the retirement home had Thompson transferred by ambulance to the local emergency department. Thompson was admitted to hospital and the next 10 days were uncertain and dispiriting for Thompson. It took the wind out of his sails. He felt unsteady and confused, and he lacked interest in common routines such as the daily news.

The cardiology team assessed him as being severely compromised with a 20% ejection fraction of his left ventricle. Thompson's life as he knew it was about to change. Because of his compromised cardiac status he was abruptly informed that his driver's license would be revoked. Thompson was shocked. He felt as though his independence had been violently stripped away. How would he manage to go out for lunch, get his hair cut, or just run a few errands? While perhaps viewed as mundane activities to many, these outings framed the passing of Thompson's days. The thought of being dependent on others was hard to grasp, let alone his loss of freedom to go when and where he pleased. Also, the thought of "giving up" his beloved car was inconceivable. While the cardiologist's decision was based on sound guidelines, it underestimated the psychological and social ramifications for the patient. In the weeks following Thompson's discharge from hospital he slowly recovered physically but his emotional health suffered as he deeply grieved his loss of independence.

In addition to managing his heart failure, the clinician needed to provide Thompson with an opportunity to discuss the increasing loss of his independence and his increased risk of depression.

Understanding the patient's personality structure, in particular the defense mechanisms they use to ward off anxiety, both internal and external, can enhance clinicians' understanding of patients' varied responses to disease and illness. Defense mechanisms, which are automatic and unconscious, serve an important function in protecting the self or the ego from real or perceived danger (Schamess, 1996; Cramer, 2000, 2006; Bond, 2004; Larsen *et al.*, 2010). Patients use a variety of defense mechanisms, including more primitive or immature defenses such as denial and projection. Higher-level or more mature defenses such as rationalization and sublimation are used to ward off toxic threats to the ego and thus help patients to cope. The defenses are used to prevent ego disintegration and as such need to be respected. As Broom (1997: 66–7) observes:

> The patient defends himself against the 'intolerable' by setting in place structures that are not ideal but are actually adaptive within the patient's total economy, and we should expect resistance to any change in this. I may be imprisoned and long for freedom, but also be terrified of venturing out into a wider world. There may also be some comforts in the prison cell that those of us outside may scorn as objects to be clung to, but this may be very understandable within the patient's perspective.

The following case serves as an example of a patient's use of defense mechanisms and takes place in the context of what is normally a happy event, the birth of a child.

Case Example

When the delivery room nurse announced to 28-year-old Isabel that her baby was a healthy 8-pound boy the patient cried out: "I didn't want a boy!" She refused to hold the baby and the shocked nurse handed the baby over to his father.

A few days later, when the visiting nurse made a home visit, she found

Isabel stiffly holding her infant. She denied that there were any problems and rationalized her outburst in the delivery room as a result of exhaustion from a long labor. Over the next several weeks as the nurse continued to visit Isabel, she observed that mother and child were bonding well. Isabel's initial displeasure about the baby's sex seemed to have disappeared. Her anger was now being displaced onto her husband, Luka, whom she described as never being around or helping out with young Anthony. The source of the marital discord was apparently Luka's "obsession with work." From Isabel's perspective, Luka was "hell-bent" on proving he could successfully operate the pizza business inherited from his father – a legacy she deeply resented. Her husband was just like her father, who had never been physically or emotionally available during her childhood. "All men are the same," concluded Isabel, "never there when you need them most."

The nurse's attempts to explore Isabel's feelings during subsequent visits were met with denial and rationalization. Because mother and child were doing well, the nurse's role had been fulfilled, yet as she closed the case she had a nagging feeling that Isabel's defenses were protecting her from some deeper distress. We will return later in this chapter to Isabel's story.

An understanding of the whole person enhances the clinician's interaction with the patient and may be particularly helpful when signs or symptoms do not point to a clearly defined disease process, or when the patient's response to an illness appears exaggerated or out of character. On these occasions, it is often helpful to explore how the patient is dealing with the common issues related to his or her stage in the life cycle. Knowing that a patient has minimal family interaction or limited social supports alerts the practitioner to an individual at risk. Also, being aware of prior losses or developmental crises assists the clinician to identify vulnerable junctures in the patient's life.

Case Example

Dr Grant was perplexed. This was the sixth time he had seen his 23-year-old patient, Suzy, and her daughter, Michelle, in the last 2 months. At each visit Suzy had expressed concern about her 5-year-old daughter's health, but from the clinician's perspective Michelle's, or rather her mother's, complaints were minor, such as a sore throat or a stomachache. On each occasion Dr Grant reassured Suzy that her daughter's problem was self-limiting and would resolve quickly. Yet Suzy continued to bring her daughter to see the doctor.

Suzy and her daughter had joined the practice a year ago and, upon reflection, Dr Grant realized he knew little of Suzy's life and experiences. At the end of the next visit he asked Suzy if she would be interested in coming back alone to talk to him regarding her concerns about Michelle. She agreed and when she returned the following story was revealed.

Suzy, a single parent on welfare, was finding it more difficult to cope with the demands of her active daughter. She had become increasingly more physical with Michelle in her attempts to control her behavior and was concerned that she might unintentionally harm her when her anger got "out of control." In order to cope with the pressure and calm herself down, she had started to drink "the odd shot of vodka," which at times had led to consuming the whole bottle.

Suzy described her feelings of guilt after having struck Michelle and how these feelings added to her sense of helplessness and growing reliance on alcohol. She often ruminated about "what could have been" if her boyfriend had not "got her pregnant and taken off." Her goal had been to go to university and train as a physiotherapist; her above-average high school grades would have ensured admission into the program. Suzy was angry at herself for "wasting" her life. She felt extremely lonely and confused. Finally, she questioned her ability to be a "good" mother and in turn demanded near-perfection in her mothering skills (e.g., hygiene and child nutrition).

The doctor then asked about her early years and learned important information about Suzy's past that illuminated her current problems and concerns. Suzy, the eldest of three daughters, was raised in a rural community. Her father had held an executive position with a nearby food processing and distributing company for 30 years. He was an alcoholic who controlled his binge drinking in such a way that it did not interfere with the demands of his job. However, when intoxicated he would emotionally and physically abuse his wife. Often, Suzy and her younger sisters "got in the way" and would also suffer physical and emotional abuse from their father.

Her pregnancy had been a shameful experience for the family and became a well-kept family secret. Forced to leave the family home and small, close-knit community where she had been raised, all Suzy's supports and connections had been severed. Furthermore, her father had forbidden her to have contact with her mother and sisters. Consequently, Suzy was raising Michelle on her own, with no family support and limited social supports.

In listening to Suzy's story the doctor gained a greater understanding and deeper appreciation of the influence of the patient's past on her current behavior. Her frequent visits to the doctor and her "overconcern" about her daughter's health were being fuelled by multiple factors, both present and historical. A pattern of multigenerational behaviors and responses was now evident. Dr Grant was no longer perplexed by his patient's actions but, rather, was informed by her difficult and tragic history of abuse and alcoholism. The patient's disclosure of this important information would assist the patient and doctor in their work together – helping Suzy be the best mom she could be.

Individuals' pasts can haunt them, immobilizing their ability to act in the present and preventing their movement toward future goals and aspirations. As Fraiberg *et al.* (1975) so aptly wrote, there are "ghosts in the nursery" – demons of the past that can be dissipated by the clinician's careful and attentive listening to the patient's life story, not just his or her disease.

Finally, the normal achievement of developmental milestones by a child can often serve as triggers for the parent of unresolved issues from his or her past. Returning to the case of Isabel serves as an illustration.

Case Example

When Isabel's son, Anthony, was 2 years of age, she began presenting to her family doctor with a variety of complaints including headaches, dizziness, leg weakness, and buzzing in her ears. Each round of investigations failed to uncover a cause for her symptoms. Reassurance from her doctor that "nothing was wrong" did not alleviate her distress; rather, her symptoms intensified and the frequency of her visits increased. Finally, during one of her many visits, Isabel burst into tears, crying out: "I think I'm dying." The doctor was initially baffled by the intensity of her response, since none of her symptoms were life-threatening. She appeared to have a happy home life, with a healthy and active toddler, and a loving husband. However, clearly Isabel's ongoing presentation of multiple and unexplained physical symptoms was a signal of some deeper distress in her life.

What unfolded was a complex multigenerational story activated by the normal developmental progression of her toddler. As Anthony began to assert his autonomy and independence she felt anxious and abandoned. The root of these powerful emotions rested in the patient's own childhood and her family of origin.

Isabel was the eldest of five children, all of whom had been born in rapid succession, thus propelling her from the maternal nest. By the age of 7, she had become her mother's "little helper," assisting in the care of her younger siblings. Unconsciously, she had assumed this role in an attempt to have her own needs addressed. When this failed, Isabel turned in desperation to her father, but he was self-absorbed with his failing business and his physical problems, including chronic leg weakness as a result of having polio in his youth. Isabel's father frequently complained how the burden of providing for his family was "killing him".

Isabel's early years had been filled with abandonment and uncertainty. Now in her late twenties, these feelings had resurfaced as her son, in whom she had invested all her love and attention, was asserting his own independence. Unable to understand or describe her inexplicable sense of loss, she had voiced her feelings through bodily symptoms.

This is a difficult and multifaceted case and the patient's story was uncovered during many visits with the family doctor and this was assisted by the expert skills of a therapist. It highlights the intricate relationship between mind and body, past and present (Broom, 1997, 2000, 2007; Frankel *et al.*, 2003). While not all patients' stories are this complex, this case demonstrates how clinicians can use their understanding of the whole person to enhance patient-centered care. Learning about the patient's developmental journey helps clinicians realize that patients are more than just their diseases. As Broom (1997: 1–2) observes:

> The patient's story is, amongst many other things, a woven tapestry – of events, of perceptions of events, and of highly idiosyncratic responses to events. Many of the very significant events have to do with the vicissitudes of the patient's relationships with the world, and with other significant persons. Therefore, when a patient and a doctor collaborate together to look for the meaning of an illness, they are usually looking for the story of a person in relationship.

SPIRITUAL ISSUES

The final segment of this section examines the role of spirituality in patients' lives and how they come to terms with illness. Spirituality can be defined as "the personal quest for understanding answers to ultimate questions about life, meaning, and relationships to the sacred or transcendent which may (or may not) lead to or arise from the development of religious rituals and the formation of community" (Koenig *et al.*, 2001: 18). However, in the second edition of the *Handbook of Religion and Health*, Koenig *et al.* (2012: 38) point out that the increasing secularization of the world has resulted in large groups of people who "claim they are neither religious nor spiritual – yet rightly argue that their lives have purpose and meaning, that they experience connections with others, have high personal values, strong character, and have a variety of personal beliefs." Consequently, clinicians need to be prepared to discuss issues that give meaning to their patients' lives, whatever label they apply to these fundamental concerns.

Until recently physicians have abdicated issues of patient spirituality to the clergy (Handzo & Koenig, 2004). Physicians are hesitant to discuss religious or spiritual issues with their patients, perhaps because they feel such inquiry is outside their area of expertise or perhaps from fear of offending patients (Post *et al.*, 2000; Koenig, 2004). However, research has revealed patients' desire for their physicians' involvement in the spiritual aspects of their personhood (McCord *et al.*, 2004; Lee-Poy, 2012a).

Furthermore, physicians have expressed an interest in engaging their patients in discussions about spirituality, recognizing that this must be approached with "sensitivity and integrity" (Ellis *et al.*, 2002: 249; Craigie & Hobbs, 1999; Steinhauser *et al.*, 2006). While physicians recognize the relationship between spirituality and patient overall well-being, barriers to assessing patients' spiritual resources include lack of time, inadequate training, and a belief that discussion of spiritual issues is beyond the proper boundaries of patient care and not part of the conventional medical culture (Groopman, 2004; Milstein, 2008). Broom (1997) views the person's mind, body, and spirituality as an integrated whole; to separate off one piece for examination is to minimize, or at worst deny, the importance of the others. In Lee-Poy's study, physicians' beliefs about the importance of religion and spirituality and their comfort level were significantly associated with asking about patients' beliefs (Lee-Poy *et al.*, 2012b).

Serious illness raises questions about meaning: why has this happened, why me, what did I do to deserve this, what will become of me, what will become of my family? Such questions (which reflect our desire to make sense of our lives and our experience of illness) may have no easy answers and are unique to each person. These questions may lead to a deepening of patients' spiritual lives or, conversely, to a loss of faith based on a feeling that God has abandoned them or a sense that life has no meaning. Thus, these questions are intensely important. Yet, because they are so personal, they may not be discussed with anyone, not even family or close friends. This may leave the patient alone with these fundamental doubts and concerns at a time when they most need to share them, a challenge to all members of the health care team to be open to discuss these issues.

Dombeck and Evinger (1998: 114) describe the qualities of effective dialogue about spiritual issues:

> Moreover, in order to be a spiritual resource to another in spiritual distress, one does not have to be an expert or have answers to spiritual questions. It is enough that one listen with openness and respect by offering non-judgmental acceptance. Acknowledging the profundity of the sufferer's questions in a spirit of connectedness rather than detachment is more valuable than offering one's own answers to another's spiritual quandaries.

Curlin and Hall (2005) outline an approach to addressing spiritual issues in health care and argue that approaching spiritual questions as a technical concern between strangers misses the point. Acknowledging that some professional boundaries are important, they submit that "the divisions of labor that reinforce many professional boundaries can yield an impersonal, technical, fragmented, bureaucratic, and ultimately dehumanizing practice of medicine that undermines genuine interpersonal care and connection" (2005: 372). Discourse on spiritual issues always requires respect for the patient's ideas and beliefs and should never be subjected to coercion, but sometimes call for "persuasive negotiation" (2005: 372) to promote the patient's best interests – for example, when their beliefs are leading them to make harmful choices.

May (1991: 14) observes that there are two kinds of ethical questions in medicine:

> On the whole, medical ethics has tended to explore those moral issues that cluster around the admittedly important question 'What are we going to do about it?' but at the expense of those deep, troubling issues which patients and families often face: How can they manage – whatever the decision or whatever the event – to rise to the occasion?

He comments further:

> the latter type of problem resembles a mystery more than a puzzle; it demands a response that resembles a ritual repeated more than a technique. (1991: 4)

The following example illustrates the dilemma faced by patients struck down by illness:

> suddenly a blood clot stalls in his coronary artery; the rescue unit pulls him out of his car and wheels him into an intensive care unit. Suddenly he finds his

time even more limited than he thought. The catastrophe confronts him with problems to solve; but these problems pale before the deeper question: who and what is he now that he has suffered this explosion from within? Accustomed to commanding his world, the patient suddenly finds himself helpless in the hands of nurses down the hospital corridor; used to total obedience from his subordinates, he discovers that the very humblest of his subordinates, his own body, has rebelled against him." (1991: 5)

How does such a man come to terms with the loss of a job that gave his life excitement and meaning? Adopting a less demanding role, perhaps as a mentor to junior colleagues, and learning to pace himself may help, but these technical solutions do not address the fundamental crisis involved in losing his former identity. Such questions are at the heart of religion and spirituality and they call out for dialogue.

The following case examines the role of spirituality in a couple's attempt to deal with a devastating health event. How the case evolves highlights the importance of teamwork described in Chapters 10 and 13.

Case Example

Together they had carefully mapped out their early retirement plan. Over the years Constance and Mert had been diligent in their financial planning to ensure a solid 10 years of travel to exotic venues – adventures they had always dreamed of. Suddenly, Constance and Mert's life together was irrevocably altered and their careful plans shattered. At 60 years of age, Mert had suffered a debilitating stroke, rendering him hemiplegic. In the early days, Constance explained: "Of course our way of life has changed and his world is only what he can reach. But I'm so glad he's here." But as much as they attempted to work together in confronting and adjusting to their present situation, both Constance and Mert also described grieving the dramatic change in their relationship.

Mert felt guilt and self-loathing for the burden he placed on Constance. "If I wasn't here, Constance could go on with her life. I'm pulling her down." Over time, Mert became more uncommunicative and withdrawn. For Constance the ongoing demands of constant caregiving gave rise to negative reactions that were also damaging to the couple's relationship. An accumulation of feelings – vulnerability, irritability, fatigue, loss, and guilt – began to surface, undermining Constance's attempt to pull her husband back into their relationship.

Constance, who had throughout their 30-year marriage devoted herself to Mert, experienced his withdrawal as abandonment and rejection. While distraught because of Mert's profound disability, Constance could not quiet her anger – not at their situation but at Mert. They had been so close, so connected, such kindred spirits. How could he withdraw from her at this moment! She was disappointed that he had also turned his back on God. Their religion had been so important to both of them and now, when they most needed it, he would not discuss his feelings about his situation. When, together, they met with their family doctor to discuss Mert's management options they were sad, angry, confused, and in conflict. The doctor was overwhelmed by their powerful display of emotions. In previous contacts with this couple he had observed their very measured and clear decision making. Yet now they were in serious distress. Recognizing that they needed more time and expertise than he could offer, the doctor referred them to the social worker affiliated with the clinic.

Several sessions with the social worker, and then with a pastoral counselor, were needed to help Mert and Constance overcome the conflict-laden behaviors they were expressing. Conversations about their shared joy of exotic travel brought them back into conflict and disappointment because such opportunities were no longer possible. However, exploration of other shared interests led them to express their common belief in the healing power of their spiritual values. Their sense of connectedness increased as together they regained their shared sense of faith. Recognizing and reaffirming their shared religious commitments helped them continue to share together what gave their lives meaning, even in the face of Mert's chronic illness.

When chronic illness strikes, each partner must accept the new role of either caregiver or care receiver, and each must subsequently reconcile how this role change affects their role as a partner in a couple relationship. This necessitates revising their own, as well as their partner's, understanding and interpretation of their respective roles. When the illness is chronic and deteriorating, with no hope for improvement, couples need assistance in understanding and accepting the changes brought about by the chronic illness. They need guidance and new skills to help express and realize both their individual and their shared needs, wants, and expectations.

Health care professionals can help couples maintain and build on their strengths of reciprocity, mutuality, and concern. Supporting couples to discuss and work through feelings of guilt, anger and frustration may alleviate negative experiences and facilitate positive, reciprocal exchanges. Specific interventions, such as providing more in-home care, increasing utilization of respite services, or giving the well spouse "permission" for time out for themselves, may assist couples in shifting from instrumental needs to relationship needs.

For all couples living with a chronic illness, an intervention directed at improved communication would include dialogue between the partners that is sensitive, open, and always patient-centered, acknowledging that both partners in the dyad are patients. This will result in a more positive balance of roles and function within their relationship and strengthen the doctor's relationship with both members of the dyad, recognizing them both as a couple and as individuals.

THE PERSON AND THE FAMILY LIFE CYCLE

Patients may be parents, partners, and sons or daughters; they all have a past, a present, and a future. We are all connected on some level to a family, which in turn shapes who we are as people and as patients. Relationships and kinships bind us to one another, making us feel needed, loved, and connected. Illness can enhance or sever these essential ties in human relationships, leaving both the sick and the well feeling alone and rudderless. The journey to recovery or, at best, attainment of the status quo can be experienced as an extreme effort, and for some this is beyond the realm of possibility.

Similar to individual development, a vast literature on family theory exists to explain and understand the intricacies and dynamics of family systems. Again, it is not the purpose of this chapter to provide a comprehensive overview of this area but, rather, to highlight the important role of the family in understanding the whole person. The reader is directed to the following texts that provide clear and thoughtful presentations of the family life cycle and family systems: Walsh (2009), McGoldrick *et al.* (2010). The following are additional works that link family systems and primary care: Doherty and Baird (1986), McDaniel *et al.* (2005), Doherty and McDaniel (2010).

In concurrence with other authors (Medalie & Cole-Kelly, 2002; McDaniel *et al.*, 2005; McGoldrick *et al.*, 2010), we define family as two or more people related or connected either biologically, emotionally, or legally with a history and a future. Our conceptualization extends beyond the traditional notion of the family, encompassing unions such as gay and lesbian couples, common-law relationships, single-parent families, couples without children, and households composed of friends. While the composition and roles of the family have changed and expanded, the function of the family has remained constant

– to provide a nurturing and safe environment that promotes the physical, psychological, and social well-being of its members. In today's society this is a daunting task. The family is being buffeted by internal and external forces. The rising divorce rate, the increase in single-parent households, changes in traditional sex-role relationships, and the financial need for both parents to work all challenge the function of the family. The health and well-being of families is assaulted by problems such as child and woman abuse, suicide, and substance abuse. Families must also face the enormous strain imposed by unemployment, poverty, serious illness, and being homeless. In examining the role and influence of the family life cycle on patients' responses to the illness experience we must take heed of Candib's caution to expand our perspective beyond gender-laden perspectives (Candib, 1995). A broad definition of family must be assumed with an acknowledgment of the broader sociocultural and political influences that shape the clinicians' knowledge, beliefs, and values about the family.

The additional burden of illness, either acute or chronic, may cause severe disruption to an already overtaxed family system (Medalie & Cole-Kelly, 2002; Newman, 2008; Gorman, 2011; Chambers, 2012). Illness, either acute or chronic, is a powerful agent of change. The impact of illness on the family ranges from the devastating loss of the breadwinner role caused by a cardio-vascular accident to the riveting effect on a family when a child is diagnosed with cerebral palsy. Jack Medalie, as a young family physician practicing on a kibbutz in Israel, experienced a powerful example of the impact of illness of one member of the family resulting in illness in the caregiver – what he referred to as the "hidden patient" (Medalie *et al.*, 1999). Medalie had been making regular home visits to an elderly man recovering from a myocardial infarction and he observed the attentive care provided by the man's wife. Late one night Medalie was called to the home for an emergency. Expecting his patient may have suffered another heart attack, Medalie was surprised to see he had improved. Instead, Medalie learned that the patient's wife had committed suicide by jumping off a cliff. This is a dramatic example of the great stress that illness in the family can place on caregivers. In one study, caregivers older than 65 were 63% more likely to die than age-matched non-caregiving controls over a 4-year period and they had higher rates of multiple physical illnesses, depression, and anxiety (Schulz & Beach, 1999).

The following case illustrates how the family's response to illness can have a ripple effect among its members.

Case Example

The possibility of breast cancer had been a foreboding presence in Mia's mind since her mother died of breast cancer when Mia was in her first year of law school. In the passing years Mia had appropriately grieved the loss of her mother and became a mother herself to three sons and a daughter. Mia shared a law practice with Raymond, her husband of 20 years, and together they had built successful careers and a happy, albeit busy, home.

While Mia's diagnosis of breast cancer 1 year ago had not been completely unexpected, the news was devastating for the entire family. However, the family quickly rallied around Mia to support her in her battle against cancer. The exception was 14-year-old Alexandria – her mother's cancer rocked the foundations of her being.

Mia faced her breast cancer with her usual strong will and determination. In character with her life view, she was positive and proactive, making the necessary lifestyle changes required to tackle her cancer. Mia knew and believed that cancer research had made significant strides since her mother succumbed to the disease over 22 years ago. Treatments were much more successful and survival rates for her type of breast cancer had improved significantly. All this Mia had conveyed to her family and most pointedly to her fearful daughter.

Always a somewhat anxious child, prone to abdominal pain, Alexandria's symptoms of anxiety were exacerbated by her mother's diagnosis. In the early months, during which her mother underwent a lumpectomy and radiotherapy, Alexandria kept her growing anxiety hidden from her family. Now that her mother had returned to work part-time, Alexandria could no longer keep her symptoms at bay. Alexandria began complaining of heart palpitations and dizziness and she was biting her nails down to the quick. On a few occasions Mia had discovered her daughter plucking at her eyelashes. In Mia's mind this was the last straw. Pushing aside her guilt for being the source of Alexandria's mounting anxiety, Mia took action. Now was the time to wrap the family's love and energy around Alexandria. With her husband Raymond's support, and the wholehearted encouragement of her sons, the family stepped forward to eradicate Alexandria's debilitating anxiety. Together they attended family therapy and together they learned more about one another – and themselves. In particular, Mia came to understand how her sometimes overly enthusiastic approach to attacking her cancer may have preempted her daughter's ability to voice her concerns and fears of losing her mother – just as she had lost her own mother to cancer. In addition, Mia recognized how denying the possibility of a recurrence of her cancer would only serve as false reassurance for the already anxious Alexandria.

Together, the family gained insight into how their "fighting stance" toward Mia's breast cancer had squelched the opportunity for all of them to share their fears and worries about their future together. This was a new healing experience for Mia and her family.

Illness in the family causes a major disruption, altering how families relate, and it may ultimately impede their ability to overcome the ramifications of the illness experience. Illness may demand a change in the family role structure and task allocation. Changes in routine may be required, such as child care responsibilities or visits to the hospital. Major alterations may be needed, such as substantial home renovations to accommodate a wheelchair-bound family member or a return to the workforce to provide for the financial needs of the family.

The disequilibrium in the family resulting from illness can also alter the established rules and expectations of the family, transform their methods of communication, and substantially alter the family structure. For example, after a disabling stroke, a mother transferred her responsibilities for the care of her five children to her eldest daughter, aged 18. The daughter, in turn, quit school, assumed the full caregiver role for her siblings, and became her father's confidant as he watched his wife resign herself to her disability. The changes imposed on families by illness are limitless and are accompanied by a host of feelings: loss, fear, anger, resignation, anxiety, sadness, resentment, and dependency.

Involving the family is also important, given that over one-third of patients are accompanied by one or more family members during a visit to their doctor (Brown *et al.*, 1998; Marvel *et al.*, 1999). Family members may be as concerned as the patient about the problem or potential treatments. They can also provide important information about the patient and be an invaluable resource in the patient's recovery (Watson & McDaniel, 2000). However, as Lang *et al.* (2002) observed, involving family members in an office visit can present specific challenges, such as maintaining confidentiality and addressing family conflict. The particular needs of the patient and knowledge of the family's dynamics will assist clinicians in deciding who to involve within the family and when to approach them. The use of a genogram may help simplify a complex family structure by displaying relationships and patterns.

How families have coped previously will influence how they negotiate the impact of the illness on their family roles, rules, patterns of communication, and structures. Therefore, in understanding the impact of the illness on the family some key questions can guide the clinician's inquiry: At what point in the family life cycle is the family (e.g., starting a family, launching pad, or retirement)? Where is each member in the life cycle (e.g., adolescence or middle age)? What are the developmental tasks for each individual and for the family as a whole? How does the illness affect the achievement of these multiple tasks? What kinds of illnesses have the family experienced? What kinds of support have they mobilized in the past to help them cope with illness? Is there currently an established support network? How has the family dealt with illness in the past? Have they responded with functional or dysfunctional patterns of behavior? For example, has the family demonstrated potential maladaptive responses, such as rejection of the sick person, or overprotection that stifles responsibility for self-care?

These latter questions are important because they elicit how families may contribute to or perpetuate illness behavior in their members (Davidson *et al.*, 2012). The family may represent a safe refuge for the ill person or, conversely, the family may aggravate the illness through maladaptive responses.

The impact of the diagnosis on the patient and family will depend on the juncture in the life cycle when it occurs. For example, an adult male with a preexisting history of diabetes mellitus may find his disease has less impact on his role (as a husband and father) than a teenager who is diagnosed at the point when he and his family are struggling with adolescent issues of independence and identity. Similarly, the preoccupations and struggles of families in each stage may be vastly different – for example, how does the diagnosis of multiple sclerosis impact on the childrearing responsibilities of the family system; what meaning does the death of an adult child have on aging parents who were relying on that child for support; and, conversely, how do aging parents plan and prepare for the care of their developmentally challenged adult child?

Finally, while the illness of an individual family member reverberates throughout the family system (Saunders, 2003), the family also plays a powerful role in modifying the illness experience of the individual. There is now a strong body of research demonstrating how families affect health, ranging from maternal-infant bonding (Klaus *et al.*, 1996; Mooney, 2010) to the consequences of bereavement (Schulz *et al.*, 2003; Stroebe *et al.*, 2007). Both McWhinney & Freeman (2009), and McDaniel and colleagues (2005) provide excellent reviews of the empirical evidence documenting the significant influence of the family on the health and disease of its members.

CONCLUSION

Clinicians develop an evolving understanding of the social and developmental context in which their patients live their lives. Usually, this information is not gathered in a single encounter as part of a formal social history but rather is accumulated over many visits that can span months or years. As the patient and clinician have shared life experiences this understanding becomes richer and more detailed. With certain patients this information may help the clinician understand the patient's complex dynamics and idiosyncratic responses to illness or demands for care (Jones & Morrell, 1995; Hani *et al.*, 2007). Specific aspects of the patient's family dynamics or developmental difficulties may not necessarily be shared with the patient but guide the practitioner in the management and care of the patient. In other instances, facilitating the patient's awareness of the origin of his or her conflicts or distress may help the patient make sense of his or her struggles and pain. Finally, understanding the whole person can deepen the clinician's knowledge of the human condition, especially the nature of suffering and the responses of persons to sickness (Cassell, 2004, 2013; Schleifer & Vannatta, 2013).

Trauma, Tragedy, Trust, and Triumph: Case Illustrating Component 2*
Judith Belle Brown

Dr Catherine Lejon had met Charlene on a few occasions when she had been the "fly-in physician" to this remote and mostly native community of 600 residents. Charlene, a community health worker, had, in spite of her petite stature, presented as a formidable figure with twinkling eyes, a charming smile, and a fierce determination to "do the very best" for her people.

When Charlene became pregnant and requested that Dr Lejon take on her prenatal care, Dr Lejon was reluctant to mix a professional relationship with personal care. However, knowing how the absence of prenatal care would place Charlene's pregnancy at risk, she agreed. What Dr Lejon did not know, and would ultimately learn, was the complex history enveloping this young and vulnerable woman. Over the course of several visits, Dr Lejon discovered Charlene's story. Her parents had suffered deeply from the injustices of the residential school program, which filled her childhood with violence, substance abuse, and daily chaos. For much of her life Charlene had felt alone and

---

*   This narrative is based on an accumulation of stories over 2 decades shared by family physician students in the Advanced Patient-Centered Medicine course of the Master of Clinical Science Program in Family Medicine at Western University.

unsupported, with her father often out of work and frequently absent – leaving her mother frantic in her attempts to care for Charlene and her five siblings.

During her teenage years Charlene silently watched in horror as each of her siblings succumbed to the alcohol and drug abuse that was the scourge of her community. The exception was her younger sister, who Charlene vigilantly protected – like a mother bear watches over her vulnerable cub. Since the age of 10, Charlene had been repeatedly raped by her father during his binge drinking. She had resolved that her sister would never suffer such pain and humiliation. Charlene believed that her mother had known about the abuse but had not intervened for fear of her husband's wrath. In her mid-teens, Charlene, after one particularly violent assault by her father, had attempted suicide by hanging herself in an old shed behind the family home. It was only by chance that her eldest brother, who had retreated to the shed to smoke a joint, discovered Charlene. Neither disclosed her suicide attempt – it became a solemn secret between sister and brother.

For a time in her late adolescence Charlene experienced a glimmer of hope. Her life could be different. Her sister was no longer at risk of abuse because their father had been incarcerated for aggravated assault. Charlene now had the chance to do something for herself. At the age of 20 Charlene left her small community to attend a special native community health worker program at a community college 200 kilometers away. The course work was challenging, the big city daunting, and the isolation from her culture at times overwhelming. However, Charlene persevered – driven by a burning desire to take back to her community the important knowledge and health strategies she was accruing through her studies.

Just as Charlene was nearing graduation she received the tragic news that her eldest brother had died. His snowmobile had smashed into a tree – he had been both drunk and high on drugs. Charlene was devastated and she felt guilty – he had saved her life, but she had not saved his. However, despite her grief, Charlene's commitment to reverse the plague of alcohol and drug abuse in her community was forged.

Charlene returned home and commenced her job as a community health worker. The work was hard and often frustrating. Drugs and alcohol permeated the community and the culture. At times Charlene's efforts felt fruitless, as if change was beyond reach, but once again she persevered, accepting one small victory at a time. Charlene experienced a sense of accomplishment when she assisted a client to make alternative care arrangements for her children when she was going out on drinking sprees. Although Charlene had not eradicated her client's alcohol abuse, at least she had helped protect the children.

Charlene's sole preoccupation was her work. Her social contacts were limited by the fact that many social gatherings in the community were saturated with booze and drugs. So for some time she felt very alone and void of any significant relationships. Charlene made a conscious decision to maintain her distance from her dysfunctional family – but at times her feelings of emptiness were palpable.

When Charlene was 25 she reconnected with Ralph, now a community peacekeeper. They had known each other for many years but Charlene had been reluctant to allow the relationship to develop because of Ralph's history of binge drinking. Ralph declared he had quit drinking, he had been dry for 6 months, and, in recovery, he was a changed man with ambition. Slowly their relationship gained momentum and after a year of dating they had moved in together. Now Charlene was pregnant – she was ecstatic but Ralph seemed ambivalent. He had already fathered two children in prior relationships during his days of booze and drunken sex. Ralph was unsure if he was prepared to assume parenting responsibilities.

Dr Lejon had pieced together all this information over the early months of Charlene's pregnancy. Her story was a patchwork of sorrow, tragedy, and loss mixed with determination, fortitude, and triumph. Dr Lejon acknowledged Charlene's pain and praised her accomplishments. She also recognized how difficult it had been for Charlene to disclose her tumultuous and tragic past to a fellow professional. Dr Lejon appreciated Charlene's ability to share her concerns about Ralph's mixed feelings regarding the pregnancy. Dr Lejon wondered about Ralph's commitment to both Charlene and their unborn child. Would he relapse under the pressure of being a husband and father? The statistics were not in his favor, but perhaps Ralph would be an exception.

During her second trimester Charlene was diagnosed with gestational diabetes and started on insulin. She took this in her stride and Dr Lejon felt very confident in Charlene's ability to manage her disease. More worrisome was Ralph's nagging reticence about becoming a father. He was undeniably committed to Charlene and remained free of any substance abuse. After some gentle encouragement, Ralph began to accompany Charlene to her prenatal visits. Hearing the baby's heartbeat for the first time appeared to make Ralph's heart stop as his looming responsibilities became more tangible. Seizing on this opportunity, Dr Lejon asked if Ralph would like to have an appointment just for himself. Ralph welcomed the opportunity and, over several visits, his equally tragic life story was revealed. Like Charlene's early years, his too were shaped by violence, loss, and abandonment. Ralph's mother had been stabbed to death in a drunken brawl. Subsequently, Ralph and his three brothers had been "looked after" by a series of women who flitted in and out of his father's life. More often than not the house was filthy, with no clean clothes and barely enough food to keep the young boys fed. Ralph recounted his life story with a deep shame coupled with bitterness. Alcohol and drugs had replaced his emptiness and quieted his anger. Ralph had never been parented, hence he felt at a loss on how to become a father.

Armed with this additional information about the tangled and tragic past lives of this young couple, Dr Lejon began to formulate a plan. She could not eradicate the pain they brought from their past, but perhaps their future could be different. Limited resources in the community would be a challenge, but by working with Charlene and Ralph they would develop a plan together. Perhaps a trusted and respected elder could offer Ralph guidance and support in becoming a father. Certainly the nurses, along with Dr Lejon, could assist Charlene in her transition to motherhood. There were other options to be considered and discussed with Charlene and Ralph. The road ahead would not be easy – but now there was hope.

Charlene gave birth to a healthy baby boy and Ralph remained at her side throughout the entire labor. With moist eyes he gently held the swaddled newborn and tenderly watched as the infant latched onto Charlene's breast. In the years to come Dr Lejon would deliver two more of their children – a girl and boy. She was privileged to observe how Charlene and Ralph found solace and comfort in returning to their Aboriginal origins – which provided them both with some semblance of peace and serenity. Moreover, they fortified Charlene and Ralph's determination to give their children the opportunities and caring that they never experienced.

This story illustrates the powerful influence of family on human growth, development, and change in the midst of adversity. Further, it reveals the tremendous impact of culture and community on patients' health and well-being.

5 The Second Component: Understanding the Whole Person, Section 2 – Context

Thomas R Freeman, Judith Belle Brown, and Carol L McWilliam

Whoever would study medicine aright must learn of the following subjects. First he must consider the effect of each of the seasons of the year and the differences between them. Secondly . . . the warm and the cold winds. . . . the effect of water on the health must not be forgotten . . . Then think of the soil . . . Lastly consider the life of the inhabitants themselves. (Hippocrates, 1986)

INTRODUCTION

Consideration of contextual factors in clinical practice is a hallmark of the patient-centered clinician (McWhinney & Freeman, 2009). It is understood that, just as the meaning of a word depends on the context of the sentence in which it resides, so too, the meaning of health and illness varies with the surrounding circumstances. In the clinical world, information only becomes useful knowledge when it is placed in the context of a particular patient's world. To ignore context will lead to errors in both the interpretation of findings and the therapies recommended. A clinician will want to remember that just as the body is made up of a number of interlocking systems, the individual, too, exists within larger systems, including family, community, and ecology. Complexity theory recognizes that the internal rules of elements of units in a system change with context, and this is one factor that leads to the unpredictability of complex systems (Plsek & Greenhalgh, 2001).

Taking into account contextual variables in arriving at an understanding of the patient reflects the dynamic tension between two notions of ill-health that have existed since antiquity (Aronowitz, 1998; Crookshank, 1926). The ontological or structuralist viewpoint is that diseases are specific entities that have an existence separate from the sufferer. The task of the clinician is to correctly categorize the disease that is afflicting the patient, based on the symptoms, signs, and investigations. Therapeutics will, naturally, be directed at eliminating or mitigating the disease entity. The environmental or physiological or holistic or ecological view, on the other hand, sees ill-health as the outcome of an imbalance or failure of the organism to adapt to the environment. Genetic, epigenetic, and early childhood experience all play a role in the adaptability of the organism (Karr-Morse & Wiley, 2012). In this sense, the environment is understood to include the social, psychological, and economic realm, as well as the physical environment. In this approach, diagnosis involves arriving at an understanding of these many factors and their interplay with respect to the patient's propensity for health and illness. One arrives at a diagnosis of the person rather than a disease category. Therapeutics then, in the ecological approach, is multifactorial and interdisciplinary in nature. In the twentieth century, these two views, the structuralist and the environmental, assumed separate pathways. The structuralist view dominates allopathic medicine and focuses on the individual patient using powerful diagnostic and therapeutic tools. The environmental view became the focus of public health and focuses on whole populations (Reiser, 2009). To some extent the environmental view has also been incorporated into whole-person medicine. Using this approach, Candib (2007) has reframed the obesity and diabetes epidemics as involving a number of complex factors including genetics, physiology, psychology, family, social, economic, and political issues. It takes into account "fetal life, maternal physiology and life context, the thrifty genotype, the nutritional transition, health impact of urbanization and immigration, social attributions and cultural perceptions of increased weight and changes in food costs and availability resulting from globalization." In some ways the public has been quicker to embrace some of the principles of the environmental approach than mainstream medicine has been, evidenced by the rise in interest in approaches outside of allopathic medicine.

> Even when caused by a toxin, by a microbe, or by the dysfunction of an organ, illness is a fluid process that changes as we change, enigmatic, insubordinate, subjective. It captures bodies, minds, and emotions, remains at its deepest level inaccessible to language, and alters under the influence of non-medical events from divorce to climate change. What biomedicine finds hard to recognize or to accept is that different observers – patient, spouse, doctor, pastor, insurance provider, hospital administrator, epidemiologist, to name a few – examining the same illness from their separate perspectives will observe different aspects of its truth. (Morris, 1998: 5)

Recent understandings about the lifetime effect of the socio-environmental context at key developmental times in childhood, have served to emphasize that context at critical times in people's lives can have long-lasting effects

(Guy, 1997; Smith *et al.*, 1997; Blane *et al.*, 1997; Karr-Morse & Wiley, 2012). Much attention continues to be directed toward the broader determinants of health, adding to the usual concern about biologic and genetic determination, consideration of healthy childhood development, gender, income, social status and education, physical and social environment, lifestyle, social support networks, employment, working conditions, and health care (Egan *et al.*, 2008; Ottawa Charter for Health Promotion, 1986; Wilkinson &Targonski, 2003). Many of the broader determinants of health, including the childhood experience of income inequality (Gupta *et al.*, 2007), social status, limited social cohesion, and related experiences of high incidence of childhood deprivation and abuse have been linked to lifestyle patterns (Lynch *et al.*, 1997; Smith *et al.*, 1997), psychosocial factors (Walker *et al.*, 1999; Kinra *et al.*, 2000; Anda *et al.*, 1999), and physical, emotional, and cognitive health and development over the life course (Graham & Power, 2007) that contribute to chronic disease later in life. Other research has linked income inequality (Kawachi *et al.*, 1999b), social status (Lantz *et al.*, 1998; Smith *et al.*, 1997), limited social cohesion (Seeman, 1996), and related factors including high incidence of childhood deprivation (Evans *et al.*, 2000; McEwen, 2000; Power *et al.*, 2000) directly to increased incidence of chronic disease and to chronic disease-related morbidity and mortality (Bosma *et al.*, 1999; Kawachi *et al.*, 1999b). Neuroscientists suggest that adaptation to stressful life challenges, such as those that accompany these broader determinants of health, activates the neural, neuroendocrine, and neuroendocrine-immune mechanisms to maintain homeostasis through change. They also suggest that an "accumulated burden of adversity" (Alonzo, 2000) ultimately overtaxes the body's adaptive capacity, predisposing one to disease processes (McEwen, 1998).

A useful categorization of the layers of context is provided by Hinds *et al.* (1992). This comprises four nested, interactive layers distinguished by these three characteristics: (1) the degree to which meaning is shared, whether individual or universal; (2) the dominant time focus, past, present, or future; and (3) the speed with which change can occur within the layer. The four layers of context are then (1) the *immediate context* focused on the individual, in the present time, and rapid changes may happen or be effected; (2) the *specific context* oriented to the individual, including consideration of the immediate past as well as the relevant present, and again change can be rapid; (3) the *general context*, including both the personal and the cultural dimensions and past as well as current variables, and change, while possible, is slower to effect; and (4) the *metacontext*, which is generally shared, although rarely articulated in a clinical encounter unless explicitly sought. It is socially constructed and predominately past-oriented. Only very slow change is possible in the meta-context. The clinician's task is to help the patient arrive at a shared meaning of the events, a finding of common ground or understanding that is mutually agreed upon.

Meaning comes from a purposeful interaction with various layers of the context. Each layer can act as a source of prediction and explanation but, generally speaking, the immediate and specific layers of context tend to be more predictive while the general and metacontext are more explanatory in nature. However, either of these layers can affect a patient's health and/or perception of health. Changes in context have been found to be associated, for example, with exacerbations of previously stable chronic disease states (Cortese *et al.*, 1999). Therefore, clinicians will try to take into account contextual issues in helping patients to arrive at a meaning for the symptoms. Similarly, practitioners will attend to contextual issues in contemplating health promotion and disease prevention strategies. The patient's context includes not only the physical and interpersonal environment of the person but also, increasingly, global factors affecting health and health care. Globalized risk factors increasingly demand attention – for example, the H1N1 pandemic; the spread of HIV/AIDS; forced migration (Papadopoulos *et al.*, 2003); immigrant status (Papadopoulos *et al.*, 2003; Lai *et al.*, 2007); international and national provincial/state and local health-related policy; programming and interventions to minimize or eliminate such threats to the health of individuals, communities, and the population at large.

Health promotion and disease prevention invite – indeed, demand – that the "whole person" be understood with a broader lens, encompassing "community" and the larger societal context. As knowledge of the broader social determinants of health has evolved, the paradigm of individualized responsibility for and focus on health, health promotion, and disease prevention no longer suffices. Thus, primary care professionals will question whether society at large, the health care system in general, and the local community provide individual patients with the options they need for optimal health. Practitioners must explore these larger contextual components with patients. For example, are the foods that constitute a healthy diet available and affordable? Does their community context enable them to exercise safely? Does air or water pollution place their health at risk? Do their living accommodations and work circumstances undermine their health?

Contextual circumstances that potentially jeopardize individuals' health should be of concern to the entire health care community, not just to the public health sector; for example, primary health care will have to attend to these factors (Betancourt & Quinlan, 2007; Collins *et al.*, 2007), particularly as the new epidemic of chronic disease has replaced infectious disease as the primary threat to health (Betancourt & Quinlan, 2007; Navarro *et al.*, 2007).

PROXIMAL AND DISTAL FACTORS IN CONTEXT

A broader, less detailed categorization of context than the one suggested by Hinds *et al.* (1992) defines those factors that are proximal and those that are distal to the patient. Proximal factors correspond most closely with the immediate and specific categories listed in the previous section, whereas distal contextual factors are more closely aligned with the general and metacontext categories. To a great extent, the boundaries between these categories must be understood to be artificial.

Proximal Factors in Context

Proximal factors include family, financial security, education, employment, leisure, and social support. These are examined here, supported by research evidence.

Family

People linked by blood, marriage, or close emotional attachment constitute a family. The field of family systems theory sees the family as a mutually inter-acting system that functions as an emotional unit. The interaction of family issues and health and illness was covered in Chapter 4. As Scarf (1995: xxii) so eloquently states, the family unit can be viewed as

> a great emotional foundry, the passion-filled forge in which our deepest reali-ties – our sense of who we are as persons, and of the world around us – first begins to form and take shape. It is within the enclave of the early family that we learn those patterns of being, both of a healthy and a pathological nature, which will gradually be assimilated into, and become a fundamental part of, our own inner experience.

Financial Security

The inverse relationship between household income and all-cause mortality is well established (Kitagawa & Hauser, 1973; Pappas *et al.*, 1993; Kaplan & Neil, 1993). Even after controlling for known biological risk factors, social status, which is in large part determined by income levels, has been shown to be inversely related to mortality. These observations were made even where the low-income people in the study were relatively well paid compared with the general population, suggesting that there are factors other than access to health care at work (Marmot *et al.*, 1987). Individuals living in socioeconomically deprived areas are more likely to suffer from depression and multimorbidity and to have poorer outcomes than those in affluent areas (Jani *et al.*, 2012). The effect of socioeconomic status is only partially mediated by financial stress, self-esteem, mastery, social support, smoking, alcohol consumption, and physical activity (Cairney, 2000). However, it can be mediated by patient-centered care (Jani *et al.*, 2012).

Education

There is a strong positive association between the number of years of schooling and mortality (Feinstein, 1993). The highest rates of obesity are found in those populations with the lowest education (Drewnowski & Specter, 2004). Furthermore, there is a positive association between education and a healthy diet (Kant, 2004). In the United States, noncompletion of high school is a greater risk factor than biological factors for development of many diseases (Winkleby *et al.*, 1999). While education is also positively associated with income, the effects of these two variables appear to be independent.

Employment

Taking an occupational history ensures that the clinician is aware of potential toxic or other dangerous exposures to the patient. The workplace can be the source of stress as well. Also, it must be kept in mind that lack of employment has been recognized as having adverse effects on health. On a deeper level, as pointed out by Cassell (1991: 164), "To know someone's occupation is to learn something about his or her social status, education, specialized knowledge, responsibilities, hours worked, income, muscular development, skills, perspective on life, politics, housing – and much more."

Leisure

It has been shown that even activities that do not necessarily enhance physical fitness improve all-cause mortality in the elderly (Glass *et al.*, 1999). Involvement in various leisure activities improves mood and widens one's social network.

Social Support

It has long been recognized that there is a positive link between the strength of social support and the health of the individual (Berkman & Syme, 1979;

House *et al.*, 1988). Individuals with healthy social networks are more resistant to illness and tend to have better coping strategies. However, it is the quality of the relationships that seems to matter the most, not just the quantity. Social contacts can be a source of stress as well as support (Corin, 1994). Aware clinicians will make sure that they get frequent updates on the nature of their patients' support systems. The availability or absence and nature of resources such as family (De Bourdeaudhuij & Van Oost, 1998; Ford-Gilboe, 1997) and social support groups (Pavis *et al.*, 1998; Sherwood & Jeffery, 2000), as well as health promotion programs (Burke *et al.*, 1999; Feldman *et al.*, 2000), health literacy (Williams *et al.*, 2002), and health promotion and disease prevention services, may enhance or detract from the individual's potential for health.

The following case example demonstrates how the proximal factors of a patient's life context affected her response to her diagnosis and subsequent treatment.

Case Example

Ruth Walker, aged 48, was at her wits end. The recurrence of her breast cancer was too much to bear. It was not that she feared for her life or was anxious about the imminent treatment; rather, she was overwhelmed by her life circumstances. Ruth's husband, Albert, had been on disability for the past 2 years after severely injuring his back at the car seat factory where he worked. Although he was able to walk short distances, Ruth had to help him out with daily activities such as dressing, bathing, and preparing meals because of his limited mobility. Because of his constant care needs, Ruth had given up her part-time job at a local convenience store. Ruth's job had been her one outlet; her customers and workmates had been her sole source of social support. Also, now finances were very limited as the Walkers struggled to survive on Albert's meager disability pension. Tanya, their 21-year-old daughter, had recently moved back home with her 10-month-old son Kyle, after separating from her husband. While Tanya was actively seeking employment she could not afford daycare and consequently she had asked her mother to look after Kyle. Ruth, bound by her strong family ties, had agreed.

Ruth was extremely angry and felt powerless; she felt that she did not have any control over her current situation. Everyone around her seemed to have problems and was counting on Ruth to be the support they needed. Ruth felt like she had no life of her own since she had remained at home to care for her disabled husband, and although she loved her grandson, now she had to take care of him too. Ruth was an only child and her parents had died when she was in her teens, hence her little family was invaluable to her, but at the same time she was feeling the burden of their care. Thus it was not surprising that when the surgeon began to discuss various treatment options Ruth became openly angry. "I can't believe that this is happening again! I have a husband and grandson to take care of – and now this. How can I possibly take care of everyone else and still get through this? I have to take the bus to get here and I can't afford that every week! What will I do?"

For this patient her life circumstance (including family problems, financial difficulties, and limited social supports) made her own health concerns a low priority. These immediate and specific contextual issues would need to be addressed as well as her health concerns.

Distal Factors in Context

Unquestionably, the world of both individuals and communities as "patients" is exceedingly complex. Understanding the distal context requires that consideration be given not only to the social determinants of health and the global prevalence, incidence, and spread of disease but also to the challenges and opportunities for health care contained within the agendas, legislated regulations, and policies of international, national, provincial/state, municipal, and professional organizations. Increasingly, these contextual factors dictate or inform health promotion, disease prevention, and disease treatment priorities and directions, as well as guide both individual and community primary health care directions.

Distal factors as examined here include community, culture, economics, health care system, sociohistorical factors, geography, the media, and ecosystem health. These correlate with general context and meta-context as defined by Hinds *et al.* (1992).

Community

The concept of community refers to a group of people recognizing some commonality, whether that is based on geography, religion, ethnic background, profession, or leisure interests. Taking a community approach to health and disease means identifying the conditions that cause or are associated with diseases and collective ways of coping with them. Even if economically deprived, communities that have a sense of identity and belonging are generally healthier than those that do not. The feeling of belonging to a neighborhood may be more important than interpersonal support for the mental health of the elderly (Roux, 2002).

Culture

With globalization, the cultural diversity of many populations has become a characteristic of the early twenty-first century. Increasing diversity of medical practitioners also reminds us that cross-cultural issues are bidirectional. Both of these trends call for the development of a culturally flexible patient interaction style. How patients conceptualize and interpret their illness is strongly determined by the culture in which they reside. Cultural norms and values influence how patients experience health and illness, how they seek care, and how they accept medical interventions (Kleinman *et al.*, 1978). As McWhinney and Freeman (2009) note, cultural differences are not only based on ethnicity but also include subcultural groups defined by age, social status, sex, sexual preference, education, occupation, and religion. One might add, as well, that some disease states or disabilities help to define subcultures with strong identities – for example, AIDS or deafness (Sacks, 1989). In North America, "truth telling" with respect to diagnosis and respect for patient autonomy is the norm, but in some cultures there is greater emphasis on being family centered, physician centered, or even family-physician centered in decision making (Searight & Gafford, 2005).

There are several features to consider for each of the five aspects (health, disease, illness, person, and context) of the whole person in the patient-centered clinical method. The very experience of illness, what constitutes illness, and what to do about it are culturally laden (Juckett, 2005). Accepting the need to receive medication to manage a chronic condition or, conversely, turning to complementary and alternative medicine can be influenced by culture (Britten, 2007). Another example, described by Desjardins *et al.* (2011) is how culture affects serious mental illness, in the manifestation of the disease, "how it is experienced and how it responds to care" (2011: 99). The final example is how conception, pregnancy, and childbirth are vastly different across cultures and how they require practitioners to be sensitive to the needs of their female patients (Culhane-Pera & Rothenberg, 2010).

Although disease categories are part of the conventional medical model, they are not immune to the influence of culture (Aronowitz, 1998). The conventional medical model and the scientific method are both products of Western culture, thus, those working within Western culture have "filters" that affect how they understand and manage diseases (Juckett, 2005).

Other factors contributing to variation in health beliefs and practices of different cultural groups include (1) perceptions about illness causation, (2) perspectives on treatment or curing practices, (3) attitudes and expectations of health care facilities and resources deemed most appropriate for the problem, and (4) specific behaviors and reactions to pain and illness sanctioned by the prevailing culture (Schlesinger, 1985).

A move from one culture to another involves major upheaval and loss that can have serious effects on self-esteem, self-coherence, and health (Sawicki, 2011; Pottie *et al.*, 2005). The immigrant experience is often made complicated by significant persecution and physical trauma in the country of origin (Pottie *et al.*, 2005). Language barriers make it even more difficult to articulate needs and to receive support (Derose *et al.*, 2007).

There are different cultural responses to transitions in the family life cycle such as pregnancy, labour, childbirth, and care of the elderly and dying. Cultural differences in family roles and rules may come into conflict with the expectations of the doctor. Just as it is important to recognize the role of culture in health and illness on the one hand, it is also important to avoid stereotyping on the other hand. Culture does not explain all differences and it should not be used to explain what may be social status or socioeconomic differences. It is important not to stereotype individuals, as there are often more differences between people in the same culture than there are among cultures.

Clinicians will want to learn strategies to bridge the cultural gap and they will want to determine from patients what they think is going on and what other treatments or practitioners they are consulting. It may be useful to explain to a new patient that in caring for the patient it is important to understand more about the home situation and their native country; clinicians can point out that they need to understand better the patient's culture. Distinguishing between cultural humility and cultural competence is important here (Trevalon & Murray-Garcia, 1998). It may be appropriate for the clinician to ask the patient for tolerance if he or she says or does something that would be inappropriate in their native land, so that that the mistake is not repeated. Some patients may be more accustomed to an authoritarian relationship with a physician and so may find such disclosure difficult at first.

Case Example

Thomas R Freeman

Maria presented to her new family physician principally to discuss her chronic headaches. These were typically felt behind the eyes and across the forehead. Her previous physician had extensively investigated them and even consulted a headache specialist. They had classified them as atypical migraine headaches, although none of the standard treatments had helped very much. Her physician noted that she looked very worried and always had a deeply furrowed brow. He asked her about her family and learned that she, her husband, and their two sons had emigrated from eastern Europe. Her husband was having great difficulty finding steady employment and while she missed her home, their two sons were accommodating well to their new country and had many friends. Recognizing the role that the stress of being a new immigrant may play in the cause of her headaches, her physician asked her to return with some photos of her former home and to tell him more about their life there. She gladly complied with this request and on her return visit brought pictures of their former house, their wedding, and the children's early lives. She spoke longingly of what she had left behind, but when she was done, she smiled and thanked her physician for the interest shown. After that visit, the frequency of headaches markedly declined.

Economics

The link between socioeconomic status and health has been well recognized and explored (Feinstein, 1993; Braveman *et al.*, 2010). Even in situations with universal access to medical care, job classification was found to be more predictive of cardiovascular death than the standard risk factors of cholesterol level, blood pressure, and smoking combined (Pincus *et al.*, 1998). More recently, debate has focused on the observation that societies that tolerate wide differences in average income, from the lowest to the highest, have poorer overall aggregate health scores than societies that demonstrate smaller differences (Daniels *et al.*, 2000; Kawachi *et al.*, 1999a). However, the presence of a strong primary care sector mitigates these adverse effects (Starfield, 2001; Starfield *et al.*, 2012). Globalization of the world economy has been identified by some as creating wider economic disparities both within and between countries, resulting in significant numbers of individuals who are marginalized. The concept of core and periphery is invoked to describe (1) those close to the center of economic activity, the entrepreneurs, and (2) those who, because of lack of ability or opportunity are not entrepreneurs and are relegated to the periphery. In general, those at the periphery are found to engage in "retreatist" behavior, characterized by increased smoking, alcohol consumption, and suicide (McMurray & Smith, 2001). This has been the fate of indigenous people on many continents.

Health Care System

It is important that the clinician remain aware that the health care system as a whole, including the practitioner and his or her relationship with the patient, is an important part of the context. This is particularly true for patients with chronic illness who spend much of their time interacting with various components of the larger system. Overall health care organization has a profound effect on whether a patient accesses health care, which health care provider is sought, and what is done about his or her problem. The clinical context can be a source of great frustration to the practitioner as well as the patient, with various barriers to accessing appropriate care. In some situations, staffing and resource problems place pressure on clinicians to change, sometimes in ways that are detrimental to patient care. These include shortened consultation times, compromised continuity of patient care, and an unfortunate focus on the disease model.

Sociohistorical

To some extent, our concept of diseases and the experience of ill-health are born of particular social and historical circumstances (Kelly & Brown, 2002). This is true of our social construction of diseases (Aronowitz, 1998; Gilman, 1988), and it is no less relevant to the social and historical factors of the individual. For example, the illness experience of type 2 diabetes mellitus in a North American Aboriginal is so different from an urban-dwelling Caucasian that it is a challenge to state why we give it the same name. These differences are, in part, a reflection of the social history of these two individuals.

The impact of social, economic, and health policy is reflective of a country's approach to the distribution of power (Starfield, 2001). There are numerous examples of groups of people who have been marginalized, sometimes over prolonged periods of time, resulting in chronic patterns of poverty and ill-health that span generations. Being aware of the history of medical experimentation on black people helps the clinician understand the reluctance of some people of color to seek medical help (Candib, 1995). Changes at the macro level in the history and sociocultural environment are translated into stress on the individual, which can then lead to increased susceptibility to ill-health. The particular manifestation of the illness will be determined by an individual's genetic makeup and environmental pressures. Early childhood experiences, for example, have been shown to be predictive of susceptibility to many chronic diseases later in life, including obesity, hypertension, and cardiovascular disease. On the other hand, social and cultural meanings and values can modify, perhaps mitigate, an individual's response to these stressors (Corin, 1994).

Geography

The field of medical geography is defined as "that discipline that describes spatial patterns of health and disease and explains those spatial patterns by concentrating on the underlying processes that generate identifiable spatial forms" (Mayer, 1984: 2680). Since the late nineteenth century this approach has evolved from the position of environmental determinism (the consideration of the physical impact of the geography on health) to a position that views human health as being interwoven with the entire biosphere (Meade, 1986; Meade & Emch, 2010). The latter line of thinking was instrumental in the recognition of the importance of the ecosystem in health and illness. Geographic information systems have been developed to assist in health care planning, stimulated by the changes in the financing of care brought about by the managed care approach. These systems make possible the linking of health outcomes with geostatistical data (Parchman *et al.*, 2002) and serve as a bridge to considering the wider role of environmental and ecological pressures on human health and well-being.

The Media

For large parts of the world, the media, comprising print materials, television, and the Internet, has become a pervasive promoter of a monoculture. Some have raised the alarm about the media as a disease agent (Oxford Textbook of Medicine, 2002). By promoting a high-consumption, materialistic, violence-prone lifestyle that challenges traditional social structures and values, the content of the worldwide media may undermine those dimensions of context that serve to sustain health. On the other hand, health promotion programs are greatly facilitated by information technology. Patients now attend health care professionals with much greater awareness of their health and options available for disease management, health promotion, and disease prevention and this can be viewed as a positive development. Moreover, mass media can influence health attitudes and beliefs in both subtle and obvious ways, and may either enhance the patient's potential for health or detract from it (National Research Council, 1989).

Mary T: Case Illustrating Component 2

Sonny Cejic and Sara Hahn

Mary was 15 when she presented to her family physician with a history of chronic depression and passive suicidal thoughts. Her visit was prompted by progression of her symptoms, particularly anhedonia, lack of motivation for studying, and panic attacks. On further exploration of possible reasons for progression of her symptoms, Mary revealed that there were multiple recent stressors in her life, including reemerging peer relationships that triggered past traumatic memories. Over the course of several appointments, Mary hesitantly revealed that in elementary and middle school she was emotionally and physically bullied by a number of her peers. In particular, one traumatic experience occurred when a male individual, whom Mary trusted and considered a friend, sexually assaulted her. A number of peers participated in the incident by holding her down and physically assaulting her. Following this, Mary was taunted and tormented to the point that she changed schools. She blamed herself for what happened, which subsequently led to chronic low self-esteem and impairment of her ability to develop trusting relationships. Within the past year, one of the male perpetrators of that incident reconnected with Mary through a social media website to apologize for his participation. Mary ignored his message and did not accept his apology. Several months later, Mary learned that this male perpetrator committed suicide. Mary experienced immense feelings of guilt, increased suicidal thoughts, and began to self-harm by cutting. Furthermore, around the same time, there was intense media coverage of a number of cases in North America involving bullying and sexual assault of adolescent girls, with social media becoming a vehicle for "shaming and blaming". Unfortunately, these cases triggered Mary's traumatic experience and worsened her depression and anxiety. After several individual counseling sessions, in addition to antidepressant therapy, Mary's mood and panic attacks dramatically improved.

Ecosystem

Since the publication of Rachel Carson's book *Silent Spring* and spurred on by widely reported ecological disasters such as the destruction of the nuclear power generator at Chernobyl in the former Soviet Union and the tragedy in Bhopal, India, there has developed a greater awareness of the impact of environment on human health. The medical literature now devotes regular attention to environmental issues (Speidel, 2000; Ablesohn *et al.*, 2002a, 2002b; Marshall *et al.*, 2002; Epstein, 1995; Patz *et al.*, 1996). Ecosystems and their impact on health is a recognized area in medicine (Dakubo, 2010). Clinicians must now take into account the way in which air pollution and environmental toxins affect their patients. There is much greater interest in the ways that climate changes can affect human health (McGeehin & Mirabelli, 2001).

Ecosystem health problems have gradually shifted from local issues to more global issues. As urban pollution increases and higher smoke stacks are constructed, acid rain becomes a regional and even a transnational problem. The worldwide dimensions of ecosystem health problems are truly staggering, with 3 billion people malnourished, 2 billion people living in water-stressed areas, and 1.4 billion exposed to dangerous levels of outdoor air pollution.

Complex relationships exist between physical conditions, ecology, and human health (Garrett, 1994). For example, the outbreak of hantavirus in the southwestern United States in 1994 can be understood as occurring in a particular environmental context, as follows. The effects of El Niño caused increased rain in the region, which resulted in increased desert vegetation. Under these conditions, the population of deer mice (*Peromyscus maniculatus*) multiplied, with the result that humans came into greater contact with the urine and fecal material left by the mice. This material contained a particularly virulent form of hantavirus, later named Muerto Canyon virus, that proved to be the third most lethal virus ever found in the United States (after HIV and rabies). In this way, complex environmental changes led to a set of conditions conducive to disease in humans.

The thinking fostered by the ecosystem health approach is a reminder to focus on relationships as well as individual units and, in that respect, it is consistent with the basic concepts of patient-centered medicine.

Community-Oriented Primary Care

Community-oriented primary care began with the work of Sidney Kark and others (Gieger, 1993; Susser, 1993) and has been recognized as a method of informing and integrating the practice of medicine with knowledge of the community. As it has evolved since the work of these pioneers, community-oriented primary care is now considered to comprise four steps: (1) defining and characterizing the community, (2) identifying and prioritizing the community's health problems, (3) developing interventions to address the health problems, and (4) monitoring the impact of programs implemented (Nutting, 1990). The techniques of community-oriented primary care are attempts to recognize contextual factors of the community as a whole rather than the individual patient. Nevertheless, such knowledge serves to improve the clinician's understanding of the problems encountered in clinical medicine.

CONCLUSION

Being patient-centered involves being aware of the many layers of contextual nuance in which both patient and clinician reside. In arriving at a shared understanding or common ground, meaning can only occur within a particular set of circumstances or context.

"Doctor, I Need You to Give Me a Test to Check if I Am a Lesbian": Case Illustrating Component 2

Darren Van Dam and Judith Belle Brown

The question took a moment to register with Dr Burgess – it was not the kind of request he was accustomed to hearing from a patient. Mrs Singh, aged 45, was a relatively new patient to his practice, and Dr Burgess was still getting to know her, having only met her twice before.

"I'm sorry, Mrs Singh, I'm not sure what you are asking. What sort of test do you mean?" Dr Burgess asked. Looking at the tiny woman seated before him, Dr Burgess was struck again by how timid she was, a first impression that had been made weeks before when they first met. Mrs Singh and her husband had recently immigrated to Canada, arriving from India to accompany their eldest daughter during her pursuit of higher education. It was not an easy move, as their youngest daughter had remained in India with family members, because her parents believed she was too young to be uprooted from her home. Mrs Singh shifted slightly in her seat, eyes downcast, apparently struggling to find the words to explain her request. Her command of the English language was quite good, but Dr Burgess couldn't help but wonder if there was some nuance of meaning that was creating a misunderstanding.

However, the timid woman in his office was determined in her request, and despite repeated attempts by Dr Burgess to clarify what he felt was surely a cultural or linguistic misunderstanding, she did not deviate from this request – she needed a test to determine if she was a lesbian. Beyond this, she was less clear – probing questions from Dr Burgess failed to shed any light on what kind of test the patient was seeking, and when the discussion turned to talk of lifestyle choices, including sexual orientation, for which there was no specific test, Mrs Singh became somewhat withdrawn. Recognizing that this encounter was not going to provide a quick answer to a challenging question, Dr Burgess asked Mrs Singh to return later that week for a special appointment to discuss the issue in more depth.

The encounter stayed with Dr Burgess for the rest of the day and the struggle to understand his patient occupied his thoughts. In previous visits, he had not observed the conflicted and emotional woman of today's encounter. When Dr Burgess had met her the first time she appeared shy and quiet but otherwise relatively content to be in Canada. Mrs Singh had been accompanied by her husband who did most of the talking for the pair. This was consistent with Dr Burgess's expectations based on his previous experiences with their culture. However, Mrs Singh did speak when spoken to directly, and there did not appear to be any indication of disharmony in the martial relationship.

Mrs Singh's subsequent visit had been somewhat more instructive, as she came to discuss the struggles she was having since her arrival in Canada; finding employment was difficult (she had been a teacher in India), and a sense of place in the community continued to elude her. Mrs Singh had left that visit seemingly content with a printout of numbers and addresses for organizations offering assistance to new immigrants.

Later that week when Mrs Singh returned, she again had an air of distress about her, fidgeting in her seat and having trouble making eye contact. She denied any specific distress, but again repeated her request for a test to determine if she was a lesbian. With more time available during this encounter, Dr Burgess began to probe the context behind her concern. He asked about her marriage with her husband – it was good, no concerns. He asked how she was proceeding in making some connections with her community but nothing had changed. Mrs Singh remained isolated and adrift. He asked after her daughters . . . and Mrs Singh paused. Sensing that this might be an area to delve into, Dr Burgess questioned further.

Mrs Singh explained that she had recently returned from a trip home to India to visit her youngest daughter. While she was vague about the details, it seemed that during this trip some friends had implied that her daughter might be gay. Mrs Singh's eyes glistened as she sat quietly, this revelation hanging in the air between them, and the outpouring began. The guilt she felt for leaving her daughter behind; the fear that her actions had led to this culturally unacceptable possibility; and, above all, the dread that there was something wrong with her that she had passed on to her daughter – that it was in some way her fault. "Please doctor, you have to give me the test. If I am lesbian, I need to know so I can help my daughter," beseeched Mrs Singh.

Once again Dr Burgess felt ill-prepared to handle his patient's request. He repeated their discussion from earlier in the week, stating that there was no "test" for sexual orientation, as it was not something another person could tell her, but something that she had to decide for herself. Dr Burgess's explanation appeared to deflate Mrs Singh, the hope that she came into the office with that day draining from her as visibly as water being poured from a jug. Mrs Singh's loss felt palpable and Dr Burgess tried to reassure her. He suggested that perhaps if she spoke with her daughter Mrs Singh might find some reassurance and that all was not as bleak as she feared. Mrs Singh seemed not to hear – she had retreated completely from the conversation, and as Dr Burgess watched her walk down the hall with a downcast head, he was left wondering what he could have said or done differently to reassure his forlorn patient.

Weeks passed, and Dr Burgess heard nothing further from Mrs Singh. It was some time after that when he noticed Mr Singh's name on the day sheet. He looked forward to this encounter, hoping to hear that the situation at home was going well and that Mrs Singh had found a place in her new community.

"I am concerned about my wife, doctor," lamented Mr Singh, "she left our home because she says it is haunted. She refuses to talk to me or tell me where she is staying. I think her schizophrenia is back."

Dr Burgess was completely at a loss. A detailed story ensued. Mrs Singh had been diagnosed with schizophrenia many years ago in India, which had been well controlled by medication. However, Mrs Singh had stopped taking her medication prior to coming to Canada. Her husband thought that she was doing well, so well that he didn't even think to include this information as part of her history during that first visit to the office. However, over the past few months Mr Singh began to notice some of the old symptoms returning – she was once again becoming withdrawn, suspicious, accusing him of mistreating her – even to the point of calling the police. Shortly thereafter Mrs Singh left the family home without warning and her husband had not seen her since.

Understanding the whole person and finding common ground with a patient can sometimes be very challenging and even more so when cultural differences muddy the waters. Attention to cultural sensitivity is also an important aspect of developing a strong patient-doctor relationship with patients from different cultural backgrounds. However, care must be taken to not allow that particular lens to obscure other important signs and symptoms a patient may be exhibiting. Dr Burgess devoted a considerable amount of time in trying to understand his patient's experience from a cultural perspective, but in doing so may have been overly reassured in assuming what was the cause of her distress, and in doing so missed some of the symptoms signaling the return of his patient's schizophrenia.

6 The Third Component: Finding Common Ground

Judith Belle Brown, W Wayne Weston, Carol L McWilliam, Thomas R Freeman, and Moira Stewart

It's a most terrifying feeling to realize that the doctor can't see the real you, that he can't understand what you feel and that he's just going ahead with his own ideas. I would start to feel that I was invisible or maybe not there at all. (Laing, 1960)

A central goal of the patient-centered clinical method is finding common ground with patients about their health problems – achieving a consensus with patients on a plan for addressing their medical problems and health goals that reflects their needs, values, and preferences and is informed by evidence and guidelines. This goal is realized by first exploring the patient's experience of health and illness and, at the same time, the signs and symptoms implying disease. This evolving understanding is placed in the context of the patient's personhood, family, other significant relationships, and the environment in which they live. This complex process is accomplished through collaboration between clinician and patient based on trust, caring, and mutual respect.

Finding common ground is often mistakenly understood as the final step in the clinical method, only occurring after all the information about the patient's problems is obtained and sorted out by the clinician. However, we suggest that finding common ground must begin at the beginning. It is a process based on a relationship in which patients are treated as partners in exploring their health and health problems and deciding on treatment. As described by Tuckett *et al.* (1985), it is a meeting between experts – the physician is the expert in the biomedical aspects of the problems and the patient is the expert in his or her experience of health and illness and how illness is interfering with the achievement of his or her aspirations in life. While a skilled and often detailed collection of biomedical data is obviously essential for understanding the patient's medical problems, it is incomplete without an equally detailed understanding of the person who is suffering from the problems. A "checklist" approach emphasizing biomedical data or a perfunctory review of the patient's ideas or concerns will give a clear message that the doctor is preoccupied with the biomedical task of diagnosis. Trying to switch gears at the end of the interview, by inviting the patient's perspective on a menu of treatment options offered by the physician, will be challenging. Having spent most of the interaction as a passive source of medical information, it is difficult for patients to engage in a conversation in which their ideas, values, and preferences occupy center stage.

In this chapter we will examine the third interactive component of the patient-centered method, Finding Common Ground. This will include a brief review of the research demonstrating the importance of patients and clinicians finding common ground; a description of finding common ground; and strategies to assist the clinician in finding common ground, such as motivational interviewing and shared decision making. Finding common ground is the process through which the patient and clinician reach a mutual understanding and mutual agreement in three key areas: (1) defining the problem, (2) establishing the goals and priorities of treatment, and (3) identifying the roles to be assumed by both the patient and the clinician. Achieving common ground often requires that two potentially divergent viewpoints be brought together in a reasonable plan. Once agreement is reached on the nature of the problems, the patient and clinician must determine the goals and priorities of treatment. What will be the patient's involvement in the treatment plan? How realistic is the plan in terms of the patient's perceptions of his or her health, disease, and illness experience? Does the plan address all the impediments to pursuing the life goals and purposes that really matter to the patient? What are the patient's wishes and his or her ability to cope? Finally, how do each of the parties, patients and clinicians, define their roles in this interaction?

THE IMPORTANCE OF FINDING COMMON GROUND

In a paternalistic model, health care professionals are in charge – they make decisions on behalf of their patients that they believe are in the patient's best interests without involving them. Over the past 40 years paternalism has gradually lost ground as patients' rights have gained support (Chin, 2002; Tauber, 2005; van den Brink-Muinen *et al.*, 2006). Although there is general agreement in the literature that patients should be better informed regarding their medical condition, and be offered choices and be asked their opinions about all decisions concerning their health care (Levinson *et al.*, 2005), clinicians still fall short of this ideal. "Not being properly informed about their condition and the options for treating is a very common source of patient dissatisfaction worldwide" (Coulter, 2009: 159). For over 30 years research has documented how doctors have failed to find common ground (Korsch & Negrete, 1972; Stewart & Buck, 1977; Starfield *et al.*, 1981; Coulter, 2002; Fong & Longnecker, 2010). In a study of primary care physicians and surgeons, Braddock *et al.* (1999) reviewed audiotapes of informed decision making and found that discussion of alternatives occurred in 5.5%–29.5% of interactions, discussion of pros and cons in 2.3%–26.3%, and discussion of uncertainties associated with the decision in 1.1%–16.6%. Physicians rarely explored whether patients understood the decision (0.9%–6.9%).

Studies exploring physician prescribing behaviors and patients' use of medication also report a paucity of finding common ground (Stevenson *et al.*, 2000; Britten *et al.*, 2000; Dowell *et al.*, 2002, 2007). For example, in a qualitative study, Britten *et al.* (2000) found that 14 categories of misunderstandings in relation to prescribing (e.g., conflicting information, disagreement about attribution of side effects) were inextricably connected to an absence of patients' expressions of their ideas, expectations, or preferences. Patients' lack of participation in the consultation was also evident in their inability to respond to "the doctors' decisions or actions" (2000: 484). This study revealed that an essential precursor to finding common ground was an exploration of the patient's illness experience (i.e., FIFE, described in Chapter 3). However, Dowell *et al.* (2002) found that when a consultation process included an exploration of their illness experience and finding common ground, previously nonadherent patients were assisted in following their medication regimen.

Another study highlighting the centrality of finding common ground is Stewart *et al.* (2000), who found that the most important association with good outcomes was the patient's perception that the physician and patient had found common ground. These outcomes included patient recovery from discomfort and concern and better emotional health 2 months after the encounter. As well, there was a 50% reduction in diagnostic tests and referrals. The importance of finding common ground is also reinforced by the findings of Tudiver *et al.* (2001), who explored how family physicians made decisions about cancer screening when the guidelines were unclear or conflicting. Central to the physicians' decision-making process to screen or not screen was finding common ground with patients.

Street and Haidet (2011) studied physicians' awareness of their patients' health beliefs and found that physicians had a relatively poor understanding. For example, physicians generally underestimated how much patients perceived value in natural remedies or preferred being a partner in their care. However, in consultations where patients asked more questions, expressed concerns, and stated preferences and opinions, physicians had a better understanding of patients' health beliefs and values. "Such understanding forms the foundation for formulating therapeutic plans that patients are more likely to follow, since such plans take into account the patient's perspective on how the illness works and what therapies are feasible, given their unique circumstances" (2011: 25).

A further set of studies provide additional support to the importance of finding common ground in the clinical encounter. Three separate research teams examined women's experiences regarding the following: the important health issues of prenatal genetic testing, specifically maternal serum screening (Carroll *et al.*, 2000); hormone replacement therapy (Marmoreo *et al.*, 1998); and the use of complementary/alternative medicine in the treatment of breast cancer (Boon *et al.*, 1999). While the medical circumstances explored in the studies were both diverse and distinct, the participants' needs and expectations regarding the decision-making process reflected a collective voice. Faced with a serious decision regarding their health, one that could have positive or negative implications on their future health and well-being, participants expressed a consistent chorus of desiring an active role in the decision-making process and ultimately in finding common ground (Brown *et al.*, 2002). Of importance in all three studies was the sharing of information between the patient and the clinician. This finding is similarly reinforced by the work of McWilliam *et al.* (2000) with breast cancer survivors, who described the inextricable link between building a relationship with their physician(s) and having the opportunity to share information as they strived to reach common ground regarding treatment of their breast cancer.

In summary, research indicates how physicians still fail to find common ground with patients but at the same time it also reveals how finding common ground is important for both patients and physicians – it is the lynchpin of the patient-centered clinical method.

DEFINING THE PROBLEM

Seeking an understanding or explanation of worrisome symptoms is a fundamental human response to illness. Most patients want a "name" or label for their disease to help them gain some sense of control over what is happening to them (Kleinman, 1988; Wood, 1991; Cassell, 2004) "adding meaning to the patient's experience" (McWhinney & Freeman, 2009: 165). When patients can assign a label to their problems it helps them understand the cause, what to expect in terms of the course or time line of the problem, and what will be the outcome (Cooper, 1998). It also assists them in regaining some degree of mastery over what may have been a frightening symptom. Some patients may develop quite magical notions of what is happening to them when they become ill. It may seem better to have an irrational explanation of the problem than no explanation at all. Other patients will blame themselves for the problem rather than see the disease as something beyond their control.

> To have a diagnosis is to have a vision of what one is up against, no matter how terrible the possible future: "Better the devil you know than a devil you don't know." Enduring a long period when one's diagnosis is uncertain can be a painful and frustrating experience. Even when a doctor only "suspects" something, patients and families want to know what it is. (Hodges, 2010: 160–1)

The initial presentation of Hanna to her doctor as described in the case at the end of Chapter 3 serves as an illustration of this.

Patients have usually formed some ideas about their problems before presenting to the doctor. They have commonly consulted family, friends, and often the Internet to gain some understanding of what is happening to them. Failure to elicit the patient's perspective may jeopardize agreement on the nature of the problem(s). Without some agreement about what is wrong, it is difficult for a patient and a clinician to agree on a treatment protocol or plan of management that is acceptable to both. It is not essential that the practitioner fully agrees with the patient's formulation of the problem, but the practitioner's explanation and recommended treatment must at least be consistent with the patient's point of view and make sense in the patient's world.

Problems develop when patient and doctor have quite different ideas of the cause of the problems. For example:

- The patient dismisses her back pain as aging and osteoarthritis, yet the doctor is concerned that it may represent metastases from her breast cancer.
- The practitioner has diagnosed hypertension, but the patient insists that his blood pressure is probably only elevated because he is working overtime on a big assignment at work and refuses to see his blood pressure as a problem.
- The parent of a 6-year-old child thinks there is something seriously wrong because the child has frequent colds: six a year. The clinician thinks this number is within normal limits, and that the parent is overly protective of the child.

In defining and describing the problem it is essential that practitioners give the information in language patients can understand, thus complex medical terms and clinical language should be avoided. If patients are intimidated by medical jargon it may limit their ability to express their ideas and concerns or to even raise important questions. Failure to elicit these patients' expressions may result in a failure to find common ground. Gill and Maynard (2006) suggest that the "canonical organization" of the medical interview powerfully structures the interaction, thus making it hard for patients to insert their ideas or for physicians to even hear them. Doctors are so busy collecting information to sort out the diagnosis that they resist being "sidetracked" by the patient's ideas.

> Although in some cases doctors do evaluate patients' explanations immediately in information-gathering contexts, they typically stay on course when this option is provided and continue to collect data from patients without outwardly indicating that they heard patients insert their analyses into the conversation. Thus, as in previous research, we find that physicians may leave patients' explanations unassessed or even unacknowledged. However, this is at least partly due to both participants' orientation to the overall organization of the medical interview. (Gill & Maynard, 2006: 117)

To counter this unspoken rule about what information is to be collected in medical interviews, patients need to be encouraged to ask questions and not fear being ridiculed or embarrassed for not knowing or not understanding technical terms and procedures. Just as active listening is key to exploring the patients' health and illness experiences, it is also central to finding common ground. Thus it is important to understand and acknowledge patients' perspectives on their problem. The format in which the patient's history of his or her illness is collected determines what information is gathered and also shapes the nature of the relationship between patient and physician and the role of the patient. If the history is simply the result of answers to a series of questions – an interrogation – the patient's role is to be a source of information in response to the physician's lead. However, if the history is acquired by listening intently to the patient's story of his or her illness, the information is rich with personal details and values and the patient has a more important role in constructing his or her medical history. But it's not that simple. Patients are often uncertain about their story and sometimes fearful of what it might mean; they may need assistance in putting it into words. Howard Brody refers to the "joint construction of narrative" in which physicians assist in writing the story.

> The physician who takes stories seriously will . . . adopt as a working hypothesis that the patient is asking a question like the following: "Something is happening to me that seems abnormal, and either I cannot think of a story that will

explain it, or the only story I can think of is very frightening. Can you help me to tell a better story, one that will cause me less distress, about this experience?" If this formulation seems overly wordy, a shorter form of the patient's possible plea to the physician might be, "My story is broken; can you help me fix it?" (Brody, 1994: 85)

From this perspective, taking the patient's history is more like a conversation in which the history is co-created. The clinician's role is to be curious, asking questions for clarification, following the patient's lead, and sometimes suggesting another viewpoint (Launer, 2002). Often the patient's story will reveal the diagnosis. Osler's oft-quoted aphorism reminds us: "Listen to the patient, he is telling you the diagnosis" (Osler, quoted by Roter & Hall, 1987: 325). Also, a narrative approach usually provides insights into the patient's experience of his or her illness – how it is affecting the patient's life; how the patient has made sense of it; the patient's feelings, especially his or her fears about the illness; and the role the patient hopes the physician will play. However, sometimes physicians must ask questions to fill in gaps in the patient's story, to explore cues to possible diagnoses and to clarify aspects of the patient's illness experience. It is also important to attend to the relational aspects of the interaction:

> patients value positive relationships with health professionals not only (or not mainly) because of the benefits of task-related information exchange and choice but also because it matters to them that they feel cared for as individuals and respected as part of the care team. (Edwards & Elwyn, 2009: 20)

In the care of patients with chronic diseases, once the diagnosis has been established, follow-up visits concentrate on therapy. History taking will focus on how the treatment is changing the story – has the patient been able to follow through on the therapeutic plans, are the symptoms improving, are there any side effects of treatment, are there any new problems, and, most important, are the impediments to the achievement of important life goals and purposes addressed adequately? In addition, effective care of patients with chronic diseases is dependent on skilled self-management (Lorig & Associates, 2001a; Lorig, 2003; Lorig & Holman, 2003; Holman & Lorig, 2004). The following case example demonstrates the value of collaboration between patient and physician. By acknowledging and respecting the patient's perspective, the doctor encouraged the patient to contribute to a shared understanding of her problem and take an active role in developing a more effective approach to the treatment of her depression.

Case Example

Faye struggled. Some days felt interminable, while others were barely within Faye's meager control. Faye struggled to mother her 7-year-old son, Cody, as a single parent; she struggled to keep a roof over their heads and food on the table; she struggled to maintain her quota as a sales representative for a local flower distributor – a loss of income would be catastrophic. However, Faye's greatest struggle was her depression. Her depression was a demon Faye could not conquer. It swept over her, delivering Faye to a fearful and uncertain place she could not manage alone.

Dr Adria was more than familiar with his 28-year-old patient Faye. He knew and empathized with her multiple struggles – how each day was a monumental effort to make a step forward – to merely survive. Yet, there was some underlying frustration, given his many failed attempts to find common ground with Faye. Various antidepressant medications had been prescribed, but each one had resulted in an undesired outcome – drowsiness, weight gain, agitation. From a pharmacological perspective Dr Adria was at a loss how best to treat Faye. Nothing seemed to address her overwhelming depressive symptoms without some negative consequence or adverse reaction. Dr Adria was uncertain about how to proceed with Faye's care. At the same time, he too struggled to address all the other complex dimensions of Faye's life – often unspoken but evident in her haggard profile.

The chaotic presentation in the office with her son, Cody, was particularly worrisome. Did this little boy's "hyperactivity" warrant an official diagnosis and intervention or was it rather a reflection of his mother's chaos – both internal and external? These questions sat suspended before Dr Adria.

On a few rare occasions Faye had shared her frustrations in caring for Cody – how when his behavior would escalate, so too would hers. The resulting yelling match left Faye feeling depleted and guilty about her poor parenting skills. As a consequence she often avoided disciplining Cody, for fear that such confrontations would lead to more angry outbursts from both of them. Faye blamed her inability to parent on her persistent fatigue, indecision, and irritability – all part of her depression.

With some further probing, Dr Adria discovered that Faye despised being on medication and the stigma associated with depression. Faye believed she should be able to cope on her own and her inability to do so led to further frustration and self-loathing. Faye revealed how, on several occasions, she had decreased or increased her medication – in the absence of consultation with her doctor. This new information opened the door for Dr Adria to seek common ground with his patient.

Faye's goals were to decrease her depressive symptoms and to gain an understanding of how to better approach parenting and discipline of her son. Dr Adria shared his patient's goals but realized simply telling her to be more "compliant" with the antidepressant medication had failed before and would fail again. He needed to engage Faye in tackling the problem together. He suggested that they brainstorm possible approaches to her problems. Faye realized that she had been fighting to avoid acknowledging her depression and that her "on-again, off-again" approach to the medication was not working. When she had maintained a regular dose she had felt better, so it made sense to try this again and stick to it. Also, she had read about parenting self-help groups on the Internet and asked Dr Adria if there was a similar program that he would recommend in her community. Dr Adria supported Faye's suggestion and provided a referral. Dr Adria also wondered aloud if Faye was interested in resuming journaling, as in the past she had found this to be helpful in sorting out her many struggles; Faye agreed that this would be a good idea. Faye suggested that it might be helpful to maintain regularly scheduled visits with Dr Adria in order to monitor her progress with their agreed-upon plan. Faye's struggles were not over yet – but they both felt more confident. They had reached common ground and together they could move forward.

DEFINING THE GOALS

Once the patient and clinician have reached a mutual understanding and agreement about the problems the next step is to explore the goals and priorities for therapy; if these are divergent it may be a challenge to find common ground. For example:

- The patient requests genetic testing to alleviate her fears of having breast cancer, while the doctor knows there are no present risk factors or family history to warrant such tests.
- A patient, suffering from unremitting back pain demands an MRI, yet the doctor feels that this is likely mechanical back pain that will resolve spontaneously.
- The doctor advises the patient to take a number of medications following his myocardial infarction to prevent a recurrence, yet the patient declines, believing that diet and exercise will suffice.

If clinicians ignore their patient's expectations and ideas about treatment and/ or management, they risk not understanding their patients, and the patients in turn will be angry or hurt by this perceived lack of interest or concern. Some patients will become more demanding in a desperate attempt to be heard; others will become withdrawn and will feel abandoned. Patients may be reluctant to listen to their clinicians' treatment recommendations unless they feel that their ideas and opinions had been heard and respected.

Timing is important. If the physician inquires about the patient's perspectives too early in the interview, the patient may think that the doctor doesn't know what is going on and is avoiding his or her responsibility to make a diagnosis. On the other hand, if the practitioner waits until the end of the interview, time may be wasted on issues unimportant to the patient. The clinician may even make suggestions that will have to be retracted. Practitioners need to actively engage their patients and explicitly inquire about their expectations. For example, a clinician might say, "Can you help me to understand what we might do together to get your diabetes under control?" Often, it is helpful to pick up on patients' cues that hint at their feelings, ideas, or expectations. For example, "I have had this back pain for 3 weeks now and none of the pain medication you recommended has helped. I just can't bear the pain!" The clinician should avoid becoming defensive in trying to justify previous advice. Instead, it is more helpful to address the patient's frustration and the implied message that something must be done: "You sound fed up with the length of time this pain has dragged on. Are you wondering if it is something serious or if there might be a better treatment?"

Often patients find it awkward or difficult to provide suggestions about the treatment of their diseases. Some patients may feel that their opinion lacks validity and value, while others may defer to the authority of the "expert" clinician in the decision-making process, not wanting to offend. Physicians need to encourage patients' participation with statements such as "I'm really interested in your point of view, especially since you are the one who has to live with our decision about these treatments." It is important for doctors to clearly explain the treatment options and to engage patients in a conversation about the pros and cons of different approaches. It is also important to acknowledge and address the patient's questions and concerns so that he or she feels heard and understood. In exploring the patient's thoughts about a specific plan, questions such as the following can be very useful: "Can you think of any difficulties in following through on this?" "Is there anything we can do to make this treatment plan easier for you?" "Do you need more time to think this over?" "Is there anybody you would like to talk to about this treatment?" Unfortunately this phase of the consultation, essential for establishing common ground, is often done badly because not enough time is spent on it. Physicians routinely spend only 1 minute out of a 20-minute consultation discussing treatment and planning but overestimate the time they spend by a factor of 9 (Waitzkin, 1984). Silverman *et al.* (2004) describe explanation and planning as "the Cinderella subject of communication skills teaching. Most teaching programmes concentrate on the first half of the interview and tend to neglect or underplay this vital next stage in the consultation" (2005: 141).

It is important to create a climate for discussion that makes it easier for patients to express their ideas and even their disagreements with the physician's recommendations. Patients need to feel that their opinions matter (Street, 2007). Ultimately, the patient is in control of whether or not they follow through with the plan and the clinician may only discover their disagreement in the follow-up visit. It is far better to discuss differing opinions openly in the initial visit, explore the patient's reasons for their ideas, and together look for a plan that both can accept. Because plans generated by patients are much more likely to be adhered to (Rollnick *et al.*, 2008; Miller & Rollnick, 2013), they are often preferable to plans developed solely by the physician, even if the physician's plans are based on guidelines. A plan rejected by the patient (even silently) is no plan at all. Patients may only hint at their disagreement, perhaps nonverbally, and clinicians need to be observant for any signs that the patient is not fully committed to the plan and should address the patient's concerns in a friendly and nonjudgmental manner.

Ford *et al.* (2003) note that, although most patients want to be well informed about their medical condition, not all patients wish to take an active role in treatment planning. However, once they are better informed about the treatment options and their consequences, they are more inclined to be involved in decisions about management. Two-thirds of patients in this study preferred either a shared approach or taking full responsibility, but 39% of patients felt they had not achieved their preferred role in decision making and "over half of patients who wanted to make or share decisions felt they had not been involved" (2003: 77). McKinstry (2000) conducted a study of patients' preferences for a directed or shared style of consultation using pairs of video vignettes of five common scenarios. In each scenario, one of the pairs showed the physician largely deciding on management (directed approach) and the other showed an interaction where the patient was involved in the decision (shared approach). Preferences varied by age, socioeconomic status, and medical condition. Patients over the age of 71 preferred a directed approach (72.6%) compared with those aged 15–60 (57.1%). Patients with upper socioeconomic status preferred a shared approach (52%) compared with those with a lower status (34.5%). Patients with an injured leg preferred a directed approach (85.6%) and those with depression preferred a shared approach (58.3%).

According to a Cochrane review of decision aids (Stacey *et al.*, 2011), they can be used by patients to improve their understanding of their options, the benefits and harms of each, and the values they place on benefits, harms, and medical uncertainties. This helps to prepare patients to participate more actively in discussions with health care providers. However, Nelson *et al.* (2007: 615) urge caution in using decision aids:

> they may interfere with a patient's implicit decision-making strategies, send the wrong message to patients about the goals of decision making, or lead patients to believe that they can reduce or eliminate uncertainty when confronting decisions that are by their very nature uncertain.

They suggest it might be preferable to teach people early in life how to tolerate uncertainty and ambiguity. Over the past 20 years, health coaching programs have developed in North America, Europe, and Australia (O'Connor *et al.*, 2008). Similar to decision aids, the health coach prepares patients before their visit to a physician by helping to clarify their priorities, developing their skills in raising questions and concerns, and developing their skills in presenting their opinions about investigation and management to their physician. Following the consultation with the physician, the health coach assists the patient to implement his or her management plans and to strengthen his or her self-confidence, often using motivational interviewing techniques. A number of reviews of the effectiveness of coaching showed positive effects on patients' knowledge, information recall, and participation in decision making (Coulter & Ellins, 2007).

Establishing the goals of treatment must also take into account the expectations and feelings of clinicians. Sometimes clinicians are concerned that patients may ask for something they disagree with, because they are not comfortable with confrontation or saying no. As a result, they may prefer to avoid the issue, but then finding common ground will not be achieved. Clinicians can become frustrated and disheartened when patients do not adhere to treatment protocols and management plans. But what physicians call "noncompliance" may be the patient's expressions of disagreement about treatment goals – it may be the patient's only option if he or she feels unable to discuss his or her disagreement. As Quill and Brody (1996: 765) observe: "Final choices belong to patients, but these choices gain meaning, richness, and accuracy if they are the result of a process of mutual influence and understanding between physician and patient." The following two case examples illustrate some challenges in defining the goals for treatment and/or management.

Case Example

As a 32-year-old single mother, Tabitha led an active and busy life caring for her three children, aged 7, 9, and 13, as well as working part-time as a teacher's assistant. A simple slip on a small patch of ice resulted in a broken wrist requiring extensive surgery. Her entire right arm was immobilized in a cast with "Frankenstein like" pins protruding from her arm. Her life was turned upside down; unable to perform routine tasks, she could not care for her children or work. The healing process was slow and painful. Her confidence and hope that she would recover was becoming severely tested. Tabitha felt that she had been reduced to a disease, stating: "I felt I was given no part in my care except to bring my arm in for appointments." She felt diminished and excluded in decisions about her treatment and rehabilitation. Her ability to voice her concerns and expectations became weaker, in striking parallel with her damaged limb: "I could not express how motivated I was to be included as someone who could influence my own health and healing. Also, in my view the doctor did not seem to appreciate or understand my feelings."

The serious misunderstandings between Tabitha and her surgeon arose because there was a failure to find common ground. As Tabitha later reflected: "I needed the physician to have a greater understanding of what I was concerned about and the relevance of my questions . . . No one asked me anything about what I needed."

Case Example

Mary, aged 64, smiled pleasantly as the doctor outlined the various options for dealing with her kidney failure. However, she had no intention of ever going on dialysis. The very thought of being hooked up to some machine three times a week was unbearable for Mary. Just let me die peacefully and with dignity, Mary thought.

Mary was defending herself from the terror she experienced when realizing how serious her illness was – talking about dialysis was too frightening! Until the physician could connect with some of her mixed feelings, she would not be willing to discuss the management of her renal failure.

Realizing that Mary seemed distracted, Dr O'Brien, her endocrinologist, commented: "You seem to have other things on your mind. Can you tell me how you are reacting to this kidney trouble?" Mary, caught off guard by Dr O'Brien's change in direction, paused a few moments, and replied, "Well, I don't like it one bit! But, I've had a good life and I will muddle through as best I can. I'm not ready to end my days attached to some infernal machine." Dr. O'Brien responded, "So, your independence is very important to you and whatever treatment I recommend must take that into account?" Mary nodded affirmatively, "That's for sure, Dr O'Brien."

Agreeing on those overall goals of management was the first step in treatment planning. Mary may or may not accept dialysis but it would need to be on her terms. If she sees it as a way to provide some increased quality of life she will accept the inconvenience and distress of long-term dialysis. In the future, when dialysis becomes necessary, the doctor and Mary will need to explore the pros and cons of independence, quality of life, and length of life.

PREVENTION AND HEALTH PROMOTION

Disease Prevention

Unlike health promotion, disease prevention is aimed at reducing the risk of acquiring a disease. An aging population, 83% of whom have chronic disease, and an increasing prevalence of chronic disease among all age groups both have heightened recognition of the importance of this aspect of health care. As a process, disease prevention reduces the likelihood that a disease or disorder will affect an individual (Stachtchenko & Jenicek, 1990), or, alternatively, that multimorbidity and acute episodes will transpire for those who already have chronic disease. Disease prevention strategies accordingly have been categorized as risk avoidance (primary prevention), risk reduction (secondary prevention), early identification, and complication reduction (tertiary prevention). The last three of these four will be raised again in Chapter 13. Risk avoidance aims at ensuring that people at low risk for health problems remain at low risk by finding ways to avoid disease. Risk reduction addresses moderate or high-risk characteristics among individuals or segments of the population, by finding ways to cure or control the prevalence of disease. Early identification aims at increasing the awareness of early signs of health problems and screening people at risk in order to detect the early onset of health problems. Risk reduction and complication reduction come into play after the disease has developed, with the goal being to ameliorate the effects of disease.

Whether the process of health care is to be health enhancement, risk avoidance, or risk reduction depends upon the timing of the opportunity for intervention and the patient's potential for disease at that time. Most important, both preventive care and health promotion efforts depend upon the patient's state of health and commitment to the pursuit of health.

Potential for Disease Prevention

In keeping with concern about human potential for disease, much of the literature pertaining to prevention deals with appropriate screening maneuvers (Canadian Task Force on Preventive Health Care, 1994; US Preventive Services Task Force, 2012) and establishing a practice infrastructure to bring these about (Battista & Lawrence, 1988). However, preventive care such as immunization is also of great significance. Enacting prevention in practice requires first and foremost the practitioner's explicit recommendation for the screening or vaccination and, second, attention to the patient's beliefs and attitudes. In multiple studies, the practitioners' recommendation for screening or vaccination was the most important predictor of the patient completing the disease prevention action (Lyn-Cook *et al.*, 2007; Chi & Neuzil, 2004; Kohlhammer *et al.*, 2007; Tong *et al.*, 2008). In addition, attention to the patients' beliefs and previous experiences with the vaccination are essential. The kinds of beliefs that are important to elicit include belief that the vaccine protects (Lyn-Cook *et al.*, 2007; Chi & Neuzil, 2004); belief that the vaccine could cause a cold; and a negative attitude toward the influenza vaccination (Chi & Neuzil, 2004).

Therefore, in disease prevention as with health promotion, the practitioner's explicit recommendation is key. After that, understanding the patient's definition of health, his or her beliefs and attitudes, and his or her past experiences will help the practitioner enhance health-promoting and disease-preventing behaviors (Pullen *et al.*, 2001).

The Clinical Method to Incorporate Prevention and Health Promotion into Component 3: Finding Common Ground

Mokdad *et al.* (2004) analyzed causes of death in the United States in 2000 and estimated the contribution of preventable behaviors to these deaths. They concluded that about half of all deaths could be attributed to a limited number of largely preventable behaviors and exposures – especially, tobacco (18.1% of all deaths), poor diet and physical inactivity (16.6%), and alcohol consumption (3.5%). These findings illustrate the remarkable but unrealized potential of health promotion and disease prevention strategies.

Every contact between patients and clinicians is an opportunity to consider health promotion and prevention. In the four components of the patient-centered clinical method, the exploration of health-promoting values and beliefs is considered as part of Component 1, found in Chapter 3 of this book. The activities of education, screening, and secondary or tertiary prevention are covered here as part of Component 3, Finding Common Ground. Every contact can include education on the benefits of a healthy diet and exercise. It also includes screening for health risks such as hypertension or sedentary lifestyle, and early detection of disease such as breast cancer or diabetes. In addition, it includes tertiary prevention to reduce the impact of disease on the patient's function, longevity, and quality of life. There are numerous and often conflicting guidelines that may create confusion for patients and even for their health care providers. Although, in typical medical consultations, time is short and serious medical conditions take priority, it is important to consider how to reduce the risk of new problems and to prevent patients' conditions from getting worse. Simple interventions, like making sure the patient's immunization is up to date, take little time. Assuring that the patient's nutritional needs are addressed before surgery can improve wound healing and recovery. Because many patients have medical conditions that cannot be cured, the primary goal of treatment is to minimize the impact of the disease on the patient's life. In particular, the goal is to reduce the symptoms and functional deficits that are interfering with the patient's ability to pursue his or her aspirations, goals, and purposes. Because only the patient knows what his or her aspirations, goals, and purposes are, it is essential to include the patient in any discussions and decisions about health promotion and prevention (Cassell, 2013).

The case example of Rex Kelly was presented in Chapter 3. He had coronary artery disease, a recent myocardial infarction, and a bypass surgery. Dr Wason identified symptoms of depression, which he clarified by exploring Rex's sadness about his losses and limitations and his fears about another myocardial infarction. Together they agreed it would be helpful to include Rex's wife in further discussion. In addition, Dr Wason had identified obesity and an elevated cholesterol. The doctor also gently explored Rex's health perceptions as basic groundwork for his health promotion and disease prevention plan. Dr Wason had explored Rex's sense that he was "no longer a healthy man," that family winter activities were very important to him, and that he was looking for guidance and reassurance about resuming lovemaking.

After the exploration of Rex's perceptions and risk factors, the work of finding common ground could continue. The doctor created a complete health promotion and disease prevention plan, which he will present to Rex in bite-sized portions over their future monthly visits. The plan includes the following points.

- Lifestyle modification: Dr Wason will continue to monitor and discuss with Rex his diet and exercise programs.
- Secondary prevention: Dr Wason will continue, and monitor as relevant, such medications as acetylsalicylic acid, statins, angiotensin-converting-enzyme inhibitors, and beta-blockers.
- Primary prevention: Dr Wason will present and discuss three immunizations (annual flu shots, pneumonia vaccine, and herpes zoster vaccine); as well, he will recommend colon cancer screening.

Dr Wason fully recognises the complexities of including health prevention in the ongoing contacts with Rex as he recovers from his bypass surgery.

Figure 6.1 organises the health promotion and disease prevention plan described in the previous paragraph into the conceptual framework of finding

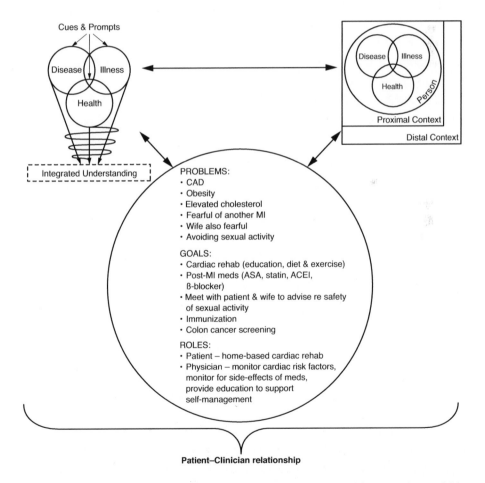

FIGURE 6.1 Finding common ground, including prevention and health promotion activities

common ground, using Rex as the example. Figure 6.1 demonstrates how prevention can be seamlessly incorporated into the care of patients with chronic conditions.

Although Dr Wason's plan was based on current guidelines, it remains tentative until discussed and confirmed with Rex and should also include consideration of alternative or additional interventions suggested by Rex. Applying the patient-centered approach allows practitioners like Dr Wason to find the methods of health promotion and preventive care that most appropriately match the patient's world – his or her health beliefs, values, preferences, priorities, aspirations, and resources. The practitioner's knowledge of this world helps in making a judgment about which health promotion or disease prevention strategy provides the most appropriate fit.

Flach *et al.* (2004), in a study comparing provision of preventive services at Veteran's Administration ambulatory facilities, found that more preventive services were provided in facilities where patients had a better opportunity to discuss issues of importance to them and where there was greater continuity of care. It may take several contacts between patient and clinician to understand what really matters to the patient and his or her wishes for health promotion or preventive procedures. Just as in the learner-centered approach to medical education, the first step is a needs assessment. This will be based partly on the patient's medical conditions, health behaviors, and health risks based on age and sex. The following three questions are helpful in gleaning the patient's perspective of health behaviors.

1. All of us at one time or another do things that aren't good for us. It might be something like not wearing a seat belt or perhaps drinking more than we think we should. What behaviours are you doing that might put you at risk?
2. Most of us forget to take our medication or follow through with diet or exercise at some point or another. What difficulties have you had with managing or treating your _____?
3. What are you doing these days that you believe is contributing to your health? (Institute for Healthcare Communication, 2010: 36–7)

The answers to these questions provide the clinician with an understanding of the patient's awareness of behaviors that might influence his or her health. However, awareness is not enough. In order to change behavior, patients must want to change, know how to change, and have the necessary environmental resources and social supports to change. Typically, people go through a number of stages in making a change – precontemplation (they are not even thinking about change or have decided not to change), contemplation (thinking about it but not changing because of strong ambivalence), preparation (having decided to change and getting ready), action (in the early phase of behaving in the new way but vulnerable to relapse), maintenance (becoming more comfortable with the change but still needing to work on it), and identification (seeing oneself as changed) (Prochaska & DiClemente, 1984; Prochaska, 2008). Identifying the patient's stage of change is a helpful step in finding common ground. People think about and experience change differently in each stage and need different help from their health care practitioners. For example, in the precontemplative stage, the clinician should ask the patient if it is all right to mention some of the reasons for concern about his or her behavior in order to advise the patient about their risks. In the contemplative stage the clinician assists the patient to consider the advantages and disadvantages of changing his or her behavior. Only when the patient reaches the preparation stage, or beyond, is it worthwhile to spend time discussing strategies that might make it easier to change. Providing detailed instruction on a healthy diet to a patient in precontemplation would be a waste of time for everyone.

Motivational interviewing is another powerful approach to collaborating with patients about behavior change. One aspect of this approach is discovering the patient's values, very akin to Component 1 of the patient-centered clinical method. The following examples of open-ended questions can be utilized.

- Tell me what you care most about in life. What matters most to you?
- How do you hope your life will be different a few years from now?
- What would you say are the rules you live by? What do you try to live up to?
- Suppose I asked you to describe the goals that guide your life, the values you try to live by. What would you say are your five most important values, maybe just one word for each to begin with. What would they be?
- If you were to write a "mission statement" for your life, describing your goals or purpose in life, what would you write?
- If I were to ask your closest friends to tell me what you live for, what matters most to you, what do you think they would say? (Miller & Rollnick, 2013: 75–6).

Questions like these will usually open up issues for patient and clinician to explore in more depth. Disease symptoms or unhealthy behavior blocking the achievement of important life goals are an obvious target for health promotion.

However, the clinician must avoid taking over the discussion; it is important for the suggestions to come from the patient. Gordon and Edwards (1997) listed a number of roadblocks that clinicians unwittingly apply when they discuss these issues with patients: warning, cautioning, or threatening; giving advice, making suggestions, or providing solutions; persuading with logic, arguing, or lecturing; interpreting or analyzing. We provide additional suggestions for using motivational interviewing later in this chapter, under the heading "Strategies to Assist Finding Common Ground."

Screening for risk factors and early disease provides additional challenges for health care providers. Generally, clinicians demand stronger evidence of benefit and safety for preventive strategies than for treatment protocols for existing disease conditions. As a rule, patients are more willing to accept the risk of side effects of treatment for a condition that is causing symptoms than the risks of a procedure that might only prevent harm in the future.

In educating patients about their health and health behaviors, it is important for clinicians to avoid providing unsolicited advice; instead, they need to listen intently for any ideas coming from patients about how they might improve their health and explore how they might be able to follow through on them. Practitioners need to ask patients about barriers, how they might overcome these barriers, and possible resources that might help. If the patient is stuck, clinicians can ask if they would like some examples about what others have done in similar situations. This approach is consistent with the learner-centered method described in Chapter 9 and with a learner-centered approach described by Rogers (1982) and many others (Falvo, 2011; Doyle, 2011; Weimer, 2013). The commonly used strategies of health education, most of which emphasize information-giving and behavior modification, make up only a small part of the process of health promotion. In order for true personal growth and change and to enhance motivation, a patient-centered approach is critical, including the exploration of the patients' health perceptions – that is, the meaning of health to them and their aspirations in life, as described in Chapter 3. Fundamental to determining common ground regarding preventive behavior is the extent to which the individual feels responsible for and in control of his or her own health. Beliefs about health risks and the degree of control one has over those risks will affect the patient's actions, as will the individual's inclination to take a proactive or reactive stance in the pursuit of health. Aujoulat *et al.* (2007) interviewed 40 patients with chronic conditions to explore the experience of powerlessness. They found that identity insecurity and disrupted identity were two major factors of powerlessness in all of the participants. They suggest that successful empowerment might occur when patients come to terms with their threatened senses of security and identity, not only with the management of their treatment. One of the primary aims of an empowering relationship might therefore be to not provide immediately choice and opportunities for participation and self-determination but to provide reassurance and opportunities for self-exploration instead. (2007: 783)

The patient's world is understood as a dynamic situation that varies with each patient at different points in time and with each health care issue. The practitioner's aim is to find the best fit with the patient's world. Sometimes, for some issues, the patient requires a health enhancement strategy. At other times, for other reasons, the patient requires prevention strategies.

Case Example

Mrs Bell:	"Doctor, my husband and I thought about having Jason vaccinated but after reading some books, we're not so sure that it is the right thing to do."
Doctor:	"Tell me about your concerns."

The Bells, responsible and conscientious parents of 6-month-old Jason were new to their family doctor's practice. The doctor was surprised to find that the child had received no immunization. A bright and well-educated couple, Mr and Mrs Bell had taken time to inform themselves on infant and baby care. They had invested in a good-quality baby car seat and were very interested in planning for the baby's future, but they were reluctant to have Jason immunized. They had been aware of sensational media reports of presumed vaccine adverse effects resulting in permanent neurological damage. This had left them doubtful about the benefits and risks of vaccination for their son. In contrast, their family physician saw vaccination as a basic investment in Jason's future health.

It may be difficult for a clinician to understand a patient's opposing viewpoint, given the clear benefits that have been made possible by vaccination programs. There are many reasons why the lay public may evaluate medical risks differently from the "experts." Research in the field of decision making has found that people's perceptions of risk are not determined by rational processes but that greater weight is given to risks if the issue is perceived to be involuntary, dreaded, immediate, appears to be uncontrollable, puts children at risk, or is unfamiliar (Whyte & Burton, 1982). The mass media, and recently the Internet, has played a significant role in shaping the public's perception of vaccinations and in some countries has been instrumental in the decline in vaccination rates, resulting in the resurgence of previously controlled infectious diseases (Cherry, 1984; Jacobson *et al.*, 2007; Kata, 2012). The Health Belief Model includes several variables that predict whether or not people will take action to prevent or screen for diseases. Perceived barriers were the strongest predictor of behavior; other predictors were perceived benefits and perceived susceptibility. Perceived severity was the least powerful predictor (Champion & Skinner, 2008). Parents who did not vaccinate their children thought their children had a low susceptibility to the diseases, that the severity of the diseases was low, and that the efficacy and safety of the vaccines was low (Smith *et al.*, 2004). The commonest reason for non-vaccination, expressed by 69% of parents, was concern that the vaccine might be harmful (Salmon *et al.*, 2005). Physicians providing care to unvaccinated children were less likely to have confidence in vaccine safety (Salmon *et al.*, 2008).

The Bell family had serious reservations about allowing vaccination of their child. Their family physician listened carefully to their concerns and answered them respectfully. She was able to put the small risks of vaccine side effects into perspective by comparing the published risks of adverse vaccine reactions with the risks of everyday events. After careful consideration of these points the Bells eventually decided to have Jason immunized, which proceeded without any side effects. In this case the family physician was able to find common ground with the parents and come to a mutually satisfactory agreement by recognizing that it is possible to have legitimate opinions that differ from the "experts," and then listening carefully to the concerns raised by those opinions and addressing those concerns in a forthright manner.

The strategies that clinicians employ will vary from patient to patient and from time to time with the same patient, depending on the circumstances, the life stage of the patient, the patient's priorities, and the presence or absence of health risk behavior. Deciding on an appropriate strategy ultimately means finding common ground. Of course, no strategy is pursued without the patient's informed consent (Lee, 1993; Marshall, 1996; Brindle & Fahey, 2002; Marteau, 2002). Achieving informed consent presents a particular challenge in the areas of health promotion and disease prevention. Since the benefits or risks of a preventive procedure are generally determined on societal rather than an individual level, it is not possible to predict the consequences for any one person (Hanckel, 1984). The tendency has been to weigh the benefits and potential harm of a preventive procedure (e.g., immunization) on a societal rather than an individual level (Rose, 1981). However, the physician has a moral and ethical responsibility to present the risks and psychological costs of proposed prevention programs to the patient (Marteau, 1990; Brett *et al.*, 2005; Collins *et al.*, 2011). Additionally, it must be made clear that the problems are difficult to predict in advance and that little is known about the prognosticators of health (Schoenbach *et al.*, 1983; Murray *et al.*, 2003). Even when problems and prognosticators are correctly predicted, known treatments only work for a portion of patients, and that portion cannot be identified. Thus, physicians cannot tell patients how certain they might be that the preventive treatment will produce the desired effect (Hanckel, 1984; Edwards, 2009). Paling (2003, 2006) provides advice to health care providers about how to help patients understand risks. For example, use a natural frequency format (e.g., "1 in 5 people" or "12 in 100 people") rather than percentages. Use absolute numbers whenever possible and avoid relative risks. Share uncertainty when it is genuinely unclear what should be done. Schwartz *et al.* (2009) advocate the use of tables to explain risks to patients and provide evidence that patients find them helpful in making wise decisions.

Clearly, health promotion and disease prevention necessitate increased attention to the ethical dilemmas in public health and the potential for harm (Strasser *et al.*, 1987; Guttman & Salmon, 2004). For example, Downing (2011) and Hadler (2008) argue that we have increasingly medicalized health and we have created the impression that there is a medical answer to all of life's problems. The result is an excessive use of technology and its potential for harm. Ultimately, patients have the right to choose, and in so choosing, they share the responsibility for outcomes. This, too, is an important parameter of health, health promotion, and disease prevention.

In all of the case examples so far mentioned, the clinician and patient needed to work together to find a treatment plan that was acceptable to both. This required that the goals and priorities of each be considered and perhaps reexamined. Finally, when disagreement occurs it may be necessary for the clinician to explore the deeper reasons for the patient's position, as these case examples demonstrated.

DEFINING THE ROLES OF PATIENT AND CLINICIAN

Inherent in articulating the roles to be assumed by the patient and clinician is a definition of mutual responsibility for the actions that will follow. These may be quite simple, such as: "I want to see you again in one month to check that this new medication is lowering your blood pressure." Implicit in this statement is the patient's use of the medication as prescribed and the doctor's desire for future follow-up. Certain situations, however, may be more complex and therefore require an explicit statement of the roles to be assumed by the patient and the doctor. Again, referring back to the case of Hanna (a patient with breast cancer) presented in Chapter 3, finding common ground was an ongoing process with the roles of the patient and doctor constantly shifting and changing in response to the patient's needs.

Sometimes there is profound disagreement about the nature of the problem or the goals and priorities for treatment. When such an impasse occurs, it is important to look at the relationship between the patient and the clinician, and at their perception of each other's roles. (The nature and characteristics of the relationship will be dealt with in depth in Chapter 7, while here we focus on problems in role definition.) Doctors, perhaps with a cancer patient, may see themselves wanting to bring about remission, and may expect the patient to assume the role of a passive recipient of treatment. Patients, however, may be seeking a physician who expresses concern and interest in their values and preferences, and who is prepared to treat them in the least invasive manner, viewing them as autonomous individuals with a right to have a voice in deciding among various forms of treatment. This is not such a dilemma for doctors when the various forms of treatment are equally effective, but physicians are understandably concerned when the patient chooses a treatment that the physician considers either less efficacious or even harmful.

Evolution of the patient-clinician relationship over time, as described in Chapters 4 and 7, allows the doctor to see the same patient with different problems in different settings over a number of years, and also to see the patient through the eyes of other family members. The physician's commitment is to "be present" with the patient throughout his or her illness. Patients need to know that they can count on their doctors to be there when they need them. This ongoing relationship colors everything that happens between them. If there are difficulties in their relationship or differing expectations of their roles, they will have problems in working together effectively. The following points are examples of this.

- The patient is looking for an authority who will tell him or her what is wrong and what he or she should do; the physician, on the other hand, wants a more egalitarian relationship in which clinician and patient share decision making.
- The patient longs for a deep and meaningful relationship with a parental

figure who will make up for everything the patient's own parent never gave; the doctor wants to be a biomedical scientist who can apply the discoveries of modern medicine to patients' problems.

- The physician enjoys a holistic approach to medicine and wants to get to know patients as people; the patient seeks only technical assistance from the doctor.

Finding common ground about a patient's role in the decision-making process does not necessarily imply that the patient will assume an active role. Patients' levels of participation in decision making may fluctuate depending on their emotional and physical capabilities. Thus clinicians need to be flexible and responsive to potential changes in their patient's involvement. Some patients may be too sick or too overwhelmed by the burden of their illness to actively participate in their care. Others may find decisions about treatment options too complex and confusing; hence abdicating the decision making to the clinician. When patients are receiving care from multiple health care professionals they assume different roles and relationships with each. Roles within and across the health care team may also influence the patient's care, as we discuss in detail in Chapter 13.

Sometimes a lack of role clarity or assumptions about the patient's and clinician's roles can result in ambiguity and uncertainty. The following case serves as an illustration.

Case Example

Ralph Kruppa, a 59-year-old family doctor, had suffered a myocardial infarction. The event had seriously unsettled this man, leaving him both concerned and uncertain about his future health and well-being. At the time of discharge from hospital his cardiologist suggested that Dr Kruppa look after his own warfarin, because, as a doctor, he was knowledgeable about managing the medication. Dr Kruppa, the patient, feeling uncustomarily vulnerable did not challenge the cardiologist's suggestion. He subsequently ordered more international normalized ratios on himself than he had ever done before with his patients. Four weeks after his discharge from hospital Dr Kruppa had an appointment with his family doctor, who indicated that he would monitor the patient's international normalized ratio to determine if it was too high or low and correspondingly alter the dosage of warfarin. There was no need for Dr Kruppa to be involved. The family doctor's office staff would call the patient if the dosage needed to be changed.

To himself Dr Kruppa thought: "Sure, sure the lab results will go to you – but I will also arrange that I get copies of the lab results so that I am informed about the results! I know the system and how information can fall through the cracks." Out loud he quietly replied: "Sure, whatever you think."

Neither of Dr Kruppa's physicians had asked the patient his perspective and what role he wanted to assume in the management of his warfarin. Nor had the patient's family doctor and cardiologist consulted each other; thus each physician had very different ideas about the management of the patient's warfarin. What the patient would have preferred and needed was to have the various options laid out to him as to what role(s) the cardiologist, the family doctor, and the patient might assume. The next important step would have been to ask him, "What option would you prefer and what role do you want to play?"

THE PROCESS OF FINDING COMMON GROUND

In the process of finding common ground it is the clinician's responsibility to provide his or her medical expertise in defining the diagnosis. This may be as clear-cut as: "You have a strep throat" or ultimately more complex and uncertain such as: "There are several possibilities for what your symptoms suggest and a number of options for the next steps including more testing or waiting to see how your condition unfolds. Do you have a preference?" Sometimes the patient's story starts out simply and evolves into something unexpected. For example, consider a healthy-looking 35-year-old man presenting with a recent history of a single episode of palpitations lasting 15 minutes and associated with a feeling of anxiety. The history and physical examination revealed no abnormalities but the patient was very worried and had discontinued his daily exercise program for fear it might damage his heart. He had surfed the Internet and decided he needed an electrocardiogram, stress test, Holter monitoring, and numerous blood tests. Because the tachycardia occurred right after receiving "bad news" the physician decided that the single episode of tachycardia was unlikely serious and, if the electrocardiogram was normal, nothing further was needed. After the physician explained his conclusions, the patient was somewhat relieved but he still requested additional investigation. Recognizing that the patient needed additional reassurance, the physician agreed to order a stress test but he explained the risk of a false-positive result. He was reluctant to order more tests that he considered unnecessary but he agreed to discuss this again after the stress test. The doctor explored further the story of the "bad news" and learned that the patient's best friend had recently died in a motor vehicle accident. They had often worked out together and had even run a marathon together a few months previously. Now it made sense why the patient needed all the additional investigation. Until he was convinced that his heart was OK he would live in fear that, like his friend, he was vulnerable. Although the additional testing may not be necessary from a strictly biomedical perspective, it was needed to assist the patient to get on with his life. In follow-up visits, the physician will invite the patient to talk more about his friend and his reaction to his loss. What started out as benign palpitations potentially needing only reassurance, revealed a life-altering experience requiring that the physician support the patient to come to terms with a major loss.

In exploring patients' stories (the meaning of health to them, their life aspirations, their symptoms, feelings, ideas, how illness interferes with their activities, and their hopes for treatment) physicians are able to discern a probable diagnosis and the impact of the illness experience. The therapeutic plan must address the whole story, not just the disease, and illness must be consistent with the patient's beliefs and aspirations. While explaining their understanding of the patient's predicament, it is important that physicians are open to patients' questions and alert to verbal and nonverbal cues that they are confused, upset, or anxious about what they are hearing. It is important to provide the patient with an opportunity to ask questions and offer suggestions. This must be more than simply clarifying the physician's plans but a genuine offer to reconsider and revise the approach to treatment if it is not congruent with the patient's values and preferences. Sometimes, when the physician asks, "What do you think?" some patients may respond with "I don't know – you're the doctor!" Doctors need to answer with a comment such as: "Yes and I will provide you with information and my opinion but your ideas and wishes are important in making our plan together." This is the basis of a true sharing of ideas.

The patient and clinician can then participate in a mutual discussion of their shared understanding of the problem and how it can best be addressed. At the conclusion of their discussion of treatment options and goals, it is the clinician's responsibility to clarify explicitly the patient's understanding and agreement. It is during this summation that the practitioner and patient can make specific their respective roles in achieving the mutually agreed upon treatment goals. This may be as simple as agreeing on how follow-up plans will be arranged, or as complex as a discussion of how a cancer patient in the palliative phase needs the doctor to assume a caring role rather than a curative stance.

If disagreements arise, clinicians must avoid getting into power struggles. Instead, they must listen to the patient's concerns or opinions, as opposed to dismissing the patient as obstinate or difficult. When conflicts do arise, the grid shown in Box 6.1 may be a useful tool. How do both the patient and the clinician view the problem(s), the goals of treatment, and their respective roles? Why are these divergent and can their differences be resolved? This grid also helps the clinician to check if important information is missing, such as the patient's experience of illness or specific issues relevant to the patient's unique context.

Box 6.1 Finding Common Ground

Issue	Patient	Doctor
Problems		
Goals		
Roles		

The next case example illustrates the key concepts of finding common ground: defining the problems, the goals, and the roles of the patient and doctor. It also emphasizes the fundamental importance of a trusting relationship between patient and clinician.

Case Example

When Dr Matise first met 28-year-old Lyle, the smell of alcohol and cigarettes permeated the examination room. Standing at just over 6 feet and weighing approximately 300 pounds Lyle was an imposing presence. He was unshaven and dressed in a T-shirt and torn jeans. His language was peppered with expletives. Lyle's stated reason for the visit was to have his cholesterol checked.

Lyle revealed how he was unhappy with his weight and was beginning to worry about his health. Lyle stated, "I asked my last doctor why the hell do I sweat so much and the doc said to me, 'Lyle, look at it like this, imagine a 150-pound man carrying another 150-pound man everywhere he goes . . . that's why you sweat so much.'" Lyle snorted, "Shit, what kind of an answer is that!"

His obesity had worsened over the last year after Lyle had been laid off work. He had completed ninth grade and maintained that "education isn't worth a damn unless you end up with a job that pays good money!" Indeed, Lyle had made good money; he had worked his way up from manual laborer to foreman at the steel plant. That was until the plant closed down. "Hell, I'd worked at the plant since I was 16," lamented Lyle, "those guys were like family to me." Unable to manage his mortgage payments after being laid off, Lyle had moved into a rundown trailer owned by his mother. He was now spending most of his days smoking and drinking with "good buddies" who shared a similar life perspective.

Lyle's cholesterol had never been previously investigated but he had heard "talk of cholesterol" on television. Now with his purported concerns about his own health, Lyle was curious about his own cholesterol. Lifestyle questions revealed the following. "I'm a meat-and-potatoes guy, doc!" explained Lyle. He also reported being a pack-a-day smoker since his teens and he drank a "case of 24" a week. While alcohol abuse was a consistent pattern for his father and his two brothers, Lyle did not view his own alcohol consumption as a problem.

It was readily apparent to Dr Matise that Lyle was facing many serious issues. The plant closing had resulted in his feeling bitter and angry, although Lyle denied these emotions. However, from Dr Matise's perspective, Lyle's loss of work and his home were seemingly related to an increase in his eating, smoking, and drinking. Despite his gruff exterior, Lyle seemed scared. When Dr Matise asked Lyle directly how he wanted to proceed in addressing his concerns about his weight and cholesterol, Lyle appeared reluctant to make any alterations to his current lifestyle.

From Lyle's story, Dr Matise had gleaned how his patient's past interactions with other health care professionals had been tenuous. While there were multiple health issues requiring attention, these would only be tackled when Lyle was ready and once a more firm and trusting relationship was established. For now, finding common ground would consist of focusing directly on Lyle's cholesterol, including learning what he knew about cholesterol and what steps Lyle was prepared to take in addressing this issue.

Dr Matise hoped that during future rechecks of Lyle's cholesterol he could further develop the relationship with his patient. Formation of a strong patient-doctor relationship would increase the likelihood of finding common ground regarding the many issues still confronting Lyle.

STRATEGIES TO ASSIST FINDING COMMON GROUND

The development of specific interviewing approaches such as motivational interviewing and informed decision making provide useful strategies to assist patients and clinicians in the process of finding common ground. Motivational interviewing reflects the same spirit of collaboration we encourage.

> It is not something done by an expert to a passive recipient, a teacher to a pupil, a master to a disciple. In fact it is not done "to" or "on" someone at all. MI [motivational interviewing] is done "for" and "with" a person. It is an active collaboration between experts. People are the undisputed experts on themselves. No one has been with them longer, or knows them better than they do themselves. In MI, the helper is a companion who typically does less that half of the talking. The method of MI involves exploration more than exhortation, interest and support rather than persuasion or argument. The interviewer seeks to create a positive interpersonal atmosphere that is conducive to change but not coercive. (Miller & Rollnick, 2013: 15)

Motivational interviewing began in the 1980s with a focus on addictive behaviors such as alcoholism and smoking, and it is now widely used in many settings to assist people wanting to make many types of behavioral change (Söderlund *et al.*, 2011). For example, a person may desire to be a nonsmoker but be unwilling or unable to tolerate the struggle to quit. They are often paralyzed by their ambivalence about quitting – on the one hand they recognize the benefits of quitting but on the other hand they enjoy smoking and find the withdrawal symptoms intolerable. Motivational interviewing challenges the "righting reflex," a clinician's almost automatic attempt to help people fix what's wrong by telling them what to do. Some clinicians will endeavor to frighten patients into changing by quoting fearful statistics about the harmful effects of smoking; others may try to make them feel guilty for not quitting. Although well intentioned, these approaches usually fail. "MI is about arranging conversations so that people talk themselves into change, based on their own values and interests" (Miller & Rollnick, 2013: 4).

Practitioners commonly intervene by providing information about smoking, tips on how to quit, and pharmacological aids such as nicotine patches, sticks, or bupropion. This is often helpful if it matches the patient's ideas about quitting, but the patient might have other ideas about what might work better. Effective clinicians begin by establishing rapport using interviewing methods such as open-ended inquiry, reflective listening, and empathy. Next they encourage the patient to discuss the behavior he or she wishes to change, what he or she has already tried, and what he or she might have successfully used for other behaviors in the past. They will pick up on any change talk (tentative thoughts about the need or desire to change, reasons to change, or how they might change) and help the patient explore and flesh out his or her ideas, identifying how the patient might tackle any barriers and how he or she might incorporate any helpful resources in his or her setting. The key to success is for the ideas to come from the patient, not the clinician.

Another helpful interviewing technique is to ask about the patient's confidence and conviction (Keller & White, 1997). For example, if a patient expresses a desire to get into better shape, ask about their conviction: "How important is it for you to get into better shape?" Scaling can be incorporated by asking: "On a scale from zero to ten, how would you rate its importance to you?" If the patient rates it five, the clinician could follow with: "What would it take for you to say seven or eight?" This helps to clarify the patient's values and motivation and may even generate change talk. Similarly, the clinician can ask about the patient's confidence in making the desired changes. This technique also helps the clinician decide where to concentrate his or her efforts. If the patient is strongly motivated but lacking in confidence, then the interview should concentrate on finding effective strategies for change; on the other hand, if the patient is confident he or she could change if he or she wanted to but lacks conviction, then the focus should be on exploring what would enhance the patient's motivation.

Several authors advocate the use of shared decision-making techniques in patient care (Towle & Godolphin, 1999; Charles *et al.*, 1999; Elwyn *et al.*, 2000; Elwyn & Charles, 2001; Edwards & Elwyn, 2009; Légaré *et al.*, 2010). For example, the Informed Shared Decision Making Model (Elwyn *et al.*, 1999; Godolphin *et al.*, 2001; Weston, 2001; Godolphin, 2009) provides an approach to involving patients in their own care to the extent that they wish to be involved. Using this approach, clinicians determine how much information patients desire and how they prefer learning more about their condition (e.g., discussion with their health care provider or health coach, decision aids, pamphlets, Internet, videotapes, or support groups, depending on what is available) and their preferences for their role in decision making (e.g., talking with other family members, relying on the clinician's advice, being self-reliant, comfortable with risk taking). Discussing how patients prefer to handle decisional conflict (what they do when they are confronted with opposing ideas and uncertainty) may help them to resolve such dilemmas. It is important to understand that, in this approach, the clinician is not simply a servant doing whatever the patient requests but, rather, a partner who brings medical expertise and evidence to the discussion about treatment. Towle and Godolphin (1999) contend that being explicit about these issues enhances patients' opportunities for an effective partnership with clinicians, as they explore choices together and come to a mutual decision that best matches the patients' preferences and is congruent with the best available evidence and clinical wisdom.

> In a truly shared decision, physicians and patients mutually influence each other, each potentially ending up in a place different from where they began, with different understandings than either would have reached alone. It is not a matter of who has power and who does not. It is a matter of mutual influence. (Hanson, 2008: 1368)

The strategies described here can be very useful in finding common ground, but they must always be applied in the context of patient-centered practice. As stated previously, patients may not feel well enough or confident enough to be active participants in decisions about their care. They may choose to abdicate their responsibilities and hand them over to the clinician. This is patient-centered care, as it respects the needs and preferences of the patient in that specific circumstance. However, the situation may change and this would necessitate that clinicians be responsive and flexible to the patients' involvement in the process of finding common ground.

CONCLUSION

Finding common ground requires that patients and physicians reach a mutual understanding and mutual agreement on the nature of the problems, the goals and priorities of treatment, and their respective roles. Sometimes patients and clinicians have divergent views in each of these areas. The process of finding a satisfactory resolution is not one of bargaining or negotiating but, rather, of moving toward a meeting of minds or finding common ground. Sometimes it means agreeing to differ, but always it means respecting one another.

As Boudreau *et al.* (2007) suggest, the single overarching goal of care is "the wellbeing of the patient and, more specifically, improvement in the patient's functions to allow the patient to pursue his purposes" (2007: 1196). As such, it is essential to involve patients in planning their treatment and determining priorities for care, since only the patient is aware of how his or her diseases are blocking the achievement of what matters most to him or her. Placing these considerations in the center of patient care transforms the clinical method by urging physicians to recognize that they are called on to do more than stamp out disease; they are called on to join with patients in addressing the full impact of disease on patients' lives.

Thus the process of finding common ground between the patient and the clinician is an integral and interactive component of the patient-centered clinical method. Finding common ground is the lynchpin or place of convergence, where all of the components of the patient-centered clinical method come together. To find common ground, the clinician must take into consideration all aspects of the patient-centered clinical method: knowing the patient's health, disease, and illness experience; appreciating the person and his or her life context; and constantly building on the patient-clinician relationship. As McLeod (1998: 678) cogently notes:

> When we listen to, accept, and validate the illness story, when we interpret the illness in terms of its symptomatic pathophysiology, when we explain treatment plans and prognosis, and, most importantly, when we define the patient's own role in the healing process, then trust, compassion, and a human connection between the patient and doctor becomes possible.

"I'd Sooner Take My Chances!": Case Illustrating Component 3
Jamie Wickett, Judith Belle Brown, and W Wayne Weston

Dr Santos returned to her office contemplating her current dilemma having just finished with her last patient of the day, 63-year-old Edward. She was undoubtedly between a rock and a hard place and uncertain how to proceed. Dr Santos sat down at her desk, reflecting on her past several years of caring for her patient. She was aware that Ed often felt overwhelmed with his multiple medical problems, which included peripheral vascular disease, diabetes mellitus, and coronary artery disease to name just a few. Furthermore, his list of medications filled an entire page. His "golden years" had been plagued with many medical challenges, culminating in a sudden and unexpected above-knee amputation of his left leg. Ed was never able to adapt to a prosthetic limb, was wheelchair bound, and suffered ongoing phantom limb pain.

Ed was a retired police officer living in an apartment with Cathy, his devoted wife of many years. With difficulty, Ed had accommodated to life following his left above-knee amputation. This amputation significantly changed both Ed and Cathy's daily lives in many ways. Cathy was not only Ed's sole care provider but also the breadwinner. Dr Santos sometimes wondered how Cathy managed all of her responsibilities. She knew that Ed relied on Cathy for assistance with his transfers. As a large man, the only reason that he was even able to transfer was because he still had the use of his right leg. Ed spent most of his days at home, but he looked forward to his weekly lunch out with some of his retired friends from the force. He also enjoyed his daily visits with the various health care providers who came into his home. His other social interactions were limited to appointments with the many physicians who were involved in his care. Aside from these interactions, he remained socially isolated.

Ed always came to each of his monthly appointments with Dr Santos carrying a detailed, typewritten agenda of the items he and Cathy wished to discuss. Dr Santos understood that Ed's agenda was part of his need to control the things in his life that he could, because so much of what he had been through in the past few years was out of his control. At least in their appointments he could decide which concerns he would like addressed and in which order. So when Ed and Cathy came into the office unexpectedly and without a formal agenda, Dr Santos knew that something must be wrong.

It had been 2 weeks since Ed had presented to the office with a small red bump that was just below his right knee and which was oozing profuse amounts of yellow fluid mixed with pus and blood. Dr Santos recalled being concerned that his right total knee replacement had become infected and had formed a sinus tract that was draining to the skin surface. Consequently, she had referred Ed to his orthopedic surgeon, who promptly saw Ed and confirmed that the right knee replacement had become infected.

Today, at his follow-up visit with Dr Santos, Ed recounted the details of his visit with the specialist. Ed was devastated with the news that his right total knee replacement had become infected. He had experienced multiple medical setbacks in the past few years and this was seen as yet another significant burden. The fact that something bad was happening to his "good" leg only increased his level of worry, and he felt that his other leg had now also failed him. Ever since the amputation of his left leg, Ed had been very vigilant with any symptoms or changes in his right leg. The prospect of possibly losing his remaining leg filled him with fear and anxiety. "Doc, it would be the end of my life if I were to lose my leg. Cathy would no longer be able to help me transfer and I would have to move to a nursing home!"

Although the surgeon strongly recommended that they immediately move forward with a two-stage revision, Ed wasn't ready to tackle such a "drastic" procedure. More surgery at this time seemed like "too much" for Ed and he preferred a nonsurgical approach. The complexity of the treatment decision that Ed had to make overwhelmed him and he struggled to wrap his head around it. This was highlighted when he stated, "I'd sooner take my chances and die than go through with the surgery and risk losing everything I have left. It may not seem like a lot to you, doc, but it's all I've got." Despite the threat of serious complications without surgery, Ed was adamant that he could not face surgery again.

Now that Ed and Cathy had returned home, Dr Santos took a few moments to reflect on this worrisome visit. On the one hand, she could see the benefit of the surgeon's treatment plan and it certainly made sense from a curative standpoint: take the infected hardware out, treat with intravenous antibiotics, and put in the new hardware once the infection was resolved. But Ed disagreed. Dr Santos wondered if Ed's paralyzing fear of losing his leg was preventing him from fully examining the benefits and risks of the two treatment options. She understood that losing his remaining leg was out of the question for him and he considered it worth the risk of potentially developing life-threatening complications. She wondered how she could help him to make a better-informed choice. Dr Santos noted that Cathy, who usually was an active participant in Ed's office visits, had been quiet on this occasion. Cathy had refrained from sharing her opinion about the two treatment options. Regardless, Dr Santos suspected that Cathy agreed with the surgeon's opinion but did not want to challenge her husband's decision. In the past, Cathy had shared with Dr Santos that she tried, whenever possible, to foster Ed's independence and did not want to say anything to undermine the few choices he had.

Dr Santos now knew how to proceed; she would call Cathy and Ed in the morning. Since both Cathy and Ed would be deeply affected by the treatment decision, each needed to be involved. Dr Santos' goal was to help Ed and Cathy understand that the best chance for saving Ed's leg involved surgery and that together they would all work to keep Ed at home, no matter what the outcome. Dr Santos knew that she had to free Ed from his fear and that Cathy would be her ally. This was one possible pathway to finding common ground.

7 The Fourth Component: Enhancing The Patient-Doctor Relationship

Moira Stewart, Judith Belle Brown, and Thomas R Freeman

INTRODUCTION*

We ask ourselves, why are the components of patient-doctor relationships not more widely embraced? (Stewart, 2005). Perhaps, current societal values do not, on the whole, support or nurture relationships. Our Western society, on the contrary, values individual accomplishment above community; values science over art; values analysis over synthesis; and values technological solutions over wisdom. In such a context, all of us suffer diminished capacity for spirituality and love. In medicine, these societal influences tip the balance so alarmingly that we and our students almost never see the alternative to individualism, science, analysis, and technology – almost never recognize the balance that must be sought. Willis (2002) argues that "the greatest challenge facing contemporary medicine is for it to retain . . . or regain its humanity, its caritas – without losing its essential foundation in science . . . to find a middle way."

In spite of these societal influences, the patient-doctor relationship "has been the focus of attention since the beginning of Western Medicine" (Cassell, 2013: 16).

A quote from Sir William Osler in the early twentieth century illustrates this focus:

> I would urge upon you . . . to care more for the individual patient than for the special features of the disease . . . Dealing as we do with poor suffering humanity, we see the man unmasked, exposed to all the frailties and weaknesses, and you have to keep your heart soft and tender lest you have too great a contempt for your fellow creatures. The best way is to keep a looking glass in your own heart, and the more carefully you scan your own frailties, the more tender you are for those of your fellow creatures. (Cushing, 1925: 489–90)

---

* Some of the material in this chapter is adapted from Stewart's article "Reflections on the Doctor-Patient Relationship: from Evidence and Experience" (2005).

How do doctors put into practice the concepts described by Osler?

The day-to-day tasks of medicine are accomplished through the interaction of patient and clinician during a visit, the "essential unit of medical practice" (Spence, 1960). Therefore, the language of medicine is a "language of events rather than the language of an ongoing (and flowing) process" (Cassell, 2013: 20). However, "coursing like a river underneath these discrete visits, is the ongoing relationship, manifesting dimensions more enduring than the qualities of any one visit, dimensions such as trust, caring, feeling, power, and purpose" (Stewart, 2004: 388). Loxterkamp (2008), as well, has used the river as a metaphor for patient-doctor relationships.

> It may be said that I buoyed him (the patient) at his low point, helped him through rocky times – saw around a bend in the river that he, for one dark moment, could not. Together we let the river carry us, knowing it was stronger and swifter than our solitary effort to swim ashore. (2008: 3)

Medical, nursing, and psychotherapeutic literature contains references to processes that have as a goal a strong patient-clinician relationship: a working alliance, or a therapeutic alliance. The relationship requires "skills as varied as highly technical, psychologically insightful and personally empathetic" (Cassell, 2013: 19). "The primary agent of treatment is the clinician" (Cassell, 2013: 83).

COMPASSION, CARING, EMPATHY, AND TRUST

> The doctor, arriving late and already anticipating her (the doctor's) next three moves, could deflect the ambiguity of his (the patient's) averted eyes and nervous hands by writing a prescription and moving to the next room, where a strep test has already turned positive. Or she could gamble her balancing act on five unscripted minutes that could open a can of worms.
>
> At that moment of indecision, why would a patient risk self-disclosure or the doctor relinquish the safety of higher ground? Their choice often reflects a mutual leaning towards relationship: trust that here one's true self can safely emerge; reassurance that their galloping fears will be calmed through the clinician's touch, words, and familiar surroundings; companionship that ends the exile of illness and offers a promise of deliverance to some recognizable shore; some sign that there is shelter here, and restorative good will. And mindfulness of what matters most. Why do we live? What is our sacrifice for? When is there more to cherish than the time stretched between us?

> The investment of these moments, whose consequence ripples in ever widening arcs, matters as much as any lifesaving heroics. These are the moments that make life worth saving. They unveil the worth of a living thing, an intrinsic value that can never be priced or marketed or proved beyond the affirmation of a handshake or nod of thanks. (Loxterkamp, 2008: 3)

In contrast, however, not all doctors "lean towards relationship."

> Brian McDonald, a young man in his early 20s already had two visits to the family doctor and had been diagnosed with mononucleosis. After 3 weeks he became too weak to get out of bed and the doctor made a house call to the patient's home where he lived with his parents. Even before examining Brian, the doctor stated: "If I had a room like this, I'd want to stay here all the time too!"

> Anne Montgomery, a young pregnant woman, was in her eighth month when she developed signs of toxemia of pregnancy. When entering her bedroom at her home, the doctor remarked, "So you've taken to your bed already, have you?"

The lack of respect, compassion, empathy, or support reflected in these two short narratives may have negative consequences for patients' self-respect and inner resources just when patients need them most. Our self-absorption as professionals, whether it is recognized or not, can interfere with care in so many ways. Further, arrogance among physicians is unfortunately common, possibly because of the unconscious collusion between the vulnerability of the patient needing an all-powerful caregiver and the invisible hubris of the doctor. Current emphasis on technology and efficiency in medical practice provides fertile ground for this problem to grow: "This distancing of the doctor from the patient breeds a kind of 'system arrogance', in which the patient is no longer seen as a human being but simply as a job to be done cost-effectively" (Berger, 2002: 146). Speaking of the tendency of doctors to distance, McWhinney (2012) has said:

> The temptation is to avoid the patient with very good excuses, such as by giving all our attention to the physical examination or pretending to ourselves that we have no time to visit them. But the patient is usually not deceived by such ways and means, perceiving perfectly well that we are frightened to face them. We may even be tempted to abandon the patient without explanation. Yet it is essential that we continue being present to these suffering patients.
>   If we speak of suffering, we will not be tempted to distance ourselves from

the experience. Facing a patient's suffering in this way, not from behind a barrier or as an expert practicing a certain technique, but as one person to another, is perhaps our most difficult task. But there are rewards, as when we witness the joy of recovery or emergence from despair. Not being tied to a particular disease, organ system or technology makes it easier for family doctors to step out of our abstractions and open ourselves or our patients. (2012: 88)

However, doctors may be mistaken if they think that compassionate care is more difficult and more taxing. On the contrary, sometimes our difficulty is that we fail to understand that what the patient wants is something very simple: a recognition of his or her suffering, or perhaps only our presence at a time of need, "dwelling for a moment in their pain, in their misery, not letting it float off our backs" (Scott, 2008: 318).

For generations, medical students have been taught: "don't get involved." In the conventional clinical method, the doctor is assumed to be a detached observer and prescriber of treatment. Remaining uninvolved may protect doctors from some very disturbing things, especially as they encounter the depth of a patient's suffering. However, it also has a personal price. To remain uninvolved, physicians have to build up protective shells to suppress their feelings. This lack of openness creates difficulties in relationships, not only with patients but also with colleagues. To suggest that one can remain uninvolved is also a fallacy. One cannot help being affected in some way by the encounter with suffering, even if the result is avoidance and denial.

While this book advocates for more emotional involvement of the clinician with the patient than is the case in conventional medicine, there has recently arisen the notion that too much emotional involvement can place unhealthy demands on the professional, resulting in compassion fatigue (Abendroth & Flannery, 2006). Nonetheless, the emotional element is considered part of the definition of compassion (Uygur et al., 2012; Blane & Mercer, 2011) in addition to identifying, acknowledging, and acting on suffering.

In contrast, empathy can be seen as a "necessary pre-requisite for compassion" (Blane & Mercer, 2011: 19) and, although empathy draws on a history of feeling, it has recently been defined cognitively and behaviorally as understanding the patient's situation, communicating that understanding, and acting on it in a helpful way (Mercer & Reynolds, 2002; Rudebeck, 2002).

Enid Balint and colleagues (1993) point out that for doctors it is important to move back and forth from objective observation to empathetic identification, in the same sort of weaving back and forth that we recommended in Chapter 3 and which we replicate here in Figure 7.1 (Virshup et al., 1999).

However, what is too often forgotten, with this sort of dichotomous thinking, is the injunction to integrate the elements. Cassell (2013) reminds us of the seminal quote from Feinstein (1967) that the work of a doctor requires the "oscillating" recommended by Balint but also, after that, "not just a conjunction but a true synthesis of art and science, fusing the parts into a whole" (Cassell, 2013: 81; Feinstein, 1967).

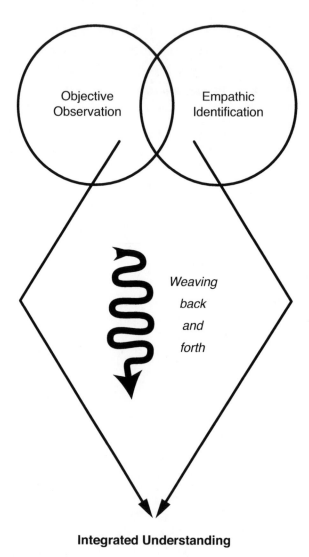

FIGURE 7.1 Connecting with patients

The following story, recounted by McWhinney (1997a: 6), illustrates this multifaceted connection.

I have never forgotten a brief experience I had as a medical student. When at home (during school holidays) I used to do rounds with the surgeon at the local hospital. After the round (one day), he was asked to see an old vagrant who was complaining of abdominal pain. The experience made a deep and lasting impression on me. The patient was exactly as one would have expected; his face red and blotchy; several days' growth of beard on his chin. For those few minutes, this old vagrant seemed to be the most important person in the world for the doctor. All his attention was focused on the old man, whom he treated with the utmost respect – a respect that showed in the way he talked and listened and the way he examined him. The word that perhaps describes it best is presence; for those few minutes the doctor was a real presence in the patient's life.

Selwyn (2008: 79) eloquently reflects on a career of almost sacred presence.

Each time I sit with a patient, it is as if everything in both of our lives has brought us to this exact moment, which can be an opportunity for the mundane or, at times, the almost sacred. Sometimes we connect only briefly, or perhaps miss each other's meaning, and continue superficially through our daily routine. But sometimes, when a certain question, phrase, or gesture opens a door, we may have a glimpse into a whole new room that is suddenly open to light and understanding. Like a glance in a crowd between strangers, sometimes everything aligns, the extraneous is stripped away, and we can look deeply into someone's soul. Random yet precise, a series of interactions, of fleeting moments that occasionally verge on timelessness. These moments can't be forced or created; the best we can do is to learn to witness, patiently, with humility, and not let ourselves or our judgments get in the way of the process – to learn to be present, attentive, and open to the story that is waiting to be told.

Perhaps the kernel of the caring relationship from the patient's point of view is trust. Breast cancer patients have difficulty understanding the vast amounts of information they need to assimilate before treatment decisions can be made, especially in their understandable state of anxiety and fear. Women with breast cancer say that they cannot make sense of all the facts and figures regarding options, unless they work with a trusted physician (McWilliam *et al.*, 1997). Trust takes time to develop in a working relationship based on respect. Trusting relationships, therefore, require personal continuity (Mercer, 2012). The sources of trust in medical practice include a just society, moral integrity, continuity of care, sharing power, compassion, authenticity, and competence

(Fugelli, 2001). "Trust is an individual's belief that the sincerity, benevolence, and truthfulness of others can be relied on. Trust often implies a transference of power, to a person or to a system, to act on one's behalf, in one's best interest" (2001: 575).

POWER IN THE PATIENT-DOCTOR RELATIONSHIP

Case Example

Janet Sutherland, a health care worker in her late thirties, recently broke her arm in a car accident. Her world was shattered, as were the bones in her arm. For 10 weeks she was unable to care for her two preschool children, or drive the car, or work. By this time, her confidence in herself was deteriorating because she felt responsible, not only for the accident but also for the fact that her bones were not healing as quickly as expected. Moreover, the confidence and trust in the family doctor were also waning, because the decisions they made together (regarding the type of surgeon she would be referred to, the type of anesthetic she would receive, and the type of follow-up care) were never realized. The information about the surgery too was conflicting. Janet expressed these fears, "Why was nothing as it should be? Why was I not recovering? Was something being hidden? Why can't I get better – I need to get better!"

The central issues of lack of control over the recovery and over the health care created a sense of powerlessness. As angry as Janet became at herself, she was doubly angry at the doctors, including the family doctor. The ebbing trust and the increasing powerlessness united in a crisis of care. It took weeks of work on the part of this patient to gain insight into her own issues. It took a new willingness on the part of all the physicians, to listen and to solve problems mutually with the patient, before both the healing of the person and the healing of the bones became evident.

Much has been made of power and control in the patient-doctor relationship in the literature in the past 30 years, culminating in a surge of interest in shared decision making (Elwyn *et al.*, 2012; Stiggelbout *et al.*, 2012). There is no doubt that the relationship that is the foundation for patient-centered care, compared with the conventional patient-doctor relationship, demands a sharing of power and control between the doctor and the patient. Shared decision-making approaches are similar but not identical to Component 3, Finding Common Ground, described in Chapter 6. The quality of a relationship within which finding common ground is possible includes a readiness of doctor and patient to become partners in care. Their encounters are truly meetings between experts (Tuckett *et al.*, 1985). However, each partnership is unique and may include permutations and combinations employing varying degrees of control along many dimensions and changing over time. One example would be the adolescent, who needs information (from the expert doctor) but who also maintains control of management (envisioning herself as expert on her life) because she yearns to be treated as an adult, but at the same time she needs guidance. An ability on the part of the doctor to remain open and alert to these shifting needs for control is an essential aspect of an ongoing partnership.

Scott and colleagues (2008) found that physicians were able to eloquently describe these shifts. One physician noted "an intuitive understanding about when and how to push patients based on assessments of patients' needs and strength of relationships." Another said "sometimes you're a coach and sometimes you're the boss and sometimes you're the sibling and sometimes you're the doctor" (Scott *et al.*, 2008: 318).

The resulting therapeutic alliance is related in complex ways to the healing of patients suffering the loss of their central purpose – that is, sense of control over themselves and their world, or loss of control of their life. We will see later in this chapter a connection between healing and key dimensions of wellness, health, and wholeness aligning this discussion with the health promotion role of clinicians. This connection between the dimensions of trust in the therapeutic alliance, the taking and giving of control, and regaining a central purpose in life is best illustrated in the following qualitative longitudinal study. Bartz (1999) characterized the evolution of relationships of nine Aboriginal diabetic patients with one physician over time, using terms such as disease-focus, misunderstandings, mistrust, detachment, and hopelessness.

> To control the environment, the doctor adopted various strategies that constrained the interactions, including use of a diabetic protocol form and a medicalized way of knowing patients. Paradoxically, these strategies produced varying degrees of mistrust, clinical nihilism, interpersonal distance, and loss of control in relationships with these patients. (Bartz, 1993)

One sees the negative implications of continued attempts to exert medical control.

Another alternative in situations of misunderstanding and mistrust may be consciously to share power, to move away from medical conversation, and to be curious about the patients' beliefs and the meaning of the situation to the patient (Charon, 2006).

> By facilitating the telling of their life-stories over time, doctors share with their patients the process whereby they reconstruct themselves through the experience of their suffering. In sharing this, doctors are also open to change, experiencing their own vulnerability and powerlessness . . . (an acknowledgement of which) may be one of the most powerful things doctors do to facilitate healing in patients, . . . the strength borne from the awareness of shared weakness. (Goodyear-Smith & Buetow, 2001: 457)

Case Example

Mrs Patrick was an elderly woman who had arthritis, irritable bowel syndrome, and a cancer of the breast 6 years ago. The doctor, in his late thirties, had been Mrs Patrick's family physician for the past year. This insightful patient and doctor found a way to accommodate her seemingly contradictory needs. On the one hand, her advanced age and physical problems left her insecure enough to require explicit reassurance. The doctor provided the reassurance after appropriate questioning and physical examination and by exploring the nature of her symptoms. On the other hand, she needed to maintain control over some aspects of her life and health; this manifested itself in her controlling the choice and the order of topics during the encounter with her family doctor. She was one of those patients who brought in a written list of her complaints. Although this family physician thoughtfully interpreted her behavior, other doctors might have been offended by her somewhat bossy manner and might have failed to see it as an important coping mechanism.

CONTINUITY AND CONSTANCY

Continuity of care is longitudinal care delivered over time within the context of a long-term relationship between patient and physician. Personal continuity is necessary for a healing relationship (Blane & Mercer, 2011). Herbert (2013: 63) described the power of continuing relationships in this way:

> Often it is the privilege of a longitudinal relationship that allows us to hear from our patients the whole story – the untold story. I have written about my patient who told me her story about being abused as a child only after she had

been my patient for many years. When I asked her why she had not told me sooner – because I had asked many times – she explained that early on she could not disclose, even when I asked in a gently and caring way, because she did not know if she could trust me. Then later, she said, she was afraid that if she told me, I would be disappointed and disgusted, and maybe withdraw from her, so she held back some more.

Continuity of relationships has been shown to accrue many benefits (Freeman, 2012). Nonetheless, in all medical disciplines and in most Western countries, policy decisions have resulted in marked disruptions in continuity of care.

Not only does the system put barriers in the way of continuity of care but also physicians themselves consciously or unconsciously close doors, or at worst abandon patients. Nonetheless, it remains the doctor's responsibility to be constant in his or her commitment to the well-being of the patient. The required commitment is not easily achieved, because the doctor may experience feelings of failure and have to encounter a patient's anger or other expressions of mistrust. Cassell (1991: 78) describes constancy in the following way:

> Constancy to the patient is necessary. Constant attention and maintained presence are not difficult when things are going well. It requires self-discipline to maintain constancy when the case is going sour, when errors or failures have occurred, when the wrong diagnosis has been made, when the patient's personality or behaviour is difficult or even repulsive, when impending death brings the danger of sorrow and loss because emotional closeness has been established. When constancy is absent or falters, too frequently, patients lose that newfound part of themselves – the doctor – that promised stability in the uncertain world of sickness arising from their relationship.

HEALING AND HOPE

The most important aspect of healing the suffering patient is "understanding suffering" (Cassell, 2013). Healers must bridge between the world of the sufferer and the well world. To begin to do this, the clinician must understand that "all suffering is unique and individual" (attend to the particulars of each patient); "suffering involves self conflict" (understand that the patient simultaneously fears rejection from his or her family while craving acceptance); "suffering is marked by loss of central purpose" (attend to the person that was before the illness so that all hope is not lost in "the redirection of purpose" solely to the medical needs such as pain relief); "all suffering is lonely" (understand that the ill experience "social deprivation and isolation even in the midst of others"). A clinician might ask, "What is there in all this that you find particularly distressing?" "Ask your questions and then be quiet and wait for the answers – and be patient" (quotes are from Cassell, 2013: 225–6).

Stein (2007: 163) too writes about the

> distance across the chasm that opens between the ill and the healthy. What patients trust about me – or any doctor – is the ability to understand that the moment they become ill they are apart, different, separate from the healthy, that relationships have changed and will change again, that life is cruel.

He enjoins doctors to welcome the revelation.

> The revelation of terror is an admission that disruption and incoherence now rule, and it is a disclosure made to a relative stranger, your doctor, who you can only hope will welcome such honesty. But such a revelation assumes your doctor can and will understand your admission in all its shadings, its context and weight. (2007: 77)

He stresses the revelation's importance:

> Doctors hold the world in place for patients . . . establish the legitimacy of their claims. We offer human contact and concern. The best we can do as doctors is to turn ourselves into a reflection of our patients' pain. The doctor's job is to make pain shareable. The impossibility of sharing . . . the pain is . . . a contributing factor in its essential horror. (2007: 53)

One patient's perspective is to encourage a courageous stance by the clinician. He, the patient, wishes clinicians would welcome uncomfortable disclosures: "I have never heard an ill person praised for how well she expressed fear or grief or was openly sad" (Arthur Frank, quoted in Stein, 2007: 139). Perhaps, our society in general needs to be more accepting of expressions of sadness. Has anyone ever said to you: "I love you for your tears"?

Stein (2007: 93) describes another courageous moment for both the patient and the clinician.

> "What if I survive and my brain does not?" I responded with chances and odds so small they were impossible to summon or calculate. We went over it again and again. I could see his mind buckle and flex, assert and cringe. But by

asking questions, patients feel less powerless, and by answering them, doctors try to alleviate terror. I know there is no drastic remedy for terror, but what patients want and need badly is, as Reynolds Price wrote, "the frank exchange of decent concern." I try never to turn away from conversation. I give looks of mild encouragement. I offer words, nothing altogether convincing, but at least amulets of hope.

If offered in an emotionally connected way, such attention and conversation is experienced by the patient as consolation and comfort; it makes the suffering more bearable and it marks a transition to a more hopeful place (Scott *et al.*, 2008; Frank, 2004). "If therapeutic relationships possess a certain unquantifiable magic, it is the magic of hope . . . Hope hinges on the presence of another and the reassurance that yes, we are knowable" (Loxterkamp, 2008: 2575).

In an ongoing patient-clinician relationship the process of healing has been described as following certain paths. For a group of patients who suffered alcoholism and/or suicide attempts but survived, the steps in their healing relationships were listening, trust, willingness to change, acquisition of life skills, and control (Seifert, 1992). For a group of chronically ill older persons, the process, akin to health promotion, included trust, connecting, caring, mutual knowledge, and mutual caring (McWilliam *et al.*, 1997). One sees a synergistic benefit to both patient and clinician in these accounts of healing.

SELF-AWARENESS AND PRACTICAL WISDOM

It would not be surprising to find that clinicians working in our instrumental society (and in health care systems much more prone to rules and accountabilities than a decade ago), feel a little embattled, perhaps running against the predominant current. Cassell (2013), as well as Kinsella and Pitman (2012), express their alarm and quickly suggest solutions highly relevant to this book. The question becomes: "To what extent can the capacity to disengage from . . . an overactive mind, contribute to how practitioners might reframe the problems of practice and discern wise action in practice?" (Kinsella, 2012: 43).

Cassell (2013) described a key dilemma for a clinician – that is, when a clinician is meeting a patient he or she doesn't "like." He tries to reframe the mindset from "I don't like, to introspection" or what was it "about that patient that got to you?" (2013: 110). In order to answer such a question, or even to ask such a question, one needs time to reflect. As well, "this requires paying attention to your own words, mannerisms and presentation to the patient," and for this, one needs "the skill of a quiet mind" (2013: 111).

A similar dilemma and reflection was presented by Miksanek (2008), whose paper described a series of "difficult" patients – they were difficult in that they did not permit him to practice in a manner approved by the rule-oriented health care system. Frank (2012), in reviewing and applauding the clinician (Miksanek), noted that, although discouraged, the clinician was courageous in showing constancy and ongoing commitment to these patients. Furthermore, the clinician also took time to reflect on the dissonance arising from the fact that his practice was out of step with the current system's expectations.

In the face of such anomalies how can a professional react? We offer two themes in response to this question: mindfulness and practical wisdom.

Scott *et al.*'s (2008) study of healing revealed that

> Mindfulness, a constant awareness of the encounter at multiple levels . . .

> Is this a story of shame and they need you to listen? Is this a story of fear and they need you to be there with them? Is this a story of blame . . . or self-blame and they need to hear that it wasn't their fault? I mean, what is the story? So what role do they need you to be in? (2008: 319)

To hear the story, the clinician is advised to remain silent while at the same time giving attention, maintaining a stable focus and having clarity (unbiased perception) (Back *et al.*, 2009). It is recommended that this "receptive stance holds back . . . analytic thinking, in favour of a more contemplative process, in which the mind acts more like a receptor, receiving ideas images and feelings and being moved by them" (Kinsella, 2012: 41).

Whatever the source, self-awareness and self-knowledge are as imperative to current practice as they were decades ago. As Howard Stein (1985a) observed, "one can truly recognize a patient only if one is willing to recognize oneself in the patient." McWhinney (1989b: 82) had a similar message: "We cannot begin to know others until we know ourselves. We cannot grow and change as physicians until we have removed our defences and faced up to our shortcomings."

TRANSFERENCE AND COUNTERTRANSFERENCE

All human relationships – and in particular, therapeutic relationships – are influenced by the phenomena of transference and countertransference. Thus any discussion of the patient-clinician relationship that excluded these important psychological processes would be remiss. We do not intend to provide the reader with a detailed examination of transference and countertransference, but, rather, with a brief description. We feel that this is essential in order to define the parameters in which many of the dimensions (i.e., compassion, power, constancy, healing, and self-awareness) of the patient-doctor relationship frequently occur.

Transference is a ubiquitous phenomenon that is pervasive in our daily lives and happens outside of our conscious awareness (Schaeffer, 2007; Murdin, 2010; Berman & Bezkor, 2010). Transference is a process whereby the patient unconsciously projects, onto individuals in his or her current life, thoughts, behaviors, and emotional reactions that originate with other significant relationships from childhood onward (Schaeffer, 2007; Murdin, 2010). In other words, past experiences that an individual has held in his or her unconscious are projected "onto a new experience, acting like a kind of colored filter which changes the appearance of the experience" (Murdin, 2010: 9). This can include feelings of love, hate, ambivalence, and dependency. The greater the current attachment, such as a significant patient-clinician relationship, the more likely that transference will occur. Transference, while often perceived as a negative phenomenon, actually helps build the connection between patient and practitioner. Frequently, clinicians are intimidated by the concept of transference, which has its roots in psychoanalytic theory, viewing it as something mysterious and to be avoided. As Goldberg (2000: 116) notes, "Many physicians intuitively and successfully use positive transference manifestations without necessarily being aware of them, negative, hostile transference manifestations in the patient may be more problematic." However, knowledge of the patient's transference reaction, either positive or negative, assists the clinician in understanding how the patient experiences his or her world and how past relationships influence current behavior.

Transference can occur during any stage of the patient-clinician relationship and be activated by any number of events. For example, when the capabilities of seriously ill patients are impaired or when patients are overwhelmed by the ramifications implied by a specific diagnosis, they may respond to their clinician in an uncharacteristic manner. They may return to a position of dependency and neediness, which is more a reflection of unresolved past relationships than of their current relationship with the clinician. During this time of crisis, patients may seek the care and comfort that was absent in the past. Conversely, they may respond by becoming distant and aloof, indicating the return to a stoical stance adopted in their early years when they were forced to assume a position of pseudo-independence and self-sufficiency. Take, for example, the story presented in Chapter 4 of Isabel, whose early years were plagued by disappointment and abandonment. Would her transference reaction be one of hostility and distancing behavior toward the clinician to avoid rejection again? Conversely, would Isabel exhibit a positive transference in response to the trust, empathy, and caring she experiences in the relationship with her clinician? Indeed, her transference reactions may fluctuate depending on her degree of vulnerability and sense of safety in the therapeutic relationship.

A clinician's inadvertent failure to respond to a patient's need or request may evoke unwarranted anger or hostility. Again it is imperative to understand the genesis of the patient's response, which may originate from years of feeling misunderstood and uncared for. Exploration of patient's transference provides explanation and prediction. Furthermore, understanding the patient's transference reactions enhances the clinician's capacity for caring and can provide an emotionally corrective experience.

Like transference, countertransference is an unconscious process that occurs when the clinician responds to patients in a manner similar to significant past relationships (Schaeffer, 2007; Murdin, 2010; Hayes *et al.*, 2011; Jiménez & Thorkelson, 2012). Practitioners need to be alert to what triggers certain reactions – that is, unresolved personal issues, stress, or value conflicts. It is here that self-awareness, coupled with the ability for self-observation during the consultation, is paramount.

Sometimes countertransference is illuminated in the moment of the patient-doctor encounter and can enhance the empathetic connection. On other occasions it is more elusive, lodged in the clinician's unconscious, but ultimately revealed, as Oldham (2012) describes:

> All of us have memory moments that seem indelible – scenes from our professional lives that are easily recalled and linked to strong emotions, either pleasurable or painful . . . The woman I remember in particular was in severe congestive heart failure. Even sitting up, her breathing was labored, and she had severe dependent edema. She looked at us with a pleading and desperate expression, saying very little since it made her short of breath to talk. She was told that things looked about the same and that the team would check on her again the next day. After leaving the room, we were told, in short, that she was dying and that nothing more could be done. This was one of my first really hard lessons in medicine, and the image of her struggling either to live a while longer, or entreating us to end her misery (I couldn't tell which) has never left me. It never occurred to me until much later that the intensity of my reaction to this patient was related to the fact that my father was at the time, slowly dying of cancer.

Internal manifestations of countertransference are reflected in the practitioner's emotional responses, such as anger, sadness, boredom, anxiety, fear, arousal, envy, and gladness (Schaeffer, 2007; Murdin, 2010; Hayes *et al.*, 2011); whereas, behavioral or external manifestations of countertransference include not listening attentively, interpreting too soon, misjudging the patient's level of feeling, becoming too active in giving advice, becoming overly identified with the patient's problem, gaining vicarious pleasure in the patient's story, engaging in power struggles with the patient, running late, running overtime, or covering the same material with the patient over and over (Schaeffer, 2007; Murdin, 2010).

The origins and significance of practitioners' countertransference are as varied and complex as their patients. As noted earlier, we all struggle with unresolved issues from our past. For example, the clinician who finds himself repeatedly giving advice to depressed female patients may be attempting to rescue the patient from her sorrow in a way similar to how he responded to his own mother's chronic angst. The constant inability to listen to a patient's painful story of failed relationships may relate to parallel experiences in the clinician's own life. The demanding and obstinate behaviors of a patient may in turn activate behaviors on the part of the physician such as running late, avoidance, or engaging in power struggles, all responses that may have been characteristic of the doctor's relationship with her domineering father.

Almost 30 years ago, Stein (1985b: xii) observed "how rarely the issue of physician countertransference was addressed in medical school, residency training, or continuing education." Unfortunately, this remains the case today, as recently reported by Jiménez and Thorkelson (2012), and it is perhaps reinforced by the lingering belief that some countertransference reactions are "shameful and unprofessional" (Schaeffer, 2007: 74). While historically, countertransference was perceived as a negative phenomenon that needed to be "managed" and at best eradicated, more recent conceptualizations of countertransference indicate how clinicians' successful understanding of their countertransference reactions can assist them in both understanding their patients and the therapeutic relationship (Hayes *et al.*, 2011; Schaeffer, 2007). Schaeffer (2007: 28) writes: "Countertransference opens the door to 'a slice of life': the client's life, the therapist's own life, and the life that client and therapist share in the therapeutic process."

The primary tool for effectively using transference and countertransference to aid and deepen the patient-clinician relationship is self-awareness. Such self-knowledge is a requirement for the doctor's accurate recognition of both transference and countertransference. Self-evaluation and working with others may help practitioners gain valuable insights which will ultimately strengthen relationships with patients and also increase their own comfort and satisfaction in their provision of care (Goldberg, 2000).

Case Example

"Why is this woman so frustrating?" Dr Fournier blurted out loud! Alone in her car she felt embarrassed, but at the same time relieved by her outburst. After leaving her home visit with Mrs Cirenski, she felt exasperated and unsure about how to best move forward in the care of her 85-year-old patient. Following the persistent requests of Mrs Cirenski's son, also a patient of Dr Fournier's, she had accepted this elderly woman into her practice just over a year ago.

From the beginning the situation had been challenging. Mrs Cirenski had multiple chronic conditions, including congestive heart failure, chronic obstructive pulmonary disease, diabetes, and arthritis. In the past few months there had been several admissions to hospital – now she was once again at home. It had taken some time to untangle Mrs Cirenski's complex medical problems, and for the most part Dr Fournier had felt as if she had been lurching from one health crisis to the next. Just when Dr Fournier thought her patient's health had stabilized and the appropriate treatment regimens were in place, the bottom fell out again. Mrs Cirneski was diagnosed with a recurrence of her breast cancer – she was riddled with metastases.

As Mrs Cirneski rapidly declined, office visits evolved into home visits. However, these too were often chaotic and difficult to navigate. Her little bungalow was often crowded with neighbors and friends who had come to sit with Mrs Cirneski and bring her plate after plate of her native food. Frequently, one or more of her 11 grandchildren would be at their grandmother's bedside, brushing her hair or poring over photo albums that bore witness to Mrs Cirneski's life and family. On one hand Dr Fournier deeply appreciated the outpouring of support being showered on her patient; on the other hand, trying to "doctor" in this utter confusion unsettled her.

Dr Fournier was baffled by her emotional response to this warm and well-loved woman. No other patient in her practice elicited similar distress. As Dr Fournier pulled into the office parking lot she resolved to discuss her concerns and confusion about her patient with a colleague. Late that day, following a busy afternoon treating coughs and colds, fevers and rashes, muscle sprains and headaches, Dr Fournier shared her struggles with one of her partners.

As Dr Fournier began to recount her story of caring for Mrs Cirneski her eyes welled up with tears and her heart began to ache. Initially taken aback by this uncharacteristic emotional response, it dawned on Dr Fournier how Mrs Cirneski's life had many parallels to her own Grandmamma.

Like her patient, Mrs Fournier's grandmother had emigrated from her homeland, married, raised a large boisterous family, and been a pillar in her community, overcoming many language and cultural hurdles. Her grandmother had also suffered from many health issues, similar to Mrs Cirneski. However, the startling revelation, as Dr Fournier's story tumbled out, was how she had been abroad at the time of her Grandmamma's final illness and eventual death. Dr Fournier had not returned home for her grandmother's funeral – a decision she had always regretted.

Through her tears and muffled sobs, Dr Fournier began to understand the emotional challenges she faced in caring for this woman who very much resembled her beloved Grandmamma. This insight offered Dr Fournier a deeper appreciation of how she could truly care for her patient and be with her until the end – amidst all the joyful chaos.

CONCLUSION

The interactive components of the patient-centered clinical method occur within the ongoing relationship. The relationship serves the integrating function and is accomplished through a sustained partnership with a patient that includes compassion, caring, empathy, trust, sharing power, continuity, constancy, healing, and hope.

The following two narratives describe the evolution of the patient-doctor relationship and, while they are remarkably different, both stories share common elements: trust, constancy, caring, and healing. This first case illustrates a young doctor learning about healing from firsthand experience.

When We First Saw Eye to Eye: Case Illustrating Component 4
Clarissa Burke

In my first month of clerkship, I was on call overnight for the internal medicine service. I was summoned to the emergency department to assess a 70-year-old lady with severe back pain and a history of general decline in the weeks prior to her admission. I remember hearing those words, "in decline," and wondering what that meant. Was she mentally declining? Physically? Was she even at that moment dying in the emergency department? Would I be able to handle such a situation?

To my relief, upon arriving at her bedside, I was met by a lovely lady, whose pleasant demeanor and smiling face put me at ease immediately. Ah, what a pleasure! No stricken face, no cries of pain, none of those terrifying situations that I feared my still tender sensibilities would be stretched to handle. As I went about my business of gathering information about this lady – her age, her medications, her past medical history – I learned that she had been through chemotherapy for breast cancer 2 years earlier. "This couldn't be a recurrence of the cancer?" she asked. The emergency room physician had suggested that the back pain may be due to metastatic disease, but further imaging was yet to be done. I tried to reassure her, and to my own eyes, she appeared so well that it seemed improbable. Yes, she had back pain, and she had been losing weight, but surely there could be other reasons?

Unfortunately, those reasons were not to be. The next 2 days revealed that her breast cancer had returned, and had spread to her spine, causing a painful compression fracture. She would remain in hospital under the care of the internal medicine team and receive radiation therapy to reduce the activity of the cancer. Despite this news, her outlook remained positive. We developed an upbeat rapport, and I looked forward to seeing her every day. We would greet each other with cheerful hellos, and she would update me on how well she had eaten. I came to know her daughter, who visited nearly every day, and learned about her two grandchildren, who were her greatest pride. For the following week I remained as her primary contact with the internal medicine team, and I would happily report back to the team about her improving pain control and weight gain. This must be what practicing medicine is like, I reflected, she has a serious illness and we are helping her to get better and go home.

As another week went by, her progress seemed to stall. Every day her pain would break through a little more, and there was discussion of trying a round of chemotherapy. And, as her appetite dropped down again, neither of us seemed willing to admit it. I started to feel some dread when approaching her room. What would I see when I arrived? Would she continue to be headed in the right direction? Or would I be forced to notice that her energy was less and less? That the nightgowns her daughter had brought from home were swallowing her already small frame? And what could I possibly offer if the medicines we prescribed and the treatments she had received were failing?

No matter the signs that this discussion was coming, when my staff physician proposed that we should consider a palliative care consultation, it felt like a physical blow. No, I thought, this can't be. Isn't she still too well to be dying? But when the team gathered at her bedside for a family meeting and I saw the changes that had come over her, and the uneaten tray of food at her bedside, and when my eyes met hers, eye to eye . . . I knew in that moment that we would both have to be more honest with each other. I would have to accept that I wasn't going to "cure" her. And, for her part, I think it was a relief that she would no longer have to pretend that everything was going well.

Our final week together was bittersweet. If our conversations lacked some of their original spunk, they more than made up for it in her ability to express her pain, and my chance to support her during those moments. As her strength faded, I realized that my own was much greater than I had imagined. I couldn't offer her a cure, but I could be there to hold her hand as she expressed her fears of the end. I could answer her questions when she couldn't recall what her oncologist had planned. I could help her make the decision to stop having meal trays sent up – and we could even laugh together when she admitted that she had been hiding food to make it seem like she had been eating well.

I will never forget one of our final conversations. "Do you have a man in your life?" she asked. When I told her that I did, she settled back in her bed and looked thoughtful for a time. "I had a good man," she said, "and every day since he's been gone, I've missed him. So you hold on tight to your man, and love him, and be happy."

Such simple words. Said with all the weight of her lifetime of experiences. Experiences of love, of joy, of sorrow, and, finally, of peace. My throat tightened, and I saw an answering sheen of tears in her own eyes. All I could do was reassure her that I would never forget her words. How to tell her how much she had meant to me? How to tell her that she was the first person with whom I walked the road to accepting death? How to thank her for the privilege of sharing the end of her life?

Twenty-four hours later she ceased to respond to anything outside of herself, and her breathing became more shallow. It was the last day of my rotation, and my final stop on the ward was to her bedside.

Thank you, I thought. Thank you for sharing your strength when I needed it, and taking mine when it was offered.

The Flag for Undefined Pain: Case Illustrating Component 4
Gina Higgins

Sun filtering through the closed window blinds fell on perfectly coifed chocolate hair, giving it a deceptive sheen and surreptitiously lent the crisp white blouse a warmth that was meant to be suppressed. Tight, fine lines around her mouth, features held in a poker mask, and cheeks like parchment pulled tight despite the age of 35 listed on her file suggested her life had been eventful. There is a purported Chinese curse: "May you live in interesting times." A hunted, hunting look to her sharp features suggested she had experienced more interesting times than many.

"How are you today?" I asked automatically, while taking in the coil of well-controlled tension that was the lady before me. I had never met her before that visit, but I already knew something about her. I knew she was not "fine, thank you."

We danced through the medical history – negative. Medications – none. Surgical history – nil. Social history – well . . . social history was a wall of reticence. I learned about this lady through her answers that weren't and monosyllables with a tight nod or barely discernible grimace attached.

35-year-old female. No know medical history. No surgical history. No family history known. No allergies. No medications. Married, husband is an engineer. She is a stay-at-home mother of two children – aged 5 and 8. Smoker, about one pack a day, no alcohol. Daily walking up to 1–2 hours. That was the extent of the initial visit. We made the usual agreement to come back in a couple weeks for a long-overdue pap and general physical.

There is a sign I use in my charts as an indicator just for myself. It flags patients that I think are in some sort of undefined pain, generally psychiatric but not always, but I didn't yet know what it was. Another physician seeing it wouldn't take note of the sign. She warranted it.

Emily didn't come in again for a few months. When she did, it wasn't for a pap. Actually, it wasn't for anything in particular as far as I could tell. She asked to have her blood pressure checked, but had no reason for the request. I asked if there was anything else concerning her. There wasn't. I had seen the sign in the chart, but by then she would have gotten flagged again in any case.

On the third visit, she presented as before, perfectly pressed and tailored, hair and nails buffed, colored, painted. Prada handbag. Steve Madden shoes. Expression protected and held close – not blank but each reaction carefully doled out if she felt it was appropriate, to the appropriate degree. She wanted some lab work done, as she had been feeling fatigued. Review of systems was almost negative, except that she got dizzy when she stood up. I pressed. She spoke.

Granite can stand in the elements for a long time, but even granite will weather with a strong enough, and constant enough, onslaught. Sometimes granite is erected only to stand as a reef to protect sandstone.

Emily was washing away like sandstone.

Her story was told over several meetings, and punctuated by her gestures, her bearing, and very occasionally her tears.

Emily has an eating disorder. Borne in the eye of the hurricane of her life, fed by her inborn and inbred tendencies toward perfectionism and obsession, unable to control anything else, she controlled herself. Eventually, like an alcoholic or addict, she lost the ability to control her control. Instead of basking in the admiration of her friends for her petite figure, she had pushed her friends away in favor of exercise and reading cookbooks. Instead of spending time with her husband, she made excuses to go for a walk or lie in bed alone, staring at the ceiling while the waves of self-loathing crashed over her unrelentingly. She knew she was too thin, and not thin enough. She trusted no one; too many people in her past had taken the trust she offered like a fragile baby bird and crushed it underfoot. She had a tremendous capacity to love, and yet was so sick she couldn't feel even the love she had always had for her children as more than a distant guilty painful echo of a once familiar emotion.

Every waking moment, Emily suffered. She suffered alone while with her family and while with her friends, who now saw only the shell of Emily that she allowed them to, with all the substance bundled tight inside. It took weeks for her to begin to believe that she had something that wasn't her fault, that was treatable; that she deserved to be treated; that suicide wasn't the only way out for her. That day was one of the few times I witnessed her tears. Sometimes, tears can be oddly reassuring. If life can be lamented, at least it is being embraced.

Now, months into our relationship, Emily is medically stable and has gained some weight. This was not easy for her, and to say she had no setbacks would be the baldest of lies. She told me a couple of times she was having no setbacks. Pulsing like the tides between improvements and stumbles, she somehow found the energy and verve to struggle her way back to join the ranks of humanity, with all the messy, sticky emotions attached. She can now tell me about her feelings of loss. I remember how difficult it was for her to admit how she missed her eating disorder. Until she said this out loud, she had been consumed with disgust at herself for feeling this. Every time she told me about the secrets she had kept as little self-torture devices, she freed herself a little more.

There was something that Emily said once that really stuck with me. It was something that I don't think she really believed when she said it – just one of those expected phrases that get trotted out for the right occasion. She said, "I guess everything happens for a reason." I'm not sure about that, but it is undeniable that everything that happens to us through life, no matter how miserable that experience is, has the potential to do some good. Emily now appreciates the time she can spend with her children, and is enjoying that time again instead of dreading it and hating herself for being selfish and distracted (as she perceived it). She is considering leaving her husband, but I think this will be a while coming to fruition if it does at all. At least Emily is facing her problems now.

I pressed. She spoke. She told me about the most intimate version of hell she had ever glimpsed, and together we took her back toward the land of the living. She will be a long time before she will really be well.

"I understand what you must be going through. Tell me about it."

She did.

PART THREE

Learning and Teaching the Patient-Centered Clinical Method

Introduction

Judith Belle Brown and W Wayne Weston

In this part of the book, we examine how to learn about and teach the patient-centered clinical method, often illustrating this with relevant case examples. Chapter 8 explores the theoretical concepts that underlie the human dimensions of learning, with a specific view to the patient-centered clinical method. Chapter 9 explores the parallel process between being patient- and learner-centered, with a matching of each of the four components. Chapter 10 addresses some of the challenges confronted by both learners and teachers. This then leads to two chapters describing some basic and essential elements required to teach the patient-centered clinical method: Chapter 11 on practical tips and Chapter 12 on the patient-centered case report.

8 Becoming a Physician: the Human Experience of Medical Education

W Wayne Weston and Judith Belle Brown

Sir Luke Fildes'* iconic painting, *The Doctor*, shows a physician at the bedside of a seriously ill child with her distraught parents despairing in the dark shadows in the background. It depicts a mythological image of the country doctor waging war against disease single-handed, with no tools but what can be carried in the doctor's bag (Barilan, 2007; Moore, 2008; Verghese, 2008). It is a popular image of caring and compassion that appeals to our longing for a healer – a physician who will be there even when there is no cure. In her paper describing the lessons the painting can teach physicians today, Jane Moore (2008: 213) states: "Most importantly, Fildes' timeless painting, *The Doctor*, reminds contemporary doctors of the crucial importance of the relationship between a patient and the doctor and the value of a patient-centred approach."

However, there is another way to see this picture – through the eyes of a young physician. What does he or she see? A doctor, without a laboratory or CT scan to confirm the diagnosis; no drugs to cure the problem; impotent to alter the natural course of the disease; and no one to refer the patient to. It is a terrifying prospect for many graduates who avoid moving to small communities where they fear they might face situations such as this.

This is ironic because, even in large medical centers, physicians frequently confront the limits of medicine (Hewa & Hetherington, 1995; Hadler, 2008; Markle & McCrea, 2008). Ingelfinger (1980), former editor of the *New England Journal of Medicine*, stated that 90% of the time, when a patient consults a doctor, the patient's condition is either self-limited or there is no treatment that will alter the natural history of the disease. Engel (1977) highlighted the limitations of the biomedical model over 30 years ago and yet it remains the dominant model of disease today (Fava & Sonino, 2008). Often, the most important thing that doctors have to offer to their patients is themselves – their time, their understanding, and their support (Stewart, 2005; Watts, 2009).

---

* Sir Luke Fildes, *The Doctor*, oil on canvas, 1891. The painting can be seen on the Internet at http://en.wikipedia.org/wiki/Luke_Fildes (accessed January 16, 2013).

In a study of 272 patients presenting to their family doctors with head-aches in London, Canada, the Headache Study Group of The University of Western Ontario (1986) looked for what would predict a favorable outcome one year later. The best outcomes were for patients who felt they had been given sufficient opportunity to tell the doctor all they wanted to say about their headaches on the initial visit. Another predictor of good outcome was the doctor's statement that he or she liked the patient. Helman (2006), who practiced as a general practitioner for 27 years and then became a medical anthropologist, describes his experiences as a "Suburban Shaman"; he points out that what patients want is

> relief from discomfort, relief from anxiety, a relationship of compassion and care, some explanation of what has gone wrong, and why, and a sense of order or meaning imposed on the apparent chaos of their personal suffering to help them make sense of it and to cope with it. (2006: 9)

Glasser and Pelto (1980) present the dilemma for medical educators who recognize that physician effectiveness often relates to their personal qualities:

> It is rather tragic: modern physicians are a type of shaman without the proper upbringing. It is rather like being Jewish as a third generation American and not knowing how to read or sing Hebrew. It is as though we physicians do not know the prayers and chants. (1980: 24)

How can physicians learn these "prayers and chants"? What does educational theory offer to guide educators who are responsible for the development of the modern shamans? The patient-centered clinical method describes a different way of doctoring; consequently, education about the method requires a differ-ent way of teaching. In this chapter, we describe a framework that addresses this challenge – a framework that builds on the distinction between traditional conceptions of teaching and several ways of understanding the human experi-ence of becoming a physician.

TWO CONTRASTING METAPHORS USED IN TEACHING

Teaching is too complex to be explained by a single model. Medical educa-tion, like medicine itself, embraces several, sometimes opposing, theories and metaphors. Metaphors allow us to comprehend one aspect of a concept in terms of another . . . the way we think, what we experience, and what we do every day is very much a matter of metaphor. But our conceptual system is not something we are normally aware of. (Lakoff & Johnson, 1980: 3)

As such, our underlying metaphors of education will have a profound effect on how we think about teaching and learning and the respective roles of teacher and learner (Botha, 2009; Sfard, 2008). Tiberius (1986) outlines two common metaphors used to describe teaching.

- The **transmission metaphor** has dominated all levels of education, with its roots in a behaviorist tradition. In this metaphor, teaching is telling, and learning is listening. The emphasis is on the efficient *flow of information down the pipeline* to the students. Examples of this metaphor in common speech are:
  - it's hard to *get that idea across* to him
  - your reasons *come through* to us
  - teaching is the *delivery* of a specific body of knowledge.
- Students are "receptacles to be filled by the teacher" (Friere, 2006: 72) at the school as assembly line. Of course, with so much complex material to learn, in a discipline where ignorance can lead to patient harm, there will always remain a role for didactic teaching. In fact, one study comparing active versus passive learning on effective use of diagnostic tests showed no significant difference in knowledge and attitudes immediately after and 1 month after the session. Also, residents in the didactic session perceived greater educational value from the session (Haidet *et al.*, 2004).
- In contrast, the **metaphor of dialogue or conversation** has roots in the Socratic method and humanist tradition. In this metaphor, students and teachers are "inquirers, helping one another in the shared pursuit of truth . . . they are engaged in a common enterprise in which the responsibility for acquiring knowledge is a joint one" (Hendley, 1978: 144). When students and teachers are "co-creators" of knowledge they are more likely to recognize and investigate their assumptions, increase the breadth and depth of their learning, develop skills of synthesis and integration, and lead to transformation (Brookfield & Preskill, 2005). Palmer describes the fundamental personal nature of teaching: "The techniques I have mastered do not disappear, but neither do they suffice. Face to face with my students, only one resource is at my immediate command: my identity, my selfhood, my sense of this 'I' who teaches – without which I have no sense of the 'Thou' who learns" (Palmer, 2007: 10).

The dialogue metaphor recognizes that becoming a physician is more than simply learning a set of knowledge, skills, and attitudes; medical training not only teaches a body of knowledge but also changes the person. In this sense, medical education is as much about the acquisition of values and character development as it is about learning a discipline (Brent, 1981; Dall'Alba, 2009; Monrouxe, 2010; Bleakley *et al.*, 2011; Scanlon, 2011; McKee & Eraut, 2011). Unfortunately, although these issues have been acknowledged for decades, medical education is often inimical to healthy personal development (Peterkin, 2008; Paro *et al.*, 2010).

The following example illustrates the challenges inherent in the application of the dialogue metaphor. One of us (WW), many years ago, learned the hard way about the importance of personal factors in teaching and learning.

> One of my postgraduate students had a very different idea of what he wanted to learn from what I wanted to teach. He worried about being able to deal effectively with emergencies but I wanted him to learn more about interviewing and the patient-doctor relationship. We often debated about the appropriate role of family doctors, and each of us stubbornly clung to our own points of view. While he was away doing hospital rotations, he sent me a book to read – Ayn Rand's *Atlas Shrugged* – a book that he told me had meant a great deal to him during his adolescence. He thought it might help me to understand him better. I started to read it but found it so at variance with my own worldview that I could not finish it. Later, he urged me to see the movie *Chariots of Fire*. He explained that he strongly identified with the main character in the film at the point when the Prince of Wales was called in to persuade him to "bend" his strong Christian principles by running a race on Sunday. He said I was like the Prince of Wales to him. I felt he must be exaggerating and had trouble equating his struggles with the moral issues in the film. He then shared with me how he grappled to assert his identity in his conflict with his authoritarian father. Despite our attempts to understand each other, we continued to disagree about what he should learn. He eventually graduated and set up a successful rural practice. A few years later I met him at a dinner party where we immediately struck up a conversation, talking for over an hour about his experiences since graduation. He told me that I had been right – he handled emergencies without trouble but still experienced difficulty treating patients with mental problems. On his own, he was gradually learning how to help them. It was an emotional and very special meeting for both of us. We learned a lot from each other about our stubbornness and our need to be in charge. I may have been right about what he needed to learn, but I was wrong in my approach.

Through our struggles with each other, we were challenged to reexamine the roles of the physician and the goals of postgraduate education. However, more important, our encounters showed us a different way for teacher and learner to relate to one another – we had to move beyond an authoritarian model that provokes resistance to a model of dialogue that respects and incorporates the contributions of each person.

This change, this different way of relating, illustrates a learner-centered approach that is a conceptual parallel with the patient-centered method. Both approaches seek a partnership between the protagonists – patient and doctor or student and teacher – characterized by mutual respect that leads to finding common ground.

UNDERSTANDING THE HUMAN DIMENSIONS OF LEARNING

In becoming physicians, students must develop abilities in three areas: (1) gaining medical knowledge and technical competence in dealing with disease, (2) "becoming" a professional, and (3) learning to heal.

1. Gaining Medical Knowledge and Technical Competence in Dealing with Disease

This is the principal preoccupation of medical school, especially the preclinical years. Students are immersed in the biological sciences and quickly learn the value system of the medical establishment – the primary task of medicine is the recognition and treatment of disease. Consequently, everything else – communication skills as well as psychological, social, and environmental factors – may appear peripheral. As a result, when students progress through medical school, their ability to communicate effectively and empathize with patients deteriorates. This decline has been noted for decades and is a continuing problem today (Barbee & Feldman, 1970; Helfer, 1970; Cohen, 1985; Preven *et al.*, 1986; Hojat *et al.*, 2004, 2009; Woloschuk *et al.*, 2004; Bellini & Shea, 2005; Tsimtsiou *et al.*, 2007; Haidet, 2010; Bombeke *et al.*, 2010; Neumann *et al.*, 2011).

2. "Becoming" a Professional

This begins from day one of medical school; in fact, it may even begin from the time a student decides on medicine as a career. However, it is through experiences with patients, especially during the clinical clerkship when students work as part of the clinical team and have responsibility for patient care, that they begin to feel like doctors (Brennan *et al.*, 2010). The metamorphosis is dramatic:

> students are admitted into a profession where they are privy to the highs and lows of life and the human condition. Doctors see people at their best, at their worst, at their strongest and at their most vulnerable. Doctors frequently see things which most of the population will only encounter rarely. Doctors deal with situations which others can usually avoid. (Scanlon, 2011: 182)

3. Learning to Heal

Scant attention is paid to healing in medical education, except for wound healing (Weston, 1988; Novack *et al.*, 1999). Consequently, not all physicians become healers. Those who do, learn by reflecting on their experiences with patients or from their own personal encounters with illness. They discover the limitations of a narrow biomedical model and recognize that patients need more than evidence-based therapies (Benjamin, 1984; Wade & Halligan, 2004; Egnew, 2005). "To be a healer is to help patients find their own way through the ordeal of their illness to a new wholeness" (McWhinney & Freeman, 2009: 104). Cassell (1982) challenges us to recognize the distinction between physical distress and suffering: "Suffering is experienced by persons, not merely by bodies, and has its source in challenges that threaten the intactness of the person as a complex social and psychological entity" (1982: 639). He points out that treatment may be technically correct but fail to relieve the patient's suffering:

> It has been one of the most basic errors of the modern era in medicine to believe that patients cured of their diseases – cancer removed, coronary arteries opened, infection resolved, walking again, talking again, or back home again – are also healed; are whole again. Through the relationship it is possible, given the awareness of the necessity, the acceptance of the moral responsibility, the understanding of the problem and mastery of the skills, to heal the sick; to make whole the cured, to bring the chronically ill back within the fold, to relieve suffering, and to lift the burdens of illness. (Cassell, 2004: 65)

It is important to note that learning to be a healer continues after formal education is completed. The seeds may be planted during the training period but only grow and develop as physicians experience the power of the healing relationship in practice. When teachers introduce the concept of healing they need to be cautious about the expectations they place on their students. These young physicians often find the tasks of diagnosing and treating the biological dimensions of their patients' problems challenging enough; pushing them to become therapeutic instruments of healing may leave them overwhelmed. They need frequent encouragement, support, effective role modeling, and opportunities to discuss their feelings and internal struggles to adopt the healer's mantle. Ways and colleagues (2000: 13–14) describe the personal challenges posed by the clinical years of medical school:

> Many clerkship experiences can be repugnant, sad, or painful. They can stimulate difficult memories and feelings, resurface unresolved personal issues, remind you of a loved one now dead, or all of the above. These impacts may be conscious or unconscious. *Of all aspects of clerkship education, students least expect the magnitude of its psychological and spiritual impact* (emphasis in the original). We see students initially open and outgoing toward their patients become self-absorbed, isolated, or depressed during a difficult clerkship. In contrast, on the rare clerkship where they receive appropriate support and attention, students can become more self-assured and open.

In a study of healing, Churchill and Schenck (2008) interviewed 50 practitioners identified by their peers as "healers." "Eight skills emerged as pivotal from the transcripts of these interviews: do the little things; take time; be open and listen; find something to like, to love; remove barriers; let the patient explain; share authority; and be committed" (2008: 720).

To help their students negotiate these three facets of development, teachers need a conceptual framework that will guide their understanding of the human dimensions of medical education. A confluence of writings from several directions provides us with valuable insights.

- **Personal narratives**: these are stories of the *journey through medical school and residency*. A remarkable number of students have described their personal experiences and struggles during their medical education, including a former professor of medicine (Eichna, 1980), an educational psychologist (Eisner, 1985), an anthropologist (Konner, 1987), and others (LeBaron, 1981; Klass, 1987, 1992; Little & Midtling, 1989; Klitzman, 1989; Reilly, 1987; Takakua *et al.*, 2004; Young, 2004; Neilson, 2006; Jauhar, 2008; Ofri, 2003, 2005, 2010; Clarke & Nisker, 2007; Lam, 2006; Gutkind, 2010). And there are many more. Poirier (2009) surveyed 40 books like this published in the United States between 1965 and 2005. In addition, a number of self-help books provide useful insights into the struggles of student doctors (Coombs, 1998; Kelman & Straker, 2000; Myers, 2000; Ways *et al.*, 2000; Sotile & Sotile, 2002; Peterkin, 2008).

- **Developmental theory**: research by psychologists, sociologists, and medical educators on adult learning and development provide valuable frameworks for understanding the personal and professional development of physicians (Coombs *et al.*, 1986; Weston & Lipkin Jr, 1989; Carroll *et al.*, 1995; Knowles *et al.*, 1998; Pangaro, 1999; Mezirow & Associates, 2000; Forsythe, 2005; Levine *et al.*, 2006; Cranton, 2006; Merriam & Caffarella, 2007; Kumagai, 2010).
- **Mentoring**: several authors (Freeman, 1998; Murray, 2001; Buddeberg-Fischer & Herta, 2006; Humphrey, 2010; Daloz, 2012) describe the learner-teacher relationship as a mentoring relationship. This concept leads to a number of practical suggestions for improving one-to-one teaching.
- **Professionalism and professional formation**: interest in professionalism, as reflected in increased publication of journal articles and books, has grown rapidly in the past decade (Wear & Bickel, 2000; Coulehan & Williams, 2001; Inui, 2003; Gordon, 2003; Kasman, 2004; Wear & Aultman, 2006; Stern, 2006; Kenny & Shelton, 2006; Stern & Papadakis, 2006; Cruess *et al.*, 2009). Cooke *et al.* (2010) call for professional formation to be the fundamental goal of medical education. They prefer the term "professional formation" rather than "professionalism"

> to emphasize the developmental and multifaceted nature of the construct . . . The physician we envision has, first and foremost, a deep sense of commitment and responsibility to patients, colleagues, institutions, society, and self and an unfailing aspiration to perform better and achieve more. Such commitment and responsibility involves habitual searching for improvement in all domains – however small they may seem – and willingness to invest the effort to strategize and enact such improvements. (2010: 41)

In the remainder of this chapter, we will elaborate on each of these four areas.

1. NARRATIVE LEARNING: A TRANSFORMATIONAL JOURNEY

A central task of development is to find meaning in our lives and in our work. One way to do this is by telling stories.

> Narrative learning . . . offers us a new way to think about how learning occurs . . . When we're learning something, what we're essentially doing is trying to make sense of it, discern its internal logic, and figure out how it's related to what we know already. The way we do this is by creating a narrative about

what we're learning; in other words, we work to story it, to make the elements of what we do not yet fully understand hang together. We work to achieve coherence. (Clark & Rossiter, 2008: 66)

Common to hundreds of myths and legends across numerous cultures and times is the tale of the heroic quest:

> The hero ventures forth from the world of common day into a region of supernatural wonder: fabulous forces are there encountered and a decisive victory is won: the hero comes back from this mysterious adventure with the power to bestow boons on his fellow man. (Campbell, quoted in Daloz, 2012: 26)

Through the "heroic quest" of medical school, the student conquers many "fabulous forces" and becomes a physician: he or she is transformed.

Klass (1987: 18) describes her experience at Harvard Medical School in these terms:

> The general pressure of medical school is to push yourself ahead into professionalism, to start feeling at home in the hospital, in the operating room, to make medical jargon your native tongue; it's all part of becoming efficient, knowledgeable, competent. You want to leave behind that green, terrified medical student who stood awkwardly on the edge of the action, terrified of revealing limitless ignorance, terrified of killing a patient. You want to identify with the people ahead of you, the ones who know what they are doing . . . One of the sad effects of my clinical training was that I think I generally became a more impatient, unpleasant person. Time was precious, sleep was often insufficient, and in the interest of my evaluations, I had to treat all kinds of turkeys with profound respect.

Cohen (1985) describes his experience as a mature sophomore medical student after doctoral training as an educational psychologist and serving as Director of Research in Education for the Department of Medicine. One day in his physical diagnosis course, he was given 1 hour to conduct a history and physical examination on a new patient and write up his findings. His reflections on this experience illustrate how the curriculum was at odds with his learning goals:

> I was astonished by my behavior with that patient. Intensive training in interpersonal communications would not have altered how I behaved. Given the time constraint, I dispensed with small talk, barely retaining a

> semblance of amenity. I omitted my usual preventive medicine questions
> about seat-belt usage and my chronic disease questions such as problems in
> complying with his therapeutic regimen. The focus of my thinking was on the
> patient's physical signs and symptoms and the physiological reasons for them.
> (1985: 332)

Another medical student, Melvin Konner (1987), had been a professor of
anthropology prior to medical school. He describes his experiences in the
clerkship as follows:

> And of course, last but hardly least, I now tend to see people as patients. I
> noticed this especially with women. It is often asked whether male medical
> students become desexualized by all those women disrobing, all those breast
> examinations, and all those manual invasions of the most intimate cavities. I
> found that to be a rather trivial effect. What I found more impressive was the
> general tendency to see women as patients. This clinical detachment comes
> not from gynaecology but from all the experiences of medicine. During my
> medicine rotation when, on a bus, I noticed the veins on a woman's hand – how
> easily they could be punctured for the insertion of a line – before noticing that
> she happened to be beautiful. (1987: 366)

All three examples illustrate how the journey through medical school may
desensitize students to human suffering – they become more impatient and
detached. The experience of postgraduate training may be even more brutal-
izing, leaving young physicians feeling abused. There is evidence that students
who feel abused by their teachers are more likely to abuse their patients (Silver
& Glicken, 1990; Baldwin *et al.*, 1991). Such an environment is inimical to
learning to be patient-centered.

In a powerful and moving story of her internal medicine residency at
New York's Bellevue Hospital, the oldest public hospital in the United States,
Danielle Ofri (2003) describes how her experiences as a resident shaped her
development as a physician and healer. In caring for Mercedes, a young woman
with headache, Ofri was horrified to learn that, 3 days after examining her
in the outpatient department, Mercedes was in the intensive care unit, brain-
dead from an illness that never was explained. Although she was off duty and
not the attending physician, Ofri felt compelled to see the patient and arrived
shortly after the family had been informed of the hopelessness of Mercedes'
condition and was being consoled by the chaplain.

He (the chaplain) glanced at me from across the bed where he was standing with one of the sisters and he must have seen a tear welling up in my eye. He circled back to where I stood and silently reached out his arm, resting it on my shoulder. The gentle weight settled onto my shoulder blades. It absorbed into the strain of my back, melting the muscles that were clenching and smothering me. My stethoscope twisted off my neck onto the floor as I leaned into his black tunic and began to cry. His arms circled around me . . . I collapsed deeper into his chest, sobbing and sobbing. The family stared with quiet amazement as I cried uncontrollably in the arms of a strange priest. One of the sisters left Mercedes' side and came to me. She stroked my back, her fingers running along my hair. I cried for Mercedes. I cried for her family and her two little children . . . I cried for the death of my belief that intellect conquers all. (Ofri, 2003: 233)

Ofri goes on to describe how this experience changed her:

And while I was intellectually frustrated, I felt strangely emotionally complete. That night in the ICU with Mercedes was excruciatingly painful, but it was also perhaps my most authentic experience as a doctor. Something was sad. And I cried. Simple logic, but so rarely adhered to in the high-octane world of academic medicine. Standing in the ICU, the chaplain's arms around me, surrounded by Mercedes's family, I felt like a person. Not like a physician or a scientist or an emissary from the world of rational logic, but just a person . . . I still didn't know why I had initially entered the field of medicine ten years ago, but I now knew why I wanted to stay. (2003: 236)

2. DEVELOPMENTAL THEORY

Developmental theory provides a way of understanding learning, not simply as the accumulation of knowledge but as a transformational experience. Klass (1987), Konner (1987), and Ofri (2003) describe their own experiences of being changed, of no longer being able to see the world "through preclinical eyes." Foster (2011: 171) reminds us that

Becoming a medical professional is a complex and multifaceted process. It is also an irreversible transformation, one which cannot be undone. In becoming a doctor, the way that one feels about oneself and the way in which one interacts with the world are forever influenced by assuming the identity of "doctor."

Perry (1970, 1981) provides a theory of intellectual and ethical development in adults that is helpful to make sense of these changes in thinking and perceiving (Moore, 1994). According to Perry, (1981) students progress from thinking that is simplistic and "black and white" to where they recognize and can accept different points of view. In the first stage, students view knowledge as dualistic – there is one right answer, determined by the authorities. Excessive reliance on lectures and multiple-choice examinations may reinforce the dualistic stage. Students at this stage may resent teachers who use small group facilitation and learner-centered approaches because they seem to take too long to get to the one right answer; they prefer simply to be told. Next, students recognize different perspectives on issues, but lack skills to evaluate them. At this stage, they may conclude that everyone is entitled to their own opinion and all answers are equally valid. They may become cynical and nihilistic, thinking that no one knows anything for sure. Then students develop the ability to critically compare different viewpoints but may be frozen in indecision because they can see the merits of each opinion. Finally, a stage of commitment is attained in which the learners are able to tolerate ambiguity and uncertainty and are willing to act according to their values and beliefs, even when plausible alternatives are recognized. Students recognize that they must take the risk of making their own choices. Until students reach this stage, they will have difficulty taking charge of their own learning.

> Perry described three alternatives to the progression from dualism to commitment in relativism. One was "temporizing", where students' development appeared to be delayed with an explicit hesitation to proceed with the next step. Another alternative was "escape" whereby students avoided the responsibility of commitment and sought refuge in relativism. And the last one was a "retreat" to a dualistic orientation, in order to find security and avoid coping with a too challenging environment. (Friedman *et al.*, 1987: 93)

Teachers can help their students' progress by addressing the special needs at each stage. Dualistic students benefit from being exposed to alternative viewpoints to help them realize the complexity of the concepts being learned. Students in relativism benefit from learning critical appraisal skills so that they can weigh the evidence for different opinions. Teachers need to be supportive and encouraging of student development, avoid being judgmental and model a capacity "to be both wholehearted and tentative" (Perry, 1981: 96) – the willingness to make firm commitments in the face of uncertainty and opposing opinions, while remaining open to new information.

Perry's (1981) approach, consistent with constructivist theory, emphasizes the importance of students finding meaning in their own experiences. As students grow and develop, they discover new and complex ways of thinking and seeing. Perry (1981) argues that this often demands a "loss of innocence" that may be painful and difficult.

> It may be a great joy to discover a new and complex way of thinking and seeing; but yesterday one thought in simple ways, and hope and aspiration were embedded in those ways. Now that those ways are left behind, must hope be abandoned too? (1981: 108)

He cautions us that it takes time for students to come to terms with their new insights – "for the guts to catch up with such leaps of the mind" (Perry, 1970: 108). Time is needed to mourn the loss of simpler ways of thought. This may explain why development is stepwise, with occasional retreats to older and more familiar ideas, rather than steady progress.

3. MENTORING

Mentoring is an important, perhaps essential, component of medical education. In a qualitative study of medical students, Kalén *et al.* (2012) describe medical students' experiences of mentoring:

> Having a mentor gave a sense of security and constituted a 'free zone' alongside the undergraduate programme. It gave hope about the future and increased motivation. The students were introduced to a new community and began to identify themselves as doctors. We would argue that one-to-one mentoring can create conditions for medical students to start to develop some parts of the professional competences that are more elusive in medical education programmes, such as reflective capacity, emotional competence and the feeling of belonging to a community. (2012: 389)

Mentors guide students along the journeys of their lives. They are trusted because they have already made the journey. According to Levinson (1978), mentors are especially important at the beginning of people's careers or at crucial turning points in their professional lives. Mentors are people who have already accomplished the goals sought by the students. A mentor is typically an older, more experienced member of the profession who takes the student "under his or her wing." The role of the university, as a parent-substitute is reflected in our reference to the university as our "alma mater" and in the term *in loco parentis* – in the place of the parent.

In the beginning, the student often experiences the mentor as a powerful authority – a parental figure with almost magical skill. This is also a potential source of trouble in the relationship especially with students who have a previous history of problems with authority figures. It is in the context of this relationship that students grow into their professional identity. In the early stages of their intellectual and personal development, students look to the mentor as all-knowing and expect to be given the right answers to questions. They are not ready to see the mentor's clay feet. The mismatch between what students were taught in the preclinical years and what they see their clinical teachers doing is one of the explanations for the increase in cynicism during the clerkship year (Coulehan & Williams, 2001; Billings *et al.*, 2011). This common phenomenon led one author to describe the curriculum as divided into two halves – the pre-cynical and the cynical years (Simpson, 1972: 64). As the students learn and develop, they recognize that authorities are not always right and that even their mentor is human. Eventually, with a growing sense of their own professional identity, students recognize mentors as colleagues. In a recent study of medical students and residents, Brown *et al.* (2012b) found that the mentoring relationship was evolutionary and fluid in nature. Participants reported that they sought out different mentors for different personal and professional needs and at different stages of their education.

Daloz (2012) provides a valuable framework for understanding the tasks of mentors. Effective mentors provide a balance of support and challenge and, at the same time, provide vision (*see* Figure 8.1).

Challenge	Support: Low	Support: High
High	*Retreat*	*Growth*
Low	*Stasis*	*Confirmation*

FIGURE 8.1 Framework of the tasks of mentors (Daloz, 2012: 208)

Support

"Be with" the students. Let them know that they are understood and cared for. Such support promotes the basic trust needed to summon the courage to move ahead. The mentor is tangible proof that the journey can be made. Listen empathically – what is it like in the students' world; what gives it meaning; how do they view themselves; how do they decide among conflicting ideas; what do they expect from their teachers? Note the similarities between these learner-centered questions and those we suggest that doctors ask of their patients to explore the illness experience (*see* Chapter 3).

Setting aside time indicates that students' ideas matter and that they are important as people. Preparatory empathy is helpful. Before the student arrives, remind yourself what it was like to be a student starting a new rotation. Prepare yourself to respond to indirect cues. Students are generally wary at first and may not be direct with authority figures. Express positive expectations. Whenever possible, build self-esteem and confidence.

Challenge

> Mentors toss little bits of disturbing information in their students' paths, little facts and observations, insights and perceptions, theories and interpretations – cow plops on the road to truth – that raise questions about their students' current worldviews and invites them to entertain alternatives to close the dissonance, accommodate their structures, *think* afresh. (italics in the original) (Daloz, 2012: 217)

Daloz justifies this approach by reference to the work of Festinger (1957) on cognitive dissonance – a gap between one's perceptions and one's expectations – which creates an inner need to harmonize the apparent conflict and thus motivates new learning.

Medical school may teach a narrow approach to practice focused on the conventional medical model – "find the problem and fix it." When it works, this approach is impressive. However, it often fails, leading to frustration and sometimes to blaming the victim for being "difficult." In such situations, the mentor could challenge the student to reconsider their underlying assumptions about medical practice. Directly confronting the learner might sound judgmental and provoke defensiveness; instead, consider other strategies.

- Share a story of your own struggles to find a more effective approach to such patients.

- Discuss seminal readings on clinical practice – for example, McWhinney & Freeman (2009) or Cassell (2004).
- Encourage students to write about their reflections on difficult interactions and regularly discuss their ideas.
- Offer opportunities to try out different approaches, with you role-playing a patient who they struggled with.

In setting tasks, the mentor brings learners to see a world they might not otherwise have observed. Asking pointed questions, pointing out contradictions, or offering alternative points of view may help push students past the stage of dualism; encouraging them to take a stand on a difficult issue or to criticize an expert may help them to develop a commitment. Professional learning involves the construction of new frames of meaning; therefore, students need the opportunity to try out their understandings and clarify contradictions. Hearing the views of their peers is often helpful. Heat up dichotomies. Pushing different points of view and challenging students to not only comprehend the differences but also deeply appreciate contrasting points of view stimulates personal development.

Vision

Inspire learners to see new meaning in their work and to keep struggling despite confusion and discouragement. Vision sustains learners in their attempts to apprehend a fuller, more comprehensive image of the world. One way of providing vision is through being a role model for the student. Parker Palmer (2007: 2–3) presents a view of the importance of inner strength and courage in teaching:

> Teaching, like any truly human activity, emerges from one's inwardness, for better or worse. As I teach, I project the condition of my soul onto my students, my subject, and our way of being together. The entanglements I experience in the classroom are often no more or less than the convolutions of my inner life. Viewed from this angle, teaching holds a mirror to the soul. If I am willing to look in that mirror and not run from what I see, I have a chance to gain self-knowledge – and knowing myself is as crucial to good teaching as knowing my students and my subject.

Provide a framework for understanding the developmental tasks facing the individual student. Offer a vision of the role of the physician that goes beyond the enumeration of skills to be learned and which acknowledges the personal and spiritual qualities inherent in becoming a healer. Suggest a new language. According to Fowler (1981), a mentor's primary function is to "nurturize into new metaphors." They give learners new ways to think about the world. The good teacher helps students not so much to solve problems as to see them anew. To think in new ways requires learners to learn a new vocabulary and especially to develop new metaphors. Physicians may be constrained by the dominant military metaphor in medicine that implies we are always "doing battle" with disease and must adopt an aggressive, interventionist approach. To see physicians as "witnesses" to their patients' illnesses, who help give that suffering some meaning, frees physicians to be more imaginative in their approaches to healing. For example, in *A Fortunate Man*, Berger (Berger & Mohr, 1967) describes John Sassall, a country doctor working in a remote and impoverished English rural community:

> He does more than treat them when they are ill; he is the objective witness of their lives . . . He keeps the records so that, from time to time, they can consult them themselves. The most frequent opening to a conversation with him, if it is not a professional conversation, are the words "Do you remember when . . .?" He represents them, becomes their objective (as opposed to subjective) memory, because he represents their lost possibility of understanding and relating to the outside world, and because he also represents some of what they know but cannot think. (1967: 109)

> It is the doctor's acceptance of what the patient tells him and the accuracy of his appreciation as he suggests how different parts of his life may fit together, it is this which then persuades the patient that he and the doctor and other men are comparable because whatever he says of himself or his fears or his fantasies seem to be at least as familiar to the doctor as to him. He is no longer an exception. He can be recognized. (1967: 76)

4. PROFESSIONAL FORMATION

Medical education borrows the concept of professional formation from the education of clergy.

> A distinguishing feature of professional education is the emphasis on forming in students the dispositions, habits, knowledge, and skills that cohere in professional identity and practice, commitments and integrity. The pedagogies that clergy educators use toward this purpose – formation – originate in the

deepest intentions for professional service: for doctors and nurses, healing; for lawyers, social order and justice; for teachers, learning; and for clergy, engaging the mystery of human existence. (Foster *et al.*, 2006: 100)

Coulehan and Williams (2001) describe how the curriculum may lead some students to abandon the idealism that brought them into medicine. They illustrate their thesis, that "the culture of clinical training is often hostile to professional virtue" (2001: 602), by quoting from a short narrative written by a particularly gifted and socially aware student who was so worn down by the curriculum that she opted for peace as a survival strategy, putting off her idealism until some undefined future date.

> When I arrived in medical school, I was eager to get involved . . . as medical students, I was sure that we would have some clout and certainly a commitment to the well-being of others . . . However, medical school is an utter drain. For two years lecturers parade up and down describing their own particular niche as if it were the most important thing for a student to learn. And then during the clinical years, life is brutal. People are rude, the hours are long, and there is always a test at the end of the rotation . . . After a while I reasoned that the most important thing I could do for my patient, for my fellow human beings, for the future of medicine, as well as for me, was to assure myself some peaceful time . . . And rather than try to change everything that I consider wrong in the hospital or the community at large, I just try to get through school in the hope that I will move on to bigger and better things when I have more control over my circumstances. On the other hand, I do believe that habits formed now will rarely be overcome in the future. So I regret not having spoken up on more issues. But I was often too tired. (2001: 599)

Some students choose to narrow their responsibilities to developing technical competence as the best way to serve their patients. Others adopt a "non-reflective professionalism" by treating their patients as objects of technical services.

Dall'Alba (2009) cautions us to be wary of the dominant model of education that "generally appears to take for granted that the purpose of higher education is primarily the development of knowledge and skills" (2009: 64). She suggests, instead, that education should begin with a concept of care "highlighting the ontological dimension of education and its role in contributing to who students are becoming" (2009: 64). She elaborates on the central role of caring in the curriculum:

reducing the practice of medicine, social work or engineering to "skills" or "competencies" overlooks the engagement, commitment and risk involved . . . For instance, in order to skillfully engage in professional practice, health of patients must matter to medical practitioners, social workers must be concerned about the well-being of their clients and it must matter to engineers that a bridge they build will support the weight of vehicles travelling over it . . . A focus on narrowly defined skills or competencies overlooks and undervalues the ontological dimension of professional practice and of learning to be professionals. It thereby undermines the relationships among what we know, how we act and who we are. (2009: 65)

Critics of the modern professionalism movement decry the hankering for a nostalgic concept of physicians willing to sacrifice everything for the benefit of their patients, and argue for more attention to the academic environment in which students are educated (Wear & Kuczewski, 2004; Hafferty & Levinson, 2008; Hafferty, 2009). Cooke *et al.* (2010: 60) assert that professional formation is "the purpose that should guide medical education and drive the learning process." They argue for a broader conception of professionalism – not only should physicians attend to the needs of individual patients, but also they must contribute to scholarship to better understand and manage health problems, and participate in a professional community by advocating for systems-level interventions. They list three premises to guide clinical education. Each premise emphasizes the importance of alignment among the curriculum objectives, teaching methods and assessment.

- *Premise one: learning is progressive and developmental.* Learning is constantly building on what was learned before. "Knowledge is dynamic – constantly reshaped, recombined, expanded, and elaborated in ways that create new understanding or improve performance in the care of individual patients and patient populations" (Cooke *et al.*, 2010: 66). The curriculum needs to be tailored to the changing needs of students – the clinical setting should provide a learning opportunity that matches what they need to tackle next. Preceptors must balance the needs for patient safety with the needs of students and residents "to make increasingly high-stakes decisions and perform more demanding procedures" (2010: 67) as they progress through their training. Learners should gradually be given more responsibility for determining when they need help and how to obtain the additional expertise to deal with clinical problems. These are essential competencies for independent practice. The experiences of caring for patients with life-threatening diseases, debilitating chronic illnesses, delivering babies, and sitting with dying patients will have a profound transformative influence on their lives. They will not be the same people when they graduate.

- *Premise two: learning is participatory.* The development of clinical expertise occurs through participation as a member of a clinical team. Initially, learners will have responsibility for routine aspects of patient care as they observe the more experienced team members deal with the high-stakes aspects of care. Their skills will improve through watching expert role models, and through receiving coaching and feedback as they take on more responsibility for patient care in an interprofessional team.
- *Premise three: learning is situated and distributed.* Learners need experiences in a variety of clinical settings where they will appreciate the importance of the expertise of other health professionals and learn how to tap the wealth of resources in different clinical settings. Medical education too often emphasizes the central role of individual mastery, discounting the value of other health professionals and the role of the team. It is important to understand knowledge as "something that is shared or distributed among colleagues or team members and that is embedded in routine actions and technology" (2010: 70). The concept of communities of practice (Wenger, 1998) provides a valuable approach to understanding medical expertise as a collaborative process.

GUIDELINES FOR TEACHERS

- Get to know your learners, not just as a students or residents but as persons. Find out what is important to them – their family, close friends, interests outside of medicine. Do they have any major obligations or commitments (e.g., a sick parent)? What do they like to do when they are not working? What are their future plans? Share aspects of your own life. "Within the learning environment, importance needs to be placed on the development of positive teacher–student relationships, as these relationships have immeasurable effects on students' academic outcomes and behaviour" (Liberante, 2012: 9).
- As a mentor, challenge your learners to go further, while also providing the support they need for transformative learning. Help them clarify their vision of the kind of doctor they strive to become.
- Remember that students sometimes feel overwhelmed with the biomedical curriculum and may discount communication issues as a strategy to survive medical school. Help them develop their skills and comfort with the conventional clinical method so that they will not be so preoccupied with

their biomedical competencies that they have no time or energy for a more comprehensive patient-centered approach. Create a learning environment where students can disclose their areas of ignorance, their errors, and their personal struggles without fear of judgment.

- Teach by example. The power of role modeling is emphasized in the following quotation attributed to Albert Einstein: "Setting an example is not the main means of influencing others, it is the only means." According to social learning theory (Bandura, 1977; Claridge & Lewis, 2005), we often learn more by observation than from verbal instruction. In fact, many of the skills acquired in medical education are too complex to describe in words; such tacit abilities, such as clinical reasoning, must be demonstrated by a teacher or skilled peer. Additionally, the commitment to patient-centered care, modeled by a respected teacher, powerfully motivates learners to do the same.

- Help them learn how to attend to what the patient wants to talk about and to realize that listening may be more therapeutic than any biomedical intervention.

- Help them develop survival strategies to avoid becoming overwhelmed. For example, physicians need colleagues with whom they can discuss difficult or emotionally draining encounters with patients.

- Help students to reflect on their experiences and how to learn from them. This provides the tools for a lifetime of learning.

- Use the parallels in the relationship between teacher and learner to demonstrate aspects of the patient-doctor relationship. There should be the same caring and attention to the humanity of the learner that we expect the learner to demonstrate with patients. Cavanaugh (2002: 992) summarized the research on the importance of creating a caring environment for medical education and concluded: "Role modeling, mentoring and coaching can effectively incorporate caring principles and practices to facilitate the transmission of caring attitudes and behaviors in aspiring physicians."

- Remember how stressful medical education can be and attend to the personal struggles of students as well as to their learning needs. Learning to be a doctor involves a profound change in identity, which may be difficult for some students. Watch for signs of unhealthy coping strategies, or frank mental illness, and be prepared to intervene. Faculty, like students, have a tendency to deny the seriousness of these problems and may assume the student is "just having a bad day." Don't procrastinate; explore the problem promptly and sensitively and be prepared to provide modified work responsibilities or sick leave and the appropriate professional help.

CONCLUSION

Learning to be a patient-centered doctor challenges young physicians to develop their skills and, more importantly, themselves. The task can feel overwhelming at times and may awaken feelings of vulnerability and inadequacy as students grapple at the growing edges of their abilities. Their teachers must be responsive to their struggles and address the learners' needs and concerns. Teachers must model, in their behavior with students, the quality of interaction they expect students to demonstrate with patients.

We have woven several strands of educational thought that provide the fabric of the dialogue metaphor of education. Medical education is a journey guided by a wise mentor who is sensitive to the issues involved in human development and the unique challenges of becoming a physician. At the same time, teachers must be skilled in the use of a variety of teaching strategies illustrated by the transmission metaphor – for example, able to teach specific interviewing and history taking skills (Sfard, 2008). Combining this repertoire of teaching methods into a seamless whole will provide the learning environment needed to foster the human dimensions of medical education. It is only in such a setting that the patient-centered clinical method can be mastered.

A Messenger: Case Illustrating Becoming a Physician
Barry Lavallee and Judith Belle Brown

The silence of Doris' inner suffering still haunts me. It reaches into a place I thought was well concealed and I am shocked at the occasional eruption within me as I encounter patients such as Doris. Intuitively, I always knew that working with my own people was right. I understood many things that others might find repulsive. I was not afraid of scabies, snotty noses, an unclean elder, and I was not shocked to hear that Mrs Wolf's children were all in care. Looking beyond the physical appearance and understanding the origin of social chaos requires patience, compassion, and empathy.

As a third-year medical student, I became friends with a physician who attended our local Aboriginal church. Cliff was unlike my regular supervisors; he understood Aboriginal people and he had faith in their spiritual strength. I accepted his offer to do clinical work and study at the inner-city clinic where he worked. After all, this was the area where I had spent most of my childhood. Classic epidemiological parameters defined this patient population; most were Aboriginal, economically disadvantaged, uneducated, and most times were in a survival mode.

In Cliff, I had finally found a teacher with whom I could explore all my fears, worries, anxieties, and triumphs. No longer did I have to pretend that I was not one of them. I could be myself, although I was unsure what that meant. I bathed or showered every day, I knew who my parents were, and I had a connection to a community. I had a past, present, and a future. I saw a variety of patients, many of whom, as I found out in time, were related to me. Cliff and I looked beyond the physical scars marking a violent life and searched for meaning, truth, and dignity in those we treated.

Sniffing solvents to induce an emotional coma was common in that inner-city community. I saw many patients whose reality was permanently affected by such organic elixirs. No problem, I thought. As children, my siblings and I saw many of our friends turn to sniff to escape their painful worlds. "Sure, I can handle these patients," I reassured myself. One afternoon, I was called into the treatment room to see a patient with multiple ulcers to her legs and arms. I walked into the room and there sat Doris, a young Aboriginal woman engulfed with the all-too-familiar sweet and caustic smell of sniff.

I approached her as I have been taught in medical school. "Hi, my name is Barry and I am a medical student. How are you?" There was no response. Perhaps she was still high or maybe she didn't hear me, I wondered. Her eyes remained fixed on the floor, locked in a world known only to her. I moved closer and repeated myself. Again, there was no reply. I looked over at the nurse and she just raised her eyebrows and shrugged her shoulders as if to say, "I don't know." I was uncomfortable. "Where do you live . . . where is your family . . . when did you first notice the sores . . . have you seen someone else for this problem?" She didn't answer any of the questions. I left the room to speak with the nurse. "She comes here occasionally and all we know is that she lives on the streets and hangs around Main Street," she replied.

I quickly examined her, ordered a few tests and realized that I felt just as helpless as she looked. Her acquiescence to my examination, as I understand today, mirrored that to "her station in life." Perhaps, she thought of herself as just another "dirty Indian"? How often had she been beaten down? She breathes, moves her limbs, and I know the nurse obtained a blood pressure, but something is missing. I thought to myself. What happened to you? What set of circumstances makes you express your pain with such cruelty? My heart raced and fear began to overwhelm me.

Cliff walked into the room. I started to tell him her story and then, suddenly stopped as the burning tears raced down my cheeks. I swallowed with difficulty and as if to challenge the reality of the situation, I gazed upon her again. A physical form resembling a young woman sat on that examining table, yet this human was devoid of emotion, spirit . . . but the most painful reality was to witness the lack of hope in her eyes.

"I don't understand," I said to my supervisor. Cliff looked at me and seeing how powerless I felt in the face of such suffering and indignity quietly said, "Sometimes, all you can do is just pray for understanding."

Today, I recognize what transpired during that important moment in my life. Doris helped me recognize the very demons I had lived with for so long. My journey had begun. I knew the pain one feels when all your life you wish your skin was a different color. The confusion one feels upon hearing the ancient and melodic language of your loving grandparents and then to have the same relatives call it the language of the "savages." I remember having my skin scrubbed so hard that it bled. As if, somehow, the daily cleansing removed me from that shameful category of "dirty Indians." The heartache my siblings and I felt when we were told to stay away from "those Indians" . . . the words conveyed with disgust and hate by my mother as she picked the nits from our hair. My parents never really understood the attraction we had for children of our own race, in that white world of our childhood. Mostly, I knew the confusion it created in my soul as I attempted to balance the love I felt for my family with the hate I had for who we were. Doris spoke to me back then, as she does today, and the power of her message will reverberate within my spirit forever.

In your silence and through you suffering Doris, I have found hope. I am left with a vision . . . and, in that vision, I see our ancestors. Their beckoning leads me toward the future. The wall of silence is broken and a dignity made of truth, faith, and respect takes its place. I am free . . . and I stand firm. Doris, as a sign of my gratitude, I will burn sweetgrass in your honor and keep you in my heart.

9 Learner-Centered Teaching

W Wayne Weston and Judith Belle Brown

> I am a little embarrassed to tell you that I used to want credit for having all
> the intelligent insights in my classroom. I worked hard to learn these facts . . .
> I secretly wanted my students to look at me with reverence. I now believe that
> the opposite effect should occur – that the oracle, the locus and ownership
> of knowledge, should reside in each student and our principal goal as teach-
> ers must be to help our students discover the most important and enduring
> answers to life's problems within themselves. Only then can they truly possess
> the knowledge that we are paid to teach them. (Flachmann, 1994: 2)

In this chapter we describe a learner-centered approach to medical education,
a conceptual model for teaching that parallels the patient-centered clinical
method. In the same way that patient-practitioner relationships have changed,
so have the relationships between learners and teachers. These parallels provide a framework to understand the changing roles of teachers and learners
in medical education. This framework also serves as a tool – learners' experiences of their relationships with their teachers help them understand their
relationships with patients. For example, when teachers interact with learners as autonomous adults with a key role in important decisions about their
education, they illustrate the kind of relationship teachers expect learners to
develop with patients. Analogous to the patient-centered clinical method, the
learner-centered method comprises four interactive components (*see* Box 9.1
and Figure 9.1).

1. Needs assessment: exploring both gaps and goals
2. Understanding the learner as a whole person
3. Finding common ground
4. Enhancing the learner-teacher relationship

This approach to teaching is consistent with a number of current concepts of
learning. The principles of adult learning, first described by Lindeman (1926),
popularized by Knowles and colleagues (2011), and elaborated by numerous authors (Merriam *et al.*, 2007; Galbraith, 2004; Stagnaro-Green, 2004;
Merriam, 2008), emphasize an individualistic and developmental perspective.

Box 9.1 The Learner-Centered Method of Education: The Four Interactive Components of the Learning/Teaching Process

1. Needs assessment: exploring both gaps and goals:
   - *gaps* – requirements for completion of training
   - *goals* – special interests and areas of discomfort.
2. Understanding the learner as a whole person:
   - *the learner* – personal background, current situation, and developmental issues
   - *the context* – opportunities and constraints of the learning environment.
3. Finding common ground:
   - priorities
   - teaching/learning methods
   - roles for teacher and learner.
4. Enhancing the learner-teacher relationship:
   - empathy, respect, genuineness
   - sharing power
   - self-awareness
   - transference and countertransference.

- With age, learners become more self-directed and actively involved in their own learning;
- Learning builds on students' previous experiences;
- Readiness to learn is closely related to the developmental tasks inherent in the learner's social or work-related role;
- Adult learners are more concerned about learning for immediate application rather than for future use;
- Internal motivation is more important than external reward;
- Adults want to know why they need to learn something. (Merriam *et al.*, 2007: 84)

Although adult learning theory has been criticized for lack of empirical support (Norman, 1999) and for focusing too much on the individual and downplaying the powerful influence of the sociocultural environment (Bleakley, 2006), it has reminded us to pay more attention to the learner's experiences and his or her aspirations. Other theories of learning – social cognitive theory, transformative learning, self-directed learning, and experiential learning – address the complexities of learning in medicine and the central role of the learner:

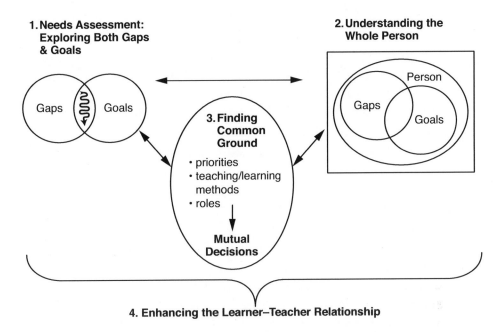

1. Needs Assessment:
Exploring Both Gaps
& Goals

Gaps   Goals

2. Understanding the
Whole Person

Person

Gaps   Goals

3. Finding
Common
Ground

• priorities
• teaching/learning
  methods
• roles

Mutual
Decisions

4. Enhancing the Learner–Teacher Relationship

FIGURE 9.1 The learner-centered method of education: four interactive components

the learner is part of a changing, complex environment, and interacts actively in the environment. The curriculum cannot any longer be viewed as something which is transmitted to or acts upon the students, be they undergraduate, postgraduate or practicing physicians; there is an important element of human agency. Moreover, in practice, the physician learner is stimulated to learn through interactions in the practice environment. (Kaufman *et al.*, 2000: 34)

This "human agency" is well described by constructivist learning theory (Tobias & Duffy, 2009) that emphasizes the central role of students in learning. Everything humans learn is strongly influenced by what they know already and that prior knowledge shapes how they construct new understandings. Consequently, a teacher's first task is to find out what their students already know. One common misunderstanding of constructivism and self-directed learning is that the teacher's role is reduced to that of a facilitator who provides encouragement and indirect guidance but does not offer any direct instruction. Bransford and colleagues (1999: 10) provide a more balanced view of the constructivist teacher:

[Students] come to formal education with a range of prior knowledge, skills, beliefs, and concepts that significantly influence what they notice about the environment and how they organize and interpret it. This, in turn, affects their abilities to remember, reason, solve problems, and acquire new knowledge . . . A logical extension of the view that new knowledge must be constructed from existing knowledge is that teachers need to pay attention to the incomplete understandings, the false beliefs, and the naïve renditions of concepts that learners bring with them to a given subject. Teachers then need to build on these ideas in ways that help each student achieve a more mature understanding. If students' initial ideas and beliefs are ignored, the understandings that they develop can be very different from what the teacher intends.

1. NEEDS ASSESSMENT: EXPLORING BOTH GAPS AND GOALS

The first step in planning any teaching or learning experience is a needs assessment – an analysis of what learners need or want to know compared with what they already know (Kern *et al.*, 2009). In the learner-centered approach, teachers and learners collaborate in defining the outcomes for learning. These are based on an assessment of two potentially divergent sets of learning objectives. On the one hand, there are the gaps in the learner's abilities based on the "official" curriculum – the core requirements for competence; on the other hand are the learner's goals and aspirations – his or her special interests, perceived weaknesses, and concept of his or her learning needs for future practice. Effective education requires learners and teachers to find common ground regarding both sets of objectives – to increase the amount of overlap in the two circles in Figure 9.1. While teachers need to respect learners' choices, they should keep in mind that their learners' aspirations might not match what they must learn to achieve competence. Because research suggests that students are often not accurate in their self-assessment (Eva & Regehr, 2008; Davis *et al.*, 2006) and may not be aware of the gaps in their knowledge or skills, teachers might need to guide students to consider different or additional choices. This is especially important in a field of study such as medicine where it is vital for learners to achieve competence.

Weimer (2003, 2013) describes a valuable approach to learner-centered teaching in which she outlines its challenges and values, common reasons for resistance by students and faculty alike, and five key strategies for implementation.

1. The teacher's role changes from authority to guide showing students how to do things not do it for them. This makes it more likely that their new learning will be connected with what they already know and will make sense to them.

2. The balance of power between teachers and learners must be more equal –
    decisions about course content, teaching methods, and evaluation should
    be shared with students, but not transferred wholesale. Research has shown
    that empowerment of students improves motivation and learning (Schunk
    & Zimmerman, 2008). However, the transfer of power must be made
    gradually as students learn to make good decisions and assume responsibil-
    ity for them.

3. Regarding content, less is more (Knight & Wood, 2005)! Attempts to cover
    everything they need to know overwhelm students and impede their learn-
    ing. Effective teachers help learners acquire the fundamental knowledge
    base they need and, more important, guide them to develop their learning
    strategies to master increasingly complex new material on their own.

4. Create learning environments that encourage students to take more respon-
    sibility for their own learning. In a review of autonomy support in medical
    education, Williams and Deci (1998: 303) report: "Research suggests that
    when educators are more supportive of student autonomy, students not
    only display a more humanistic orientation toward patients but also show
    greater conceptual understanding and better psychological adjustment."

5. Student assessment should be fair, equitable, and robust, with an emphasis
    on feedback to support learning. Involving students in determining the
    methods of assessment and in self- and peer assessment enhances learning
    and may improve self-assessment. The assessment system should inform
    learners about their strengths and gaps and guide their ongoing learning
    plans to assure that they are competent at the time of graduation.

In the past, the transmission perspective on teaching, based on behavioral
theories of learning, dominated medical education. Because there is so much
to learn and medical error is often blamed primarily (and falsely) on ignorance,
medical faculty may feel compelled to use a didactic approach. The recent
worldwide adoption of a competency-based model of medical education reinforces our preoccupation with content and standards. Abraham Flexner in his
first book, *The American College* (1908), and again in his famous report on
medical education (1910), criticized the overreliance on the lecture method.
On the other hand, a teacher who is a master of the content and a skilled presenter provides invaluable guidance to medical students, especially when they
are being introduced to a new and complex topic (Pratt & Associates, 1998).
However, sometimes teachers try too hard to teach concepts that students are
not ready to learn:

> In general, our instructional policies and practices do not make students thirsty. Rather, we tell students that they are thirsty – that they should be drinking. They remain unconvinced and so (mostly out of concern for them) we force the issue. We use rules, requirements, and sticks to try to hold their heads in the watering trough. Most do end up drinking, but a lot of them never figure out why water is so important. A few drown in the process. (Weimer, 2002: 103)

The learner-centered approach shares many features with self-directed learning (Tough, 1979; Cheren, 1983; Grow, 1991; Spencer & Jordan, 1999; Norman, 2004; Merriam, 2007; Poole, 2012). An early champion of self-directed learning, Malcolm Knowles (1975: 18), defined it this way:

> In its broadest meaning, 'self-directed learning' describes a process in which individuals take the initiative, with or without the help of others, in diagnosing their learning needs, formulating learning goals, identifying human and material resources for learning, choosing and implementing appropriate learning strategies, and evaluating learning outcomes.

Cheren (1983) agrees with Knowles that self-directed learners often ask for help and points out that self-direction in learning is not an all-or-none phenomenon but, rather, a continuum with varying degrees of learner autonomy. Greveson and Spencer (2005) warn us to be cautious about overzealous promotion of self-directed learning, a concept based more on rhetoric than evidence. Planning a learning experience involves answering a series of questions – what are the gaps in my knowledge and abilities, what are the priorities for my learning, how is the learning to be accomplished, how and by whom is the learning to be assessed (Doyle, 2011)? Learners who are completely self-directed will answer these questions on their own. However, often this task is too daunting, especially for students who are unfamiliar with the content to be learned. "So much work is required to exercise complete control over every aspect of a learning project that it is not practical or worth the effort to try to exercise all that control all the time" (Cheren, 1983: 27). For these learners, the questions will need to be answered by the students in consultation with their teachers. There are many reasons to begin by determining students' deepest felt concerns about what matters most in their education. This enhances motivation (Svinicki, 1999; Svinicki & McKeachie, 2011) and personal responsibility for learning. Furthermore, it gives them practice in self-assessment – a critical skill for lifelong learning. However, students may not be aware of all the requirements for competent practice and may have blind spots regarding their own abilities. Addressing these issues is a paramount responsibility of their teachers who must have a clear conception of the knowledge and skills needed for competent practice and the skill to assess students on each of these. In addition, teachers must be able to articulate these learning needs in a manner that is constructive, practical, and makes sense to their learners.

Grow (1991) provides a useful staged model of self-directed learning that matches the teacher's role with the stage of independence of the learner. In stage 1, the learner is "dependent" and needs an authority or coach. Lectures may be appropriate for this stage, especially for new and complex material or when time is limited. The stage 2 learner is "interested" and benefits from guided discussion and goal setting. In stage 3, the learner is "involved" and does well with a facilitator who encourages the student to participate as an equal. The stage 4 learner is "self-directed" and does best with individual work or a self-directed study group. The teacher acts as a consultant.

Teachers will help students understand what is important for practice, not by threatening them with difficult exams, but by providing opportunities to experience the need to know. The research on motivation is clear – except for rudimentary procedural skills, extrinsic rewards do not incentivize learning. In fact, external rewards are more likely to reduce motivation and performance (Pink, 2011). Positive motivating experiences can take many forms: stories of teachers' own struggles to learn; role-play with simulated patients; seminars with previous students who discuss the evolution of their own understanding of their discipline; discussion with patients about qualities they most admire in physicians. Helping students to reflect on their experiences with patients (what went well and what might have been more effective) encourages them to consider what additional skills they need and how they might improve.

Case Example

Dr Jacques Boisvert was a first-year family medicine resident in Dr Mary Denzin's community family practice, where he had been observed frequently over the past month during patient encounters. Jacques had consistently demonstrated a conscientious approach to the workup of patients; his case presentations and records were an accurate representation of what he had done; he correctly assessed his need for assistance; and he was not hesitant to seek help appropriately. His patient Joseph Yong, aged 68, returned for a follow-up regarding his type 2 diabetes and a new problem of right shoulder pain. Dr Denzin was generally satisfied with Jacques' clinical skills relevant to the assessment and management of diabetes and had observed him care for other patients with poorly controlled diabetes. She was less comfortable with his abilities regarding musculoskeletal problems. In briefing Jacques before seeing the patient, Dr Denzin commented: "I am confident in your skills in dealing with Joseph's diabetes and helping him regain his control of his diabetes. I will leave it to you to tell me if you need any assistance with managing Joseph's diabetes. I remember a few weeks ago you mentioned you would like to learn more about musculoskeletal problems. Would you like me to join you with Joseph when you are ready?" Jacques was encouraged by Dr Denzin's appraisal of his skills in the management of diabetes and relieved that he would be able to learn more about the assessment of shoulder pain.

In a survey of third-year medical students, Hajek and colleagues (2000) assessed their common concerns about communicating with patients and compiled a list of 15 issues, ranked in order of importance from the students' perspective:

- The patient starts crying or becomes angry with me
- The patient is in pain or emotional distress
- Not understanding the patient
- The patient tells me something important but wants to keep it confidential
- Not knowing the answer to patients' questions
- Appearing nervous or incompetent
- Drying up, not knowing what to ask next
- Being so concerned about what to ask next that I don't take in what the patient is saying
- Making a fool of myself or being humiliated when presenting a patient
- The patient does not want to talk to or be examined by a student
- Embarrassed about asking certain questions or by the patient's response
- The patient rambles on and I cannot interrupt them
- Unsure about shaking patient's hand. When is it all right to touch the patient?
- The patient asks me personal questions
- Unsure how to introduce myself
- Unsure how to dress, e.g., should I wear a white coat? (2000: 657)

It is ironic that student manuals frequently offer advice about dress, an issue at the bottom of students' list of concerns, but often do not address more important issues such as "drying up" and not knowing what to ask next. This list by Hajek *et al.* (2000) may assist teachers to be more attentive to students' learning needs.

In the patient-centered clinical method, it is important for the physician to acknowledge each patient's preexisting problems so that current issues will be managed in the context of all of the patient's problems. In the same way, teachers need to be cognizant of their students' prior learning experiences. Students are not blank slates. Knowledge of learners' strengths, weaknesses, and special interests accelerates the learning process and increases the potential intensity and complexity of the knowledge, skills, and attitudes that can be mastered. The curriculum can be viewed as a spiral; the same content may be encountered on several occasions but each time it is assimilated in greater depth. Sometimes such repetition is misunderstood and students complain that it seems like unnecessary repetition. They need to understand the purpose of revisiting some topics and may need to be challenged by their teachers to dig deeper.

2. UNDERSTANDING THE LEARNER AS A WHOLE PERSON

In Chapter 8 we elaborated on the developmental issues in becoming a physician; in this chapter we will focus on some of the difficulties students face during their education: stress, burnout, and mental illness. Next we will address some features of the learning environment that hamper or assist their learning and development: the hidden curriculum and medical student abuse. This framework may be helpful in analyzing the difficulties of a faltering or failing student.

The Learner: Personal Background, Current Situation, and Developmental Issues

Akin to the two important dimensions of understanding patients as whole persons (patients' stage in their life cycle and their context) there are two dimensions for understanding students as whole persons. Teachers need to be aware of the students' background, their life history and personal and cognitive development, and their learning environment.

In the same way that physicians oversimplify their patients' complex problems by focusing on the pathophysiology of disease, so too do teachers oversimplify their students' educational needs by concentrating only on their major learning deficiencies. Teachers may speak of making a "learning diagnosis" in terms of the gaps in students' knowledge, skills, and attitudes compared with the competencies to be achieved. This may be very helpful, as far as it goes, but it may fail to convey an accurate understanding of what the learner, as a person, really needs (Lacasse *et al.*, 2012a). Students are different in so many important ways: in previous life experience, courses taken, preferred learning styles, willingness to take risks, self-confidence, and resistance to change (Curry, 2002). Sir William Osler (1932: 423) commented on how individual differences in physicians determine their enjoyment of practice:

> To each one of you the practice of medicine will be very much as you make it – to one a worry, a care, a perpetual annoyance; to another, a daily joy and a life of as much happiness and usefulness as can well fall to the lot of man.

In dealing with the many stresses of medical education, pacing is important. When students become overwhelmed by the emotional intensity of a learning experience, they may need a break. Then, restored, they return to the learning environment ready to proceed with the next learning task. For example, helping dying patients come to terms with their mortality is often psychologically draining and students may need an emotional respite. This may only happen with the support and permission of their teachers. Noonan describes the value of weekly support sessions for residents:

> At a weekly house staff support meeting, led by a psychiatrist-facilitator, residents shared frustrations, discussed anxieties about their roles, and proposed solutions to their common problems. They could talk about the tragedy of death; the sometimes-irrational behaviour of patients; and the competing demands of family, friends, patients, colleagues, and teachers. Several times a year, the noon teaching conference was devoted to sharing "critical incidents". Faculty and house staff described events in their medical and postgraduate educations that left indelible and sometimes painful memories. These conferences encouraged trainees to recognize the pain that is an inherent part of practicing medicine and reassured them that they were not alone in facing uncomfortable issues. (Noonan, quoted in Coombs, 1998: 180)

Case Example

A few months ago when Dr Sunir Patel had been accepted into the Family Medicine program as an international medical graduate, he had expressed his deep appreciation and sense of privilege. It had been a long and difficult process to reach this point since immigrating from his war-torn country 5 years earlier. In recent weeks his supervisor, Dr Steinhouse, frequently observed Sunir to be pensive – often lost in thought. Somewhat baffled by his student's change in demeanor, Dr Steinhouse decided to gently explore how her student was managing. Sunir was initially surprised by his supervisor's inquiry and unsure how best to respond. After some consideration he revealed his feelings of confusion. Sunir explained: "The practice of medicine is so different here compared to my country. Back home doctors tell patients that they should do this and that and patients obey. Here we are expected to talk with patients and learn what they want and need – to be patient-centered! This is all so new for me – it is very confusing." Dr Steinhouse probed further: "Are other things different?" Sunir quickly replied: "Oh yes! Back home you would never speak directly to a consultant or a senior resident – you wouldn't even look them in the eye." Sunir sighed, "But here everyone is very friendly and helpful, which is great, but it is so different. Sometimes it is hard to know how to be."

By understanding the challenges Sunir was facing in making the transition from a very hierarchical medical system to one that was both patient- and learner-centered, Dr Steinhouse is guiding her student through this time of adjustment and change.

Even students from the same school and the same class have vastly different abilities and learning needs. It is crucial to identify these so that students are not put into situations where they are out of their depth. It is also essential to identify their strengths so that valuable time is not wasted practising skills already mastered while ignoring areas of deficiency. Students also differ in their stages of personal, cognitive, and professional development, as described in Chapter 8.

The student population has changed dramatically in most medical schools with the entrance of more women and greater ethnic diversity. These changes have the potential to alter the focus and priorities of the curriculum. Some authors have commented on the impact of the "feminization" of medicine. For example, Gilligan and Pollack (1988: 262) observe:

> women medical students in their heightened sensitivity to detachment and isolation often reveal the places in medical training and practice where human connection has become dangerously thin . . . women physicians may help to heal the breach in medicine between patient care and scientific success. For this reason the encouragement of women's voices and the validation of women's perceptions may contribute to the improvement of medical education. Since humanism in medicine depends on joining the heroism of cure with the

vulnerability of care, reshaping the image of the physician to include women constitutes a powerful force for change.

Levinson and Lurie (2004) describe how increasing numbers of women in medicine will change four domains of medicine: (1) the patient-physician relationship, (2) the local delivery of care, (3) the societal delivery of care, and (4) the medical profession itself. Women are more likely than men to go into the lower-paying primary care specialties and have been described as the "housewives" of the profession. A meta-analytic review by Roter and colleagues (2002: 756) showed that female primary care physicians "engage in more communication that can be considered patient centered and have longer visits than their male colleagues." Sandhu and colleagues (2009) reviewed studies of the impact of gender dyads on patient-doctor communication and noted that there was "less tension around power and status within same sex dyads" and that this would facilitate "data gathering and patient participation in treatment decisions . . . where more patient-centred talk occurs, and in an atmosphere of ease and equality" (2009: 353). Interestingly, male patients were more likely to discuss emotional agendas with female physicians perhaps because of the female stereotype as being more emotional and therefore the best experienced to deal with others' emotions. They acknowledge that the evidence-base on gender effects is small, there are many confounders, and more rigorous approaches are needed. Kilminster *et al.* (2007a) urge caution in interpreting the impact of feminization in medicine. Studies in different countries show contrasting results, some studies finding "differences are minimal, at best, and of little explanatory value" (2007a: 41).

Another important issue is the effect of stress, substance abuse, and mental illness on the performance of medical students. In a study of burnout in residents in internal medicine programs, Shanafelt and colleagues (2002) found 76% of respondents met the criteria for burnout using the self-administered Maslach Burnout Inventory. Other studies show similar results. Burned-out residents were more likely to self-report providing suboptimal patient care at least monthly. For example, 40% of burned-out residents, compared with less than 5% of non-burned-out residents, reported that they had "paid little attention to the social or personal impact of an illness on a patient" weekly or monthly (Shanafelt *et al.*, 2002: 363). In a similar study at seven US medical schools, burnout was associated with self-reported unprofessional behavior such as cheating on an exam, or reporting a physical examination finding as normal when it had not been done (Dyrbye *et al.*, 2010). In a study of urban family physicians using the Maslach Burnout Inventory and in-depth interviews, Lee and colleagues (2008) found 42.5% of participants had high stress levels and almost half had high scores for emotional exhaustion and depersonalization. The most-cited challenges were paperwork, long waits to access specialists, feeling undervalued, difficult patients, and medicolegal issues. Few training programs prepare their residents to effectively manage such common stressors in medical practice. However, on a more encouraging note, Shanafelt (2009: 1339) describes a number of studies showing how "enhancing meaning in work increases physician satisfaction and reduces burnout." One of these studies, involving an intensive 52-hour curriculum on mindfulness, had large and lasting improvements in burnout, mood disturbance, and attitudes associated with patient-centered care (Krasner *et al.*, 2009). Cassell (2013) describes his personal experience of discovering that getting closer to dying patients reduced the pain associated with their loss.

> I believe the answer is that my symptoms of the past and the distress so common in other physicians, and probably also in "burnout," do not come from being too close to patients, but by *not being close enough* . . . Whereas in other situations, in common with other clinicians, to avoid getting hurt I had always held back – even though I was not conscious of doing so. The pain of loss, I realized, was not a pain of loss it was a *pain or recrimination* for not doing as well by a patient as demanded by the ideal of physicianship. (2013: 187)

Several studies of substance use among medical students report worrisome levels of abuse. In a convenience sample of 16 US medical schools by Frank *et al.* (2008), 78% of medical students reported drinking alcohol in the past month and 34% drank excessively, and these proportions changed little over time. Of the excessive drinkers, 99% reported binge drinking at least once in the past month and 36% reported three or more binge episodes. Men were more than twice as likely to drink excessively. Students' perception of the importance of alcohol counseling for patients declined from 76% to 59% and only a quarter of final-year students routinely assessed their patients' drinking behavior.

In a survey at nine US medical schools, Roberts and colleagues (2001) found one-quarter of students suffered from symptoms of mental illness, including 7%–18% with substance abuse disorders. Ninety percent reported needing care for various health concerns, including 47% having at least one mental health or substance-related health issue. Although medical students recognize that medical education contributes to stress, they are reluctant to seek help. "Avoidance of appropriate help-seeking behaviour starts early and is linked to perceived norms which dictate that experiencing a mental health problem may be viewed as a form of weakness that has implications for subsequent career progression" (Chew-Graham *et al.*, 2003: 873). In a study of family practice residents, Hawk and Scott (1986: 82) reported that trying to balance both a professional life and personal life is the "most outstanding stress of all." Puddester and Edward (2008: 207) outline the importance of a formal program on wellness and coping strategies in medical school:

> While no program format has clearly been shown to be superior, most studies report multiple positive effects of formal programs, especially in those which involve students in the design and organization of the program. There needs to be more emphasis on caring for each other within the profession including instruction on how to be vigilant for colleagues under stress and how to care for physicians when they are one's patient. Students need to be formally taught about wellness and provided with coping strategies. Both the formal and informal curricula need to be consistent in emphasizing wellness, including systematic discouragement of and intolerance for student maltreatment. Finally, efforts to address the needs of physicians with disabilities and to protect those who seek help from professional and social stigma are necessary to ensure engagement of individuals at risk.

Although teachers should generally not take on the role of therapist with their students, they need to know when their students are struggling with personal issues that might be interfering with their learning, help them to recognize the problem, and direct them to appropriate professional care.

The Context (Opportunities and Constraints of the Learning Environment)

In addition to understanding the cognitive, developmental, and personal struggles of students, a whole-person approach requires the teacher to comprehend the student's learning context.

> In addition to the documented curriculum, students and teachers both become aware of the 'educational environment' or 'climate' of the institution. Is the teaching and learning environment very competitive? Is it authoritarian? Is the atmosphere in classes and field placements relaxed or is it in various ways stressful, perhaps even intimidating? These are all key questions in determining the nature of the learning experience. (Roff & McAleer, 2001: 333)

The environment of medical education strongly influences what can or will be learned. In the preclinical years of medical school, the course structure, content, and evaluation will steer students' learning. In clinical teaching, case mix, quality of teaching, and practice setting – inpatient, outpatient, primary, secondary, or tertiary – will be the principal influences. Three aspects of the clinical environment will influence the quality of the student's experience – the physical, emotional, and intellectual milieus.

1. *Physical environment*: in ambulatory teaching there should be enough space for students to see patients on their own, without slowing down the whole office, and space for private discussions and feedback between teacher and student. Patient volume and case mix should be adequate to achieve the educational objectives.

2. *Emotional climate*: students should feel safe. Although there will inevitably be some anxiety inherent in the nature of the work, and students need to feel challenged for optimal learning, students should not be placed in situations where patient safety is jeopardized. Their teachers should be excellent role models of patient-centered care, trained in best practices of clinical teaching and should include all members of an interprofessional team. Team members should interact effectively and demonstrate respectful communication. Teachers must be approachable, welcome questions from students, and provide frequent feedback to enhance learning. There should be enough continuity in the relationship between teacher and student to foster mutual respect and trust and opportunities to understand the specific learning needs of each student.

3. *Intellectual climate*: there should be time for reflection and discussion about patient care. Rapid access to learning resources such as the Internet is essential. All members of the team should model intellectual curiosity and ongoing learning from one another. It should be OK to say "I don't know" and use that as a springboard to further learning. General practice in the United Kingdom has pioneered the use of Significant Event Audit as a way for a team to review, analyze, and reflect on an incident that was "significant" to them – usually when something went wrong with patient care (Bowie & Pringle, 2008). It is an approach to learning from an event through a structured discussion by members of the whole health care team who had been involved in the event. Because such discussions can be sensitive and threatening, to use this approach successfully it is important to have strong team dynamics and good leadership (Bowie *et al.*, 2008).

It is important to remember that medical education is not just about learning a set of knowledge, skills, and attitudes; it is also about changing laypersons into physicians – a profound life-altering transformation, as we described in Chapter 8. The syllabus defines the course of study that students must digest but it does not describe the intimate personal interactions that bring about this important change. To understand how this occurs we need to examine medical school as a cultural institution.

Why do students concentrate on biomedicine and tend to disregard everything else? Where do they get the message that interviewing, medical humanities, and behavioral science are less important than traditional courses? Even in curricula that espouse a patient-centered mission, students do not take these subjects as seriously as the big biological courses. A key to understanding this puzzle is the environment for learning in medical school. One of the key features of the learning environment is the hidden curriculum, which reflects beliefs and values that may not support, and may even be at odds with, the official curriculum. The hidden curriculum is so influential because it is taught by example (Bandura, 1986). It is contagious – students "catch" the lessons of this tacit curriculum through immersion in the system especially through students' relationships with more senior learners and their preceptors. Because it is part of the unspoken culture of medical school, it is not subject to critical reflection but simply taken for granted (Hafferty, 1998; Margolis, 2001; Inui, 2003). The same phenomenon is found in all professional schools. Writing from the perspective of nursing, Bevis and Watson (2000: 75–6) describe the hidden curriculum in these terms:

> It is the curriculum in which we are unaware of the messages given by the way we teach, the priorities we set, the type of methods we use, and the way we interact with students. This is the curriculum of subtle socialization, of teaching initiates how to think and feel like nurses. It is the curriculum that covertly communicates priorities, relationships, and values. It colors perceptions, independence, initiative, caring, colleagueship, and the mores and folkways of being a nurse. It is taught by subtle, out-of-awareness things that pervade the whole educational environment: when classes are scheduled, how much time is given a subject in relationship to other subjects, how many test items are assigned a topic or whether or not a term paper is given to the area, who addresses whom in what way, how the teacher responds to students who openly differ in opinion from the teacher, how students are or are not encouraged to work together, and how teachers interact with students. All of these give the value messages to students that shape their learning in this curriculum.

Some of the lessons taught by the hidden curriculum:

- Biology trumps everything else – medicine is essentially applied biology.
- Behavioral issues are just "common sense" – it's not necessary to understand the sciences that explain behavior.
- The humanities are "nice to know" but can be ignored if time is needed to learn important subjects (and time is always needed for more important subjects).
- Feelings are dangerous and should be avoided in medical practice – they can lead to overinvolvement with patients and interfere with clinical reasoning.
- The more hours a subject has in the curriculum, the more important it is.
- Factual knowledge is more important than attitudes.
- Being able to recite the latest fact is more valued than a deep understanding of concepts.
- Acute care is more important than preventive or chronic care.

Coulehan (2006: 116) describes the necessity for role models to counter the negative influences of the hidden curriculum:

> The first requirement for a sea change . . . is to increase dramatically the number of role model physicians at every stage of medical education. By role model physicians I mean full-time faculty members who exemplify professional virtue in their interactions with patients, staff, and trainees; who have a broad, humanistic perspective; and who are devoted to teaching and willing to forego high income in order to teach. . . . Their presence would dilute and diminish the conflict between tacit and explicit values, especially in the hospital and clinic. The teaching environment would contain fewer hidden messages that say "Detach" while at the same time overt messages are saying "Engage." What trainees need is time and humanism.

One of the most disturbing and intractable problems in medical education is abuse of students and residents. Since the publication of Silver's (1982) article on medical student abuse 30 years ago, this "blight on the conscience of the profession" continues (Rees & Monrouxe, 2011: 1374). In one study, 72% of medical students reported at least one abusive experience, the most common being yelled at by faculty, residents, and other staff, reported by 54% of students (Kumar & Basu, 2000: 448). In a survey of students at 16 nationally representative US medical schools, 42% of seniors reported having experienced harassment, and 84%, belittlement during medical school. "Although few students characterised the harassment or belittlement as severe, poor mental health and low career satisfaction were significantly correlated with these experiences" (Frank *et al.*, 2006). Despite a 13-year effort to eliminate medical student abuse at the David Geffen School of Medicine at UCLA, more than half of the students still experienced some form of mistreatment during their clerkship, especially from residents and faculty. Although there was a decline, especially of verbal and power abuses, during the first 2 years of the study, there was no further decline after that. The authors suggest that the hidden curriculum, operating through role models, contributed to the persistence of abusive behavior. "In this context, the model 'see one, do one, teach one' could result in residents emulating inappropriate behaviors in their own teaching, perpetuating the widespread view that student mistreatment is a 'rite of passage'" (Fried *et al.*, 2012: 1197). Regrettably, mistreatment of learners continues into postgraduate education. In a survey of family medicine graduates from two postgraduate programs in Canada, 44.7% reported they had experienced intimidation, harassment, and/or discrimination during their 2-year residency program, most commonly verbal comments (94.3%) and punishment (27.6%) (Crutcher *et al.*, 2011).

The following incident, based on a true story, illustrates the type of harassment that remains all too common, despite numerous studies decrying such behavior by teachers. On her first day of clerkship, the medical student arrived on the ward for orientation to her inaugural rotation. While trying to introduce herself, she was initially ignored by the staff physician who was grilling the resident on the team. Finally, he turned in her direction and exclaimed sarcastically, "Oh . . . you're the 'clerkette'!" Turning back to the resident, he commented, "You'll find that clerkettes are all useless."

While the teacher's comment could be interpreted as a failed attempt at humor, most clerks would experience it as humiliating. Being in a one-down position on a new clinical team, just beginning clerkship, leaves the clerk with several unpleasant emotions – confusion, fear, anger, and perhaps even shame. If the student felt harassed by the teacher's comment, her situation is further complicated by having no recourse because of fear of retribution.

Since the well-publicized Libby Zion case (an 18-year-old patient who died in 1984 from serotonin syndrome misdiagnosed by residents exhausted by 18-hour shifts) there has been a steady attempt to reduce residents' work hours. This case drew widespread attention to the patient safety issues and adverse effects on residents of long shifts without sleep (Woodrow *et al.*, 2006). In the mid-1900s, residents and interns in the United States were on call for 36 hours starting every other night, totalling more than 100 hours per week. In 2011, the Accreditation Council for Graduate Medical Education restricted interns to 16-hour shifts and no more than 80 hours per week (Rosenbaum & Lamas, 2012). In Europe the restrictions on working hours are even stricter (Moonesinghe *et al.*, 2011). Studies on the impact of these changes are still limited and show mixed results (Institute of Medicine, 2009; Jamal *et al.*, 2011).

3. FINDING COMMON GROUND

The central purpose of the patient-centered clinical method is finding common ground – reaching an agreement with patients about the nature of their health problems, the goals of treatment, and a plan describing the roles and responsibilities of patient and clinician. Similarly, the central purpose of the learner-centered method is finding common ground – achieving a common understanding about the priorities for learning, co-planning how these goals will be achieved, and clarifying the roles and responsibilities of the teacher and learner. The other components of each model have inherent benefits; for example, as clinicians or teachers listen intently or share empathic comments, they will deepen their understanding of the other that may even have therapeutic or educational benefit. However, these other components are primarily in the service of reaching a shared decision about what is to be done to improve the patient's sense of wellness or the learner's growth and development as a clinician.

Establishing Priorities

Difficulties arise when there is a conflict between what a student wants to learn and what a teacher wants to teach. When the official curriculum reflects the realities of practice, rather than being a difficult hurdle for students to jump in order to "prove themselves," such conflict is less likely. Also, students may become frustrated when there are so many required competencies that there is no time left to address topics of particular interest or self-assessed need. A learner-centered approach does not hand over the curriculum to the students, but it does respect their intelligence, common sense, and good intentions by involving them in decisions about what to learn, when to learn it, how deeply to focus, and how to evaluate their learning. For example, the value of understanding the family situation of patients may only become relevant to students when they are faced with patients whose family dynamics are central to management.

Case Example

Raymond Zegers, a first-year resident in family medicine, had been an infrequent participant at behavioral science seminars. He argued that "most of this stuff is common sense and I need more time learning about heart failure and COPD [chronic obstructive pulmonary disease]." But then he met Pat! Pat was a 75-year-old crusty woman with metastatic lung cancer who challenged all of her health care providers. She seemed to anticipate rejection and was determined to reject them before they rejected her. Raymond could not understand why she insisted on being so difficult. Despite her rough edges, he liked her hard-nosed determination and stoicism. When he was discussing discharge plans with her, he learned that her family had sold all of her belongings and canceled the lease on her apartment. They had even sold off her clothes and jewelry. Raymond was furious at Pat's family and wondered how they could behave in such a cruel manner. He explored the family dynamics further and discovered that this was not the first time they had treated her this way. He started to understand why Pat kept people at a distance – it would be too dangerous to risk trusting anyone based on a lifetime of betrayal. The seminars on family dynamics started to have more interest for Raymond as he realized how a better understanding of family functioning could help him to provide better care to his patients.

In this case, the learner's struggle to help the patient led to his recognition of a need to learn more about family dynamics. Often, when patients are not doing well, learners blame themselves, even when they have provided appropriate care. As a result, the learner's priorities may be inaccurate. In these situations, the teacher may need to help the learner reflect on why he or she is feeling guilty and how this is affecting his or her management of the patient. The learner may need to concentrate on learning more about his or her feelings than solely about the biomedical topics the learner thinks he or she had missed. The following case illustrates how the teacher helped the resident get past the guilt that was blocking his awareness of the patient's primary needs.

Case Example

Stewart Zabian, a second-year family practice resident, after seeing his patient recovering in hospital from a myocardial infarct, wanted to focus his learning on the pharmacological management of cardiac risk factors. The resident had seen this patient in the office about a week before the infarct and wondered if he had missed some subtle warning signs. Stewart was determined to provide optimal care of his patient's cardiac problem and failed to recognize the major adjustment the patient was now experiencing. The initial reaction of his supervisor, Dr Leblanc, was to address the importance of understanding the patient's illness experience and the value of good communication in improving adherence and recovery. However, knowing that this might not match the resident's priorities, Dr Leblanc decided to explore the resident's experience with this patient. He discovered that Stewart felt somewhat guilty that he had not addressed all of his patient's risk factors before the infarct and was determined to make up for it now. Dr Leblanc asked Stewart to tell him more about the office visit – in hindsight, had he in fact missed anything important. Together, they reviewed the chart. The resident had checked the patient's blood pressure and ordered a serum cholesterol and asked about diet, exercise, and smoking. The patient had mentioned being more tired than usual but had no chest pain or shortness of breath. She was working longer hours than usual and her elderly mother was requiring more care, but she was planning to take a vacation in the near future. The resident agreed that a vacation would be a good idea and asked the patient to return in 3 months to see how she was doing. Dr Leblanc stated that he agreed with his assessment and plan and complimented him on his thorough review.

Dr Leblanc commented: "Even when we have done everything right, we can feel upset when things turn out badly for our patients. Our feelings may lead us to overreact by ordering too many tests or by not tending to the patient's other needs. You are feeling badly for your patient's predicament. I wonder how she is feeling about her current situation?" By supporting Stewart, Dr Leblanc modeled the kind of concern he hoped the resident would demonstrate with his patient. This encouraged Stewart to recognize that his preoccupation with the biomedical issues was related to vague feelings of guilt and to realize that the patient would benefit from a discussion of her personal reaction to her serious illness.

Teaching and Learning Methods

There are several studies defining the characteristics of excellent clinical teaching that support the use of a learner-centered approach (Heidenreich *et al.*, 2000; Bain, 2004; Kilminster *et al.*, 2007b; Yeates *et al.*, 2008; Sutkin *et al.*, 2008; Farnan *et al.*, 2010; Skeff & Stratos, 2010). Whether done from the point of view of learners or teachers, or both, these studies agree that clinical teachers should demonstrate the following points.

- *Clinical competence*, including demonstrating good skills, procedures and patient-care abilities. They have a humanistic orientation, stressing the social and psychological aspects of patient care. They possess an excellent fund of knowledge and are able to present information in a clear and well-organized fashion. They are prepared to share with students their struggles and success with patients as a model of continuing learning.

- *Enthusiasm for teaching.* They obviously enjoy associating with students and make themselves accessible to them.
- *Supervisory skills.* They are sensitive to patient and student needs simultaneously and involve students actively in patient care and in their own learning. Students particularly value being given increasing patient responsibility as their skills improve (Alguire *et al.*, 2008). They provide clear and appropriate direction and give frequent constructive feedback. Helpful feedback is the teacher's description of students' effective and ineffective behaviors that shows them how to improve their ineffective behaviors (*see* the outline of constructive feedback in Chapter 11). They emphasize problem solving by challenging students to discuss their thinking processes and give students an opportunity to practise skills and procedures. They are open to criticism from students, using it to enhance mutual learning.
- *Effective interpersonal skills.* They are sensitive to student concerns, such as feelings of inadequacy, and demonstrate a genuine interest in students through a friendly manner. Whenever possible, they build the self-esteem of students. In an excellent text on collaborative clinical education, Westberg and Jason (1993) describe the qualities of helpful teacher-learner relationships. Particularly effective are collaborative relationships that foster independence:

> learners are seen as valuable contributors to the teaching-learning partnership and are encouraged to be as actively involved as possible in their learning: generating learning goals, devising strategies for meeting their goals, critiquing and monitoring their progress. Collaborative teachers do not immediately force learners to function as self-directed learners if the learners are not ready for this role. Rather, they start where the learners are and help them become increasingly more independent. (1993: 92–3)

Roles of Teacher and Learner

McKeachie's (1978) outline of teachers' roles helps us understand the many and varied responsibilities of teachers. On the one hand, teachers function as facilitator, ego ideal, and person; they support and encourage students by the force of their own personality. Students incorporate aspects of their teachers into their own developing professional identity and often form close personal relationships with them. On the other hand, teachers are experts, formal authorities, and socializing agents; they are guardians of the traditions of the profession and stand as trustees who decide whether or not each student measures up for admission into the ranks. In this sense, no matter what else they represent in the minds of their students, they are powerful and sometimes intimidating authority figures. Thus, teachers wear many hats and have complex multidimensional relationships with their students. Similar challenges have been described in nursing. Clinical instructors are

> mentors who role model, counsel, and guide students; they are directors who take charge and direct the actions of the students. They are also monitors who evaluate and mark the students; they are brokers who liaison between staff and students and academia and practice. (Barry, 2006: 1)

Harden and Crosby (2000) describe 12 roles of the teacher. There are six main roles – (1) information provider, (2) role model, (3) facilitator, (4) assessor, (5) planner, and (6) resource developer – and each of these six roles represents two roles, to make a total of 12. For example, the information provider is both a lecturer and a clinical or practical teacher; the facilitator is both a learning facilitator and a mentor; the assessor is both a student assessor and a curriculum assessor. The authors acknowledge that few teachers can accomplish all roles. In fact, some roles may be in conflict with others. Cavalcanti and Detsky (2011) explain why coaches cannot be judges. The dual role makes it difficult for trainees to seek help in areas where they feel weak for fear of receiving a negative evaluation. As a result, the supervisor may have to guess about their learning needs. In addition, evaluators, as coaches, have a vested interest in the success of their trainees, thus making it less likely they will notice their trainees' deficiencies.

4. ENHANCING THE LEARNER-TEACHER RELATIONSHIP

The relational nature of good teaching is captured by Palmer (2007: 74–5):

> Most important, I learn that my gift as a teacher is the ability to dance with my students, to co-create with them a context in which all of us can teach and learn, and that this gift works as long as I stay open and trusting and hopeful about who my students are.

In a comprehensive review of the role of teacher-learner relationships in medical education, Tiberius *et al.* (2002: 463) conclude: "teacher-learner relationships have an enormous impact on the quality of teaching and learning. By some estimates the teacher-learner relationship explains roughly half of the variance in the effectiveness of teaching." In a list of influences on student achievement, Hattie (2012) places teacher-student relationships near the top with an effect size* of 0.72 based on over 900 meta-analyses. Other interventions with a similar effect size include classroom discussion (0.82), teacher clarity (0.75), and feedback (0.75). Good teachers have a desire to help their students learn which transcends the challenges that teaching creates. Teaching may interfere with clinicians' intimate one-to-one relationships with their patients. It slows them down. It exposes their weaknesses and areas of ignorance. Thus it demands a positive regard and caring for learners even when their behavior may frustrate or upset the teacher. It is essential that clinical teachers "walk the talk" – there must be congruence between the patient-centered clinical method and the process of teaching it. For example, just as patient-centered care must always be provided as part of a healing relationship, so too teaching should be in the context of care for the learner as a developing clinician and not just for their knowledge base. This commitment transcends individual learning problems or specific skills to be learned. It extends into the very being of the learners and challenges them to stretch themselves to their limits. Such learning may require students to experience painful self-discovery or to make difficult personal changes.

Case Example

Brigit Jansen had wanted to be a child psychiatrist since her youth. She had loved caring for young children and had served as an aide at a children's psychiatric facility during her teens. Brigit had also battled with bulimia throughout her late teens and early twenties; hence she was very familiar with the process of psychotherapy. Upon completion of her Bachelor of Education at the age of 22, Brigit decided to apply to medical school. It had been an uphill battle conquering the basic sciences she lacked in her undergraduate education and keeping her bulimia at bay. However, she had succeeded and now was embarking on her child psychiatry residency. Brigit was both excited and anxious. She was eager to work with the younger

---

*   Effect size = Average (post-test) – average (pre-test) / Spread (standard deviation)
     Effect size is a standardized approach to measuring the effectiveness of an educational intervention. An effect size greater than 0.4 is considered worthwhile.

children but doubted how she might relate to the adolescents, particularly the females who would have an eating disorder like hers. Yet as time went by Brigit became both skilled and assured in her work with adolescents. It was not until her rotation on the inpatient adolescent unit when she was assigned two seriously ill patients with eating disorders that she began to question her ability to work with this patient population. Their issues were too close to her own and she struggled to keep clear what were their issues and what were her own demons.

Dr Tillman had been her supervisor and mentor since Brigit had joined the residency program. While she had not disclosed her bulimia to him, she realized that it was time to share this information. Her own personal problems were beginning to affect her ability to care for her patients.

What allowed Brigit to expose her feelings about this situation was the trust, respect, and safety that she experienced in the learner-teacher relationship with Dr Tillman. She knew from her past experiences with him that he would not judge her past behavior or question her current situation. He would listen and be there for her. Dr Tillman would invite her "to wonder" what might be causing her present difficulty and how she would overcome this problem. He would respect the boundaries of the learner-teacher relationship. He would not become her therapist but remain her teacher all the while knowing when referral for further professional counseling would be important for Brigit, both personally and professionally.

Students will often defend against such self-awareness and may find themselves in conflict with their teachers over the need for change. At this stage in the development of their professional identity they often experience ambivalent feelings about their teachers: on the one hand they wish for a dependent relationship where their obligations are spelled out and clearly limited; on the other hand, they resent the imposition of control and long for independent responsibility. Their feelings may vacillate from one extreme to the other depending on the complexity and volume of patient care, fatigue, and feelings of self-efficacy. It is not surprising that intense emotions may develop in the student-teacher relationship replicating similar feelings with other powerful authority figures from the student's past. Working through this transference may enhance the student's self-understanding and prevent similar reactions from occurring in the future. It requires the development of an intimate and trust-based relationship before such intensely personal learning and growth can occur. Continuity in their relationship is the basis for establishing trust and for developing the deep understanding necessary for helping students develop as healers. These decisive personal and contextual issues, so critical in determining what will be learned, and how the teacher can help, cannot be easily communicated from one teacher to another. Supervision of psychotherapists shares many similarities with clinical teaching especially regarding the importance of the relationship between teacher and learner. Alonso (1985: 47–8) summarizes this aspect as follows:

> the development of a clinician from novice to expert is primarily an emotional, maturational process, much like the development of a child from infancy to adulthood . . . It is assumed that a transference relationship will develop between therapist and supervisor and that this transferential field will become a primary vehicle for influencing the student's clinical growth . . . there is a concerted effort to shore up and strengthen the supervisee's healthiest defences, either by reducing the ambiguity or by helping the trainee to tolerate the inevitable confusion of clinical work . . . When difficulty occurs . . . this regression is seen as a healthy and expectable rite of passage . . . In fact, the clinician who never regresses in the course of training is probably avoiding the more difficult levels of learning that occur in the unconscious merger of patient/therapist and may be keeping too great a distance between self and patient.

There are a number of teacher behaviors that contribute to the creation of an impasse with their learners: the need to be admired; the need to rescue; the need to be in control; the need for competition; the need to be loved; the need to work through unresolved prior conflict in the supervisor's own training experience; spillover from stress in the personal or professional life of the supervisor; tension between supervisor and the administration of the institution (Alonso, 1985: 83–104). This highlights the importance of a healthy and open relationship between teachers and learners characterized by empathy, genuineness, and positive regard (Rogers, 1951). Tiberius (1993–94: 3) describes the central role of relationships in teaching and learning:

> The relationship between teachers and learners can be viewed as a set of filters, interpretive screens or expectations that determine the effectiveness of interaction between teacher and student. Effective teachers form relationships that are trustful, open and secure, that involve a minimum of control, are cooperative, and are conducted in a reciprocal, interactive manner. They share control with students and encourage interactions that are determined by mutual agreement. . . . Within such relationships learners are willing to disclose their lack of understanding rather than hide it from their teachers; learners are more

attentive, ask more questions, are more actively engaged. Thus, the better the relationship, the better the interaction; the better the interaction, the better the learning.

CONCLUSION

In this chapter we have described the four components of the learner-centered method of education illustrating the many parallels with the patient-centered clinical method. Key points from this chapter are as follows.

- It is important to include learners' ideas and aspirations about what they wish to learn into all educational planning. Incorporating knowledge of learners' strengths, weaknesses, and special interests improves motivation, accelerates the learning process, and increases the potential depth and complexity of the competencies that can be mastered.
- There are two dimensions of understanding the student as a whole person: the student's life history, including personal and cognitive development, and the learning environment. Becoming a physician is a life-altering process, not just the accumulation of competencies. Stress, burnout, and mistreatment can all interfere with learning. The hidden curriculum can have a greater impact on learning than the official curriculum and sometimes it teaches a contrary lesson.
- There are three key elements in finding common ground in the learner-centered approach: (1) establishing priorities, (2) choosing appropriate teaching-learning methods, and (3) determining the roles of both teacher and learner. When teachers and learners collaborate in identifying goals and selecting learning experiences, students are more likely to be successful.
- The way teachers relate to learners will influence the way in which learners interact with patients and is central to their development as effective healers. The relationship between teachers and learners is the dominant influence in creating an effective environment for learning and development.

Being There: Case Illustrating Being Learner-Centered
Christine Rivet and Judith Belle Brown

It was Monday, a beautiful September morning when Grace, our team nurse, called me at home. She told me that my resident Sam and his wife, Helena, had just had a baby girl. But it didn't make sense – her voice was muted, unreal. "Chris, she's just beautiful. I was just at the hospital with them." Was it the shock that made her voice sound that way? It just didn't match the horror of what she was saying. Did I miss something? Was she really saying that their baby was dead?

"I think you should go over to the hospital." *No, I can't; I can't do it. Don't ask me that. I'm just his supervisor. I don't even know him that well.* He was a first-year resident from a small northern community. New to town. No family here. "You know they don't have any family or close friends here in town. Their parents haven't arrived yet." Sam had been an engineer before going into medicine. A nice guy just a few years younger than me. *What can I do? I certainly can't replace his parents or family.*

I had only met Helena a couple of times at some family medicine outings and she was very thin, shy, and delicate. She and Sam had been trying to start a family for several years. Finally Helena was pregnant and everything was going well. Sam was thrilled: even though he was off service he would drop into the family medicine center and describe the progress of her pregnancy. Last week he had told me she was 37 weeks pregnant.

"Chris?"

"What happened? I thought her pregnancy was going so well."

"I don't know. Helena stopped feeling movement and they did an ultrasound on Friday that showed that the baby had died." *They had known for 2 days?! How could they live through this?*

The hospital was only a 5-minute walk away. When I got up to the maternity floor, I walked down a long hallway to the reception where a nurse was sitting. An unfamiliar setting since I don't do obstetrics. "I'm Dr Rivet. I've been told that Sam and Helena Howell are here and that their baby has died." *I don't belong here. Don't let me go to see them. I shouldn't be allowed. I'm just his supervisor. Not family or close friend. And what can I do to help in such a tragedy?* "Yes, I'll take you. It's just down this hallway." My heart was pounding. What could I say or do? I have three young children. I can't imagine anything more horrible than losing one of my children. *I have no solutions for them – no words of comfort.*

Helena was lying in bed, her face frail and blank. There was a nurse near her and there was Sam standing in the corner. He was holding their baby in his arms wrapped like all newborns in a cocoon of blankets. He came toward me crying. "Would you like to hold her?" *No I couldn't do it. The blankets look like the blankets around all the other newborns I have ever seen but this baby is dead! I can't hold this baby.* But I nodded yes. And there she was in my arms. As light as a feather. A beautiful baby. Perfect face. Her eyes were closed. She was swaddled in so many blankets that I couldn't feel the cold of her body. *The nurses must do that intentionally.* Her skin must have been cyanotic but in my memory this baby is pink like all newborns. *I wish I could do something to help you but I'm overwhelmed by your tragedy.* Then I started to weep as I looked down at their baby.

The expression "just being there" for our patients evokes this tragic event during my early days of being a supervisor. My situation as a supervisor is not unique. All supervisors have been somehow involved in very personal life events of their residents: the sudden death of a parent, severe depression, the breakdown of a marriage. This experience demonstrates the challenges we face when we go beyond the conventional learner-teacher relationship. Yet, if we are seeking to teach our students how to extend their relationship with patients beyond the narrow biomedical approach then we must model this behavior.

10 Challenges in Learning and Teaching the Patient-Centered Clinical Method

W Wayne Weston and Judith Belle Brown

In the previous chapter, describing the learner-centered method of education, we outlined a framework for teachers applying this approach to teaching. In this chapter we present some of the common challenges faced by those who strive to learn, teach, and practice the patient-centered clinical method. In Chapter 11 we will provide practical, hands-on teaching tips to assist teachers at all levels of education.

Teaching and learning the patient-centered clinical method is demanding for many reasons. First, we will describe issues related to the nature of clinical practice and patient-practitioner communication; second, we will elaborate on challenges specific to being a teacher of the patient-centered clinical method.

THE UNRECOGNIZED COMPLEXITY OF PATIENT-PRACTITIONER COMMUNICATION

Students and clinicians have been talking all their lives; it feels natural and seems easy. Consequently, some students think they do not need any instruction on communication. And, once they have learned the basics, most students, especially postgraduate students, feel that further instruction on communication is a waste of time. They have failed to realize the complexity of patient-practitioner communication.

> Communication is a little like sex. It is a normal function and most of us think we are good at it and some are, but many aren't. Superior clinical communication is a learned skill. Speaking with patients, families, and colleagues calls for a studied blend of selective curiosity, quiet intensity, and the ability to attend to what is *not* being said. (Taylor, 2010: 53)

Communication skills are usually taught in the first 2 years of medical school, often as part of a clinical skills course, where students also learn history taking and physical examination skills. In recent years, communication courses include practice with simulated patients and, by the time they reach clerkship, most students have acquired basic skills for engaging with real patients. However, the clinical setting is more complex and unpredictable than the well-organized and structured communication lab; not only must students concentrate on applying good communication techniques such as open-ended inquiry, active listening, and empathy but also they must gather a comprehensive medical history, conduct an accurate physical examination, consider the differential diagnosis, and, together with the patient, develop a tentative plan of management. And real patients are sick – often very sick! Their illnesses may make it hard for them to provide clear answers to the student's many questions and may diminish their capacity to engage in a dialogue about treatment choices. It is not surprising that the lessons learned in the communication lab do not transfer easily to the clinical setting.

Kurtz *et al.* (2003, 2005) point out that there are three broad categories of communication skills (content, process, and perceptual skills) that students must learn to integrate when they interact with patients.

- Content skills are *"what health care professionals communicate"* – they include taking a history, conducting the functional inquiry, and performing the physical examination. They also include exploration of the patient's illness experience and finding common ground.
- Process skills are *"how they do it"* – how they build their relationship with the patient and how they provide structure to the interview. This includes the way they ask questions (whether open-ended or closed) as well as non-verbal communication, and how they pick up on patient cues. Finally, it addresses the strategies they use to attend to the flow of the interview and make the organization of the interview overt.
- Perceptual skills are *"what they are thinking and feeling"* – the intrapersonal aspects of the interaction. They include clinical reasoning skills, thoughts, and feelings for and about the patient and also include student's values, beliefs, and biases related to the patient, and awareness of distractions. This category has been expanded by the Canadian Communication Working Group to include personal qualities of the physician (authenticity, commitment, integrity, trust, and trustworthiness) that are foundational to effective interactions with patients. (Canadian Communication Working Group, 2013)

According to cognitive load theory, performance degrades when the learner is overloaded (Paas *et al.*, 2003, 2004). Cognitive load theory assumes that working memory is limited – humans can attend to only a limited number of concepts at once (Miller, 1956). An expert has learned to "chunk" concepts together to free up space in working memory, but the novice is still struggling to know what goes together. For example, a novice has a hard enough time simply attending to all the elements of the functional inquiry until, with repeated practice, they can perform without referring to a checklist. Each element of the three broad categories of communication skills is gradually mastered, separate from the others, with repetition. However, in the fast-paced and messy setting of clinical practice, even an experienced clinician can become overwhelmed by the multiple factors that must be considered simultaneously. Imagine an office visit in which the patient says to her physician: "I'm really concerned about this chest pain I've been having." And then she places her fist against her chest and the clinician notices a tear in her eye. At the same time, he hears a knock on the office door. How does the physician decide whether to first address the chest pain: "What does it feel like, how long does it last, what makes it better or worse? Are you having pain right now?" Or perhaps it would be better to explore her mood: "You seem upset; can you tell me about it?" And what about the distracting knock on the door? How can the physician handle that without losing this special moment in the interview? To top it off, he realizes he is already 20 minutes behind in his schedule and he promised to attend his son's football game after school.

Communication training focuses on one component at a time and provides opportunities to practice and receive feedback. Thus, students are able to learn the skills for taking a medical history and the process of interviewing. In some programs they will explore their personal reactions to patients and to being clinicians. Smith *et al.*, (1999) explored the importance of developing learners' awareness of interfering emotions and beliefs. For example, believing that emotions are harmful and should be avoided in medical interviews, or feeling that all interruptions are rude, that clinicians should remain in control of the interview at all times, or believing that clinicians should carefully keep their distance from patients. These beliefs could prevent clinicians from exploring difficult or painful issues, make it harder for patients to express their opinions and result in a cold interaction between clinician and patient. Novack *et al.* (1997) describe several strategies to "calibrate" physicians by enhancing personal awareness – "insight into how one's life experiences and emotional make-up affect one's interactions with patients, families, and other professionals" (1997: 502). Strategies include regular or even impromptu support group discussions, Balint groups, family-of-origin group discussions, literature in medicine discussion groups, personal awareness groups, and behavioral science/interpersonal skills curricula. Halpern (2007: 698) describes how physicians can learn to empathize with patients even when they are in conflict by "an ongoing practice of engaged curiosity. Activities that can help in this process include meditation, sharing stories with colleagues, writing about doctoring, reading books, and watching films conveying emotional complexity." Often the personal qualities, described here earlier under perceptual skills, are taught in courses on professionalism. Clinical reasoning, if it is taught at all, is usually addressed in a separate course or left to the clerkship or residency. Rarely is there time for, or attention given to, integration of all three sets of skills. As a result, students adopt a survival strategy to avoid being overwhelmed by the complexity of the patient-physician encounter; they focus on conducting a good history and establishing a credible diagnosis and appropriate management plan. It is during their clinical training where students and residents need more guidance in learning to integrate the three categories of communication skills. It is ironic that, when they need it most, so little has been offered to students after the first 2 years of medical school.

This gap is now being recognized and training is offered beyond the pre-clerkship years in some schools. Deveugele and colleagues (2005) describe a communication program in Belgium that spans all years of the undergraduate curriculum using video demonstrations, paper cases, small group discussion, and role-play with colleague students and simulated patients. Students with difficulties are identified early and provided with remediation. The key elements taught are based on the Calgary-Cambridge Guides (Silverman *et al.*, 2004). Kalet and colleagues (2004) describe the Macy Initiative, a collaborative project in three US medical schools to teach communication skills to clinical clerks. Each school tailored its curriculum to its own needs and resources. All made use of simulated patients for practicing the skills. At Case Western Reserve University, each clerkship rotation concentrated on specific communication topics – for example, surgery focused on shared and informed decision making; medicine and family medicine, on screening for addiction and chronic pain; obstetrics and gynecology, on domestic violence. A controlled study, using a 10-station Objective Structured Clinical Examination before and after the intervention, showed a significant improvement in communication skills at all three schools. Janicik and colleagues (2007) developed a communication skills curriculum in the Internal Medicine clerkship, as part of the Macy Initiative, at the New York University School of Medicine consisting of four 2-hour structured bedside rounds. Each session focused on a challenging communication issue (alcohol-related problems, different cultures, difficult patients, and terminally ill patients) and included a discussion of the topic followed by an interview with a real patient and ending with a debriefing. Students appreciated the bedside format because it taught them practical skills for caring for the patients they saw during their clerkship. Van Weel-Baumgarten and colleagues (2013), in Nijmegen, the Netherlands, developed a program to integrate communication and consultation skills. Unlike many schools, the undergraduate curriculum in Nijmegen delays teaching communication skills until near the end of the preclinical years and continues training throughout the 3 clinical years. The educational rationale was:

1. to introduce communication skills not as a separate skill but integrated with medical content;
2. to provide training just before each clerkship starts, so students can immediately practice what they have learned during training ('just in time learning'); and
3. to reinforce and further develop communication skills throughout their clinical training. (2013: 178)

Each clinical block in the curriculum included 1–4 weeks of preparation for the types of patients the students were likely to observe and participate in caring for on that rotation and ended with a 1-week classroom-based session where students reflected on issues raised during that block. Students had opportunities to practice communication and consultation skills with simulated patients focused on the clinical conditions relevant to each discipline-based block. In the surgical block, students learned their suturing skills on a simulated "bleeding" head wound in a wig the simulated patient was wearing while they practiced their skills of reassuring an anxious patient and explaining what they were doing. Ninety-eight percent of students agreed, "It is important that communication is taught integrated with medical content" (2013: 180).

Wouda and van de Wiel (2013: 51) express doubt that "expertise in professional communication can be fully attained during medical training." There are many reasons for this, including lack of curriculum time devoted to communication and the complexity of the skills to be learned. They refer to the seminal work on the development of expertise by Ericsson (Ericsson, 2008; Ericsson *et al.*, 1993) and suggest that it is only after years of practice that physicians can master the full spectrum of communication skills. In deliberate practice, unlike the way most people practice, students must avoid rote learning or settling into a comfortable routine and they must set themselves new goals that raise the bar on their abilities. They must force themselves to reflect on their performance and continually strive for improvement. The learning conditions for deliberate practice are:

(a) clear and comprehensive objectives about which skills have to be learned and how to teach them in simulated consultations, (b) stimulating learning tasks of short duration with opportunities for immediate feedback, reflection and corrections, (c) ample opportunities for repetition and gradual refinements of performance, (d) possibilities for individual students to rehearse their existing skills frequently in different sorts of consultations and to acquire new skills in challenging consultations of an increasing complexity, and (e) transfer of the learned skills into real life consultations/clinical practice. (Wouda & van de Wiel, 2012: 61)

However, if students fail to recognize the importance of learning more about communication skills, they are unlikely to exert the effort needed.

THE NATURE OF CLINICAL PRACTICE

Clinical practice often seems arduous enough when limited to the diagnosis and treatment of disease; suggesting to clinicians that they must also consider patients' perspectives on their health and illness experience, as well as the social context in which patients live their lives, may seem overwhelming. This is especially true for young clinicians who are struggling to learn their craft. Several characteristics of practice pose difficulties for learning. Hippocrates commented on this 2000 years ago in his aphorism: "Life is short and the Art long; the occasion fleeting; experience fallacious, and judgment difficult" (Adams, 1985: 697). The long hours, lack of sleep, and the personally draining nature of patient care often leave students and practitioners exhausted and emotionally spent. Physicians, in this state, may have little energy to invest in learning to be patient-centered. In the long run, we argue, patient-centered care is more rewarding for both doctors and patients. However, when doctors are harried, they are tempted to focus narrowly on the patient's presenting complaint alone and to end the visit quickly by ignoring any other concerns the patient may have. When doctors appear rushed, patients may collude in this approach by keeping their worries to themselves. This may reinforce some physicians' beliefs that most patients are primarily interested in quick solutions (Brown *et al.*, 2002).

Although there are undeniable time pressures in practice, sometimes clinicians are caught up in "busy work" to avoid the emotional demands of practice. Without a commitment to continuing personal growth and self-awareness, practitioners may not confront the reasons for their avoidance. The following case serves as an example.

Case Example

Michael Wong, a first-year internal medicine resident, described his discomfort with the recent death of his patient. He found the experience painful because, in spending time with the patient, he had developed a relationship. Unlike the deaths of other patients who had remained strangers, this patient's death touched him deeply. Michael almost wished he had not become attached and was ambivalent about allowing himself to become vulnerable again. This experience was a turning point in his education; the opportunity to discuss his feelings with his peers and teachers helped him to accept his pain as a necessary part of his learning and growth. Michael realized that protecting himself from further painful experiences, by avoiding getting to know his patients, would rob him of one of the most valued aspects of practice. He also recognized that his relationship with the patient was the most helpful element of his care.

DISCOMFORT WITH FINDING COMMON GROUND

In disease-centered interviews, doctors simplify their patients' problems by reducing them to disease categories. The focus is on the problem, not the person; the personal, social, and cultural contexts seem irrelevant to the physician's central mission of diagnosis and cure. Another way in which the interview is simplified is for both doctor and patient to agree that the doctor is in charge. The roles of doctor and patient are clear and distinct; the doctor's task is to make a diagnosis and to tell the patient what to do to recover and the patient's job is to comply with the "doctor's orders." Patient-centered interviews may be more complicated. Not only are doctors looking for disease but also they are actively seeking to comprehend their patients' suffering; in addition, doctors are striving to determine the extent to which patients wish to be involved in the decisions about what should be done and seeking to understand their preferences. Physicians may be reluctant to enquire about their patients' expectations for fear it might take too much time or they will ask for something that the doctor disagrees with; they are uncomfortable with confrontation and saying no and usually have not received any training in how to handle disagreements effectively. Also, discussing the pros and cons of different treatment options is complicated. Both doctors and patients have trouble understanding the meaning of the numbers associated with different options and their consequences, thus making it difficult to discuss the risks and benefits of different treatment choices. Gaissmaier and Gigerenzer (2008: 412) referred to this as "collective statistical illiteracy." In addition, if clinicians acquiesce to the patient's wishes and a poor outcome ensues, they worry about the threat of lawsuits. Doctors tend to see such disagreements as win-lose situations, where one opinion must prevail, rather than potential win-win situations where the ideas of both may lead to a more creative solution, especially when the textbook answer may not be the best response for the unique circumstances of the individual patient.

Physicians and patients seem to be ambivalent about shared decision making. Even in studies where physicians did not share information with patients, patients were very satisfied with their care. For example, in a study of Israeli hospitalized patients, only 39%–60% recalled receiving explanations about the risks of invasive procedures and only 8%–40% remembered a discussion about alternative options. However, 80% of patients rated overall satisfaction with decision making as good or very good (Brezis *et al.*, 2008). This might be explained by patients' lack of experience with shared decision making – having never experienced it, they would not know what they were missing. Until recently, most physicians were not trained in engaging patients in shared decision making and felt uncomfortable changing their usual practice. In a systematic review of interventions to enhance shared decision making in routine clinical practice, Légaré *et al.* (2012) found 21 studies in which only three described the professionals' adoption of shared decision making as reported by their patients. Only when the interventions included both physicians and patients did the patients report changes – that is, training physicians how to share decisions with patients, and providing tools (such as decision aids) for patients that help them sort out their options. There are a number of models for shared decision making worth studying. Towle and Godolphin (1999) point out that, since shared decision making involves both patient and physician, each must bring a set of skills into their interaction. They provide a list of competencies for both physicians and patients. Elwyn *et al.* (2012) provide a model for shared decision making divided into three steps: (1) choice talk, (2) option talk, and (3) decision talk. Légaré *et al.* (2011) describe an interprofessional model of shared decision making developed through consensus by a group of 11 team members from Canada, the United Kingdom, and the United States including four nurses, three physicians, a dietician, a psychologist, an anthropologist, and a community health specialist.

It may be particularly difficult for young physicians, still struggling to develop their self-confidence as professionals, to share power with their patients. The following example illustrates some of the challenges in finding common ground.

Case Example

Melvin Langer, aged 42, presented to Rebecca Bridge, a second-year family medicine resident, convinced that he had been misdiagnosed. At his last appointment at the clinic 2 weeks previously, he complained of symptoms similar to what he experienced with Graves' disease 10 years ago. He was adamant that this was a recurrence of his hyperthyroidism. However, he had been treated with radioactive iodine at the time of his diagnosis of Graves' disease and his most recent thyroid-stimulating hormone blood test was consistent with hypothyroidism. Based on this, Dr Bridge had diagnosed hypothyroidism and gave him a prescription for an increased dose of levothyroxine. On this follow-up visit, Dr Bridge was surprised by Mr Langer's agitation. He was normally a very pleasant and humorous individual but today he appeared angry and frustrated. When she inquired how he was doing on the increased thyroid medication, he retorted, "Not well at all! I'm feeling the same as I did when I had Graves' disease. I am convinced I have too much thyroid, not too little, so I did not take the new pills." Dr Bridge felt herself getting annoyed and defensive. She felt she had provided correct advice based on a careful assessment of his medical condition and thought to herself, "My treatment was appropriate; I don't know how I can handle his anger and noncompliance." Feeling at a loss, she consulted her preceptor. Recognizing her frustration with this patient, the preceptor helped her understand that the most important issue was the patient's conviction that the diagnosis was wrong. Until that was addressed, trying to change Mr Langer's mind about management would be futile. Resuming her interview with Mr Langer, Dr Bridge acknowledged that she had not fully explored his understanding of his symptoms. As she listened carefully to his explanation, Mr Langer became remarkably calmer. As they explored the conflict between his lab results and his symptoms, Mr Langer mentioned that he was taking diet pills that he ordered on the Internet. Dr Bridge wondered if the symptom of feeling "revved up" might be related to an unknown ingredient in the diet pills. Together they developed a plan for management over the next week. Because Mr Langer was reluctant to take an increased dose of his levothyroxine, Dr Bridge agreed that he would continue the lower dose of thyroid medication and would repeat his thyroid-stimulating hormone blood test in a week. As well, Mr Langer would discontinue his diet pills. Having now established a trusting relationship they were able to agree on a management plan.

NEED FOR SELF-AWARENESS

McWhinney (1996: 436) challenges medicine to become a self-reflective discipline:

> We can only attend to a patient's feelings and emotions if we know our own, but self-knowledge is neglected in medical education, perhaps because the path to this knowledge is so long and hard. Egoistic emotions often come disguised as virtues and we all have a great capacity for self-deception. But there are pathways to this knowledge and medical education could find a place for them. Could medicine become a self-reflective discipline? The idea may seem preposterous. Yet I think it must, if we are to be healers as well as competent technologists . . . The fault line runs through the affect-denying clinical method which dominates the modern medical school. Not until this is reformed will emotions and relationships have the place in medicine they deserve. Finally, to become self-reflective, medicine will have to go through a huge cultural change. In these changes, general practice is already some distance along the way. The importance of being different is that we can lead the way.

Clinicians who explore patients' cues to personal problems quickly find themselves discussing intensely intimate issues. When confronted with having a serious illness, patients often wonder about its meaning for them and their families. For example, it may raise fundamental questions such as: "Why me?" or "What will happen to my children if I die?" Other patients may present with symptoms that reflect their concerns about their relationships or employment. These situations may trigger questions and feelings in practitioners' minds related to their own current relationships or to unresolved issues from their families of origin. As a result, young clinicians, with little life experience, may be overwhelmed by their feelings and thus distance themselves for self-protection. Additionally, they may form relationships with some patients that unconsciously replicate troubled relationships from their past; without insight the practitioner is likely to become entangled in the same difficulties.

Because the patient-provider relationship is so intensely personal, such difficulties are inevitable at times. Students and young clinicians need opportunities to develop self-awareness. These issues must be addressed with sensitivity by the teacher, taking into consideration the student's level of comfort in discussing his or her feelings. Often this can be done in a small group, such as a Balint group (Balint, 2000; Kjeldmand *et al.*, 2004) so that all students learn from one another's insights; but sometimes this may be too threatening or overwhelming. Opportunities for one-to-one discussion also need to be available. Another approach to self-awareness is the use of narrative, as described in Chapter 8. Self-awareness is an important aspect of what Epstein (1999) describes as mindful practice. He outlines five forms of self-awareness:

> Intrapersonal self-awareness helps the physician be conscious of his or her strengths, limitations, and sources of professional satisfaction . . . Interpersonal self-awareness . . . allows physicians to see themselves as they are seen by others and helps to establish satisfactory interpersonal relationships with colleagues, patients, and students . . . Self-awareness of learning needs allows physicians to recognize areas of unconscious incompetence and to develop a means to achieving their learning goals. Ethical self-awareness is the moment-to-moment cognizance of values that are shaping medical encounters. Technical self-awareness is necessary for self-correction during procedures such as the physical examination, surgery, computer operations, and communication. (1999: 836)

He goes on to discuss the implications for teachers: "The teacher's task is to invoke a state of mindfulness in the learner, and, thus, the teacher can only act as a guide, not a transmitter of knowledge" (Epstein, 1999: 838). Kern and colleagues (2001) describe the importance of powerful experiences, which evoke strong feelings, as a stimulus for personal growth particularly if they are accompanied by introspection, a helping relationship, or both.

> Powerful experiences occur commonly in medicine but may lack optimal conditions for personal growth. To promote practitioner personal growth, medical settings may wish to explore methods to promote introspection, helping relationships, and the acknowledgement of powerful experiences when they occur. (2001: 97)

Despite the perceived importance of self-assessment during medical education and for the maintenance of competence after graduation, several studies (Kruger & Dunning, 1999; Dunning et al., 2004; Eva et al., 2004, 2012; Davis et al., 2006) indicate "humans are poor at producing self-generated summative assessments of their own performance or ability" (Eva et al., 2008: 15). For example, students' self-rating of performance was poorly correlated with supervisor ratings of physical examination skills or external tests of factual knowledge (Gordon, 1991). On average, people consider themselves to be above average – the Lake Wobegon effect (Kruger, 1999). In a study of medical students, the relationship between self-ratings and supervisor ratings declined as they progressed through medical school and, during their final year, self-ratings did not correlate at all with board scores (Arnold *et al.*, 1985). Unfortunately, weaker students are more likely than stronger students to overestimate their abilities and thus fail to recognize their learning needs. In one study of psychology students, those in the bottom 25% of their class thought they had done better on a course exam than the majority of their peers (Dunning *et al.*, 2003). Eva and Regehr (2008: 17) emphasize: "Personal unguided reflections on practice simply do not provide the information sufficient to guide performance improvements adequately." Boud (1999: 122) cautions: "It is important to note . . . that the practice of self-assessment does not imply that this engagement is an isolated or individualistic activity. It commonly involves peers, makes use of teachers and other practitioners and draws upon appropriate literature." The definition of self-assessment by Epstein *et al.* (2008) emphasizes the importance of students using a standard for comparison with their own performance. Self-assessment is "a process of interpreting data about our own performance and comparing them to an explicit or implicit standard" (2008: 5).

Several strategies can be utilized to enhance self-assessment skills. Watching a video of their interviewing improved the accuracy of students' assessment of their interviewing performance (Ward *et al.*, 2003). Reviewing a video with faculty increased the accuracy of surgical residents' self-assessment of their surgical skills (Lane & Gottlieb, 2004). The opportunity for benchmarking – reviewing the performance of other students for comparison with their own performance – improved self-assessment for high-performing students but not for poor-performing students (Martin *et al.*, 1998; Hodges *et al.*, 2001). Final-year medical students' self-assessment of their suturing ability in a simulated environment showed moderate correlation with expert assessor scores. There was no improvement in their self-assessment after reviewing a video recording of their performance. However, after viewing a video recording of an ideal performance – the "benchmark performance" – their self-assessed scores showed strong correlation with expert scores of their performance ($r = 0.83$; $p < 0.0001$) (Hawkins *et al.*, 2012).

Sargeant *et al.* (2010) describe how learners and physicians informed their self-assessments in clinical settings by utilizing data from both internal and external sources. A "gut feeling" that one is not doing well in a particular area might stimulate seeking out opportunities to learn more about that topic. However, without external feedback, many learners will not recognize their deficiencies. Because feedback from trusted, credible supervisors was notable for its absence, learners sought feedback from peers, often through informal discussions related to how they handled similar situations. The authors of this qualitative study noted the "tensions between wanting to know how one is doing and fear of learning one is not doing as well as one should" (2010: 1218). One value of portfolios is that they make it more likely that a learner will reflect on a patient event that did not go well rather than ignoring it to avoid the discomfort of recognizing ones error (Van Tartwijk & Driessen, 2009). Another important study by Mann *et al.* (2011) explores how tensions between people might hamper self-assessment – for example, worrying about damaging a relationship with a colleague or student by providing honest feedback.

Some researchers draw a distinction between summative self-assessment ("guess your grade") and self-monitoring – "moment-by moment awareness of performance during a task" (McConnell *et al.*, 2012: 320). Schön (1987) referred to this as "reflection in action." For example, experienced surgeons slow down and pay more attention to parts of a surgical procedure that are unusual or more complicated. Epstein and colleagues (2008: 5) suggest that "Self-monitoring is characterized by an ability to attend, moment-to-moment, to our own actions; curiosity to examine the effects of those actions; and willingness to use those observations to improve behaviour and patterns of thinking in the future." They suggest that these skills can be enhanced by practicing mindfulness techniques to cultivate an "observing self" (2008: 5) that helps to resist the tendency of going on automatic pilot. One way of improving the ability to stay focused and attentive to the patient is practicing paying attention to one's breathing while clearing the mind of everything else and, when the mind wanders, bringing attention back to the breathing over and over again. Clinical teachers can help students develop their curiosity, another important feature of mindfulness, by encouraging them to ask themselves reflective questions such as:

- If there were data that I ignored, what might they be?
- What am I assuming that might not be true?
- Did I avoid premature closure?
- Is there another way in which I can formulate this patient's story and /or my response?
- What are important aspects of the present situation that differ from previous situations? How might prior experiences be affecting my response to this situation?
- What would a trusted peer say about how I am managing or feeling about this situation? (Epstein, 2008: 9)

Eva and Regehr (2008: 15) suggest that students be taught the habit of "self-directed assessment seeking." Students should learn how to gather evidence about their knowledge and performance from a variety of sources (personal reflection and reading, peer assessment, review questions, Objective Structured Clinical Examinations, and feedback from patients and supervisors) and use this multisource feedback to inform their self-assessments, which can then be used to guide their ongoing learning. Weak students tend to discount feedback that is too much at variance with their self-assessments and may benefit from counseling from a peer or mentor to place the feedback in context – guidance on how to use the feedback to improve performance rather than as an assessment of their worth as clinicians (Eva *et al.*, 2012). Students at all levels might benefit from practice sessions in which they learn, with role-play, how to ask their supervisors to observe them and provide feedback. This strategy would likely be more effective than exhorting faculty to provide more feedback.

The following example describes a teaching intervention that promoted self-awareness.

Case Example

In a teaching practice, Sarah Pinchot, a first-year family medicine resident, stepped out of an interview to consult with her supervisor. This was the second time she had seen the patient for tension-type headaches. Tony Sanatani, a 45-year-old executive, was not improving and he initiated this visit in order to be referred for a CT scan. The resident was frustrated and angry with what she described as an "abuse of the system." Her attempt to persuade Mr Sanatani that the test was unnecessary terminated in a heated disagreement. Dr Pinchot felt her medical knowledge had been rejected and her professional credibility undermined. She needed to win this argument!

While the resident was describing her frustration and the standoff with her patient, the supervisor recognized Dr Pinchot's vulnerability and need for support. But, from previous knowledge of Mr Sanatani, the supervisor understood his request probably stemmed from the death of his uncle from a brain tumour 6 months ago. The teacher's task was to help the resident ventilate her feelings and then to help her explore why she had fallen into a win-lose relationship with the patient. Dr Pinchot needed to understand how both she and her patient had contributed to this impasse. Then she had to find a way to convert the struggle into a win-win outcome. The resident recognized that her recurrent conflict with authority figures led her to experience Mr Sanatani's request for reassurance as a demand for an unnecessary test and a challenge of her medical competence. Instead of exploring his fears, she reacted by defending herself. Dr Pinchot dismissed the patient's request as unwarranted and the fight was on. After realizing what had happened, Dr Pinchot was able to return to the patient, acknowledge that they had reached an impasse and ask if they could begin again. This culminated in an exploration of the patient's concerns and fears about the headaches. Following a careful neurological examination and discussion about why a brain tumour was highly unlikely, the patient was prepared to consider other causes for his headaches.

Later, Dr Pinchot sat down with her supervisor to discuss options for exploring her problem with authority figures. The supervisor's recognition of Dr Pinchot's vulnerability had prevented him from criticizing her error and engaging in a parallel struggle, which would have replicated the student's difficulties with authority. Instead, his nonjudgmental stance encouraged the development of her self-awareness.

For the most part, as physicians grow in their personal and clinical wisdom, they become more comfortable with the uncertainties of medicine and the complexities of their patients' problems; but ongoing self-reflection is essential to promote a deepening understanding of the patient-physician relationship. In an inspiring paper, gastroenterologist Michael E McLeod (1998: 678) reflects on his struggle to achieve self-awareness:

> I worked to keep my emotions and intuitions from influencing medical decisions because they were subjective and not measurable. I became adept at hiding the feelings of vulnerability and helplessness that I felt when my patients died, and those of anger and frustration with "hateful" patients . . . As a result I became increasingly isolated from my own emotions and needs; I shared less with my colleagues at work. I evolved a workaholic lifestyle with the subconscious expectation that others would figure out my needs and satisfy them because I was "doing so much." I did not take the risk of identifying and asking for what I needed. I hid behind a mask of pseudocompetence and efficiency. I let power, money, and position take the place of empowerment, love, and meaning. But because they were substitutes for my primary needs, they were never enough.

OVEREMPHASIS ON THE CONVENTIONAL MEDICAL MODEL

There are several features of medical education and professional socialization that may interfere with learning an effective clinical approach to the familiar problems presented by patients. Medical training indoctrinates students to see patients' problems as derangements of the "body-machine" and to be concerned about missing some rare but deadly disease. As a result, most students and many physicians attempt to find a disease to explain each of their patients' complaints. This may result in overinvestigation, unnecessary referral, and overprescribing. Also, patients' personal concerns may receive little attention because physicians are concentrating all of their thought and energy on ferreting out pathology. This is not surprising since, until recently, the majority of medical students' clinical experience was in large tertiary care hospitals where they were exposed to very seriously ill patients. While more education has shifted to community sites, the aging population and associated multimorbidity reinforces the focus on the conventional medical model. Despite worldwide reductions in duty hours (Woodrow *et al.*, 2006; Rosenbaum and Lamas, 2012), clinicians are still often overworked and may have little time to do anything but tend to the grave physical needs of their patients.

It is understandable that young physicians will use the framework they are most familiar with – the conventional medical model. Even experienced physicians, when stressed or overwhelmed by the problems of a patient, will often revert to a simplistic focus on conventional medical diagnosis even if they have learned and have used a more sophisticated and comprehensive patient-centered approach.

One of our students, in describing her struggle to use the patient-centered clinical method, expressed her fears that she would be mandated to relinquish the conventional medical model altogether:

> I want to remember that stuff (textbook information), you know! Not only did I work hard to learn it and to remember it for a short while, and it has helped me to fend off attendings in the past, but even without the quizzing, it is a form of security, a teddy bear of sorts. Beyond that, sometimes it's a source of pride, of excitement, of fun, of conversation with colleagues, a worldly treasure. Yeah, I know it's a treasure moths will soon destroy (to coin a phrase), but meanwhile I am trying to live in a world that demands these things!

The conventional medical model has a long history of success, it is highly respected in our culture, and it allows physicians to remain comfortably distant from patients and their problems. Also, if doctors do their best (biomedically speaking), and their patients do not improve, the physicians need feel no blame. If the patient did not "comply" with the doctor's "orders" then the lack of improvement is inappropriately blamed on the patient. Students and physicians need to learn a more appropriate clinical method, one that incorporates the power of the conventional medical model but which is not constrained by its narrow focus on disease. Such a clinical method cannot be learned all at once. Students may need to learn each component of the patient-centered clinical method separately and they will also require opportunities to practice integrating their clinical skills into a unified whole.

CONCENTRATION ON HISTORY TAKING RATHER THAN LISTENING TO THE PATIENT

Students in first-year medical school have little difficulty learning how to inquire about patients' ideas and expectations concerning their illnesses but, as they progress through medical school, they become consumed by the task of making the right diagnosis and their interviews become less patient-centered (Barbee & Feldman, 1970; Helfer, 1970; Cohen, 1985; Preven *et al.*, 1986; Hojat *et al.*, 2004, 2009; Woloschuk *et al.*, 2004; Bellini & Shea, 2005; Tsimtsiou *et al.*, 2007; ; Haidet, 2010; Bombeke *et al.*, 2010; Neumann *et al.*, 2011). This may be a consequence of the emphasis on taking a thorough history of each disease and completing a comprehensive functional enquiry. Much less attention is given to open-ended exploration of the patient's feelings and ideas. Without practice, most young doctors feel uncomfortable enquiring about patients' personal lives. Often there is concern that patients will become emotional and perhaps cry or show anger; they worry that they will open up a "can of worms" that they will not be able to handle. Physicians' training tends to make them cautious about trying new approaches with patients where they feel uncertain about the outcome; they are also reluctant to try unfamiliar techniques if they feel uncomfortable or awkward. The commonest excuse given to avoid asking about patients' personal concerns is lack of time. However, it is not efficient use of time to search for a disease that is not present or to ignore a major source of patients' distress such as their fear or concern about the possible cause and implications of their symptoms.

Alternately, when physicians are learning the patient-centered clinical method, they mistakenly equate it with a "psychosocial functional enquiry." The following example typifies this common misunderstanding.

> When a patient presented with concerns about her severe sore throat and about how long she was going to be off school the resident interrupted her story with: "Wait, I need to get to know more about your personal situation. Where did you grow up? What was your childhood like? Was there much conflict in your family?" These questions would be very useful in the appropriate context, but

in this case they seemed unconnected from the patient's practical concerns about receiving effective treatment and getting back to school as soon as possible. The physician needed to be sensitive to any cues about how this patient's home and school situation were related to her illness but was not being patient-centered by imposing a psychosocial inquiry.

TEACHER INEXPERIENCE

Teachers often go through stages in their development. They start out motivated by fear – fear that they do not know enough about the content and will be found out. Brookfield (2006: 80) describes how novice teachers sometimes feel like imposters:

> Impostership means that many of us go through our teaching lives fearing that at some unspecified point in the future we will undergo a humiliating public unveiling. We wear an external mask of control, but beneath it we know that really we are frail figures, struggling not to appear totally incompetent to those around us.

With experience, teachers move to the next stage – they are more confident now and want to show how much they know. Tompkins (1990: 654) describes this stage:

> I had finally realized that what I was actually concerned with and focused on most of the time were three things: a) to show the students how smart I was, b) to show them how knowledgeable I was, and c) to show them how well-prepared I was . . . I had been putting on a performance whose true goal was not to help the students learn but to perform before them in such a way that they would have a good opinion of me.

In the third stage, teachers are comfortable with their knowledge and skills and can focus on the learners and their needs instead of on themselves.

It takes considerable experience, first as a doctor and then as a clinical teacher, before a physician is able to integrate secondhand information about patients in order to make good decisions. To make the task even more complex, teachers are trying to assess not only the patient's problems but also the student's learning needs. To achieve this, teachers must consider many different factors at the same time. First, there are several questions about students: Did they establish a comfortable relationship with the patient that allowed the patient to mention everything he or she had in mind? Did the student pick up on all the important cues the patient gave? Did the student mention to the teacher all of his or her concerns about the patient, or did the student avoid those topics that might have disclosed his or her own ignorance? What are the student's blind spots? Unless the teacher has prior knowledge of the students or has witnessed their conduct in actual interviews with patients, it may be difficult to answer many of these questions. It is important to establish a climate of acceptance, where students are not criticized for admitting ignorance. Students need to know that the teacher is depending on the information they gather to make important management decisions; hence they must state where they are confused or uncertain so that the teacher will explore or double-check these areas.

Second, there are questions to be considered about the patients: What more information does the physician need to make a reasonable diagnosis? Why did the patient present now? What are the patient's feelings, ideas, and expectations about the problem and how are they affecting his or her life? Here, too, prior knowledge is invaluable. However, unless teachers have seen the patient-student interactions, they must depend on obtaining secondhand information from students. Here is where a patient-centered case report, described in Chapter 12, is an invaluable tool for both the learner and the teacher.

Finally, inexperienced teachers may be concerned about their reputation among their students and may feel a need to prove themselves by demonstrating their excellence as clinicians. The dilemma for physicians who are teaching a patient-centered approach is that the value system of the medical school may be at odds with this approach. As a result, excellence may be defined in terms of one's technical prowess and diagnostic acumen and may give little credit to one's ability to relate to patients.

In clinical teaching, the discussion may focus on the latest treatment for the patient's problem, leaving no time for exploring the patient's experience of his or her illness. For young students, desperate for unambiguous answers in the chaotic and messy domain of clinical practice, knowing the latest treatments for various diseases is highly valued. Because they have not yet learned how to deal with uncertainty, students may reward teachers who can provide black-and-white answers and discount teachers who urge them to address not only the patient's diseases but also the patient's health and illness experiences in the context of his or her life setting. Thus, students' needs for certainty and simplicity, coupled with the teacher's need for acceptance by peers, can have a powerful adverse influence on novice teachers.

COMPETING DEMANDS ON TEACHERS

Full-time faculty are pulled in many different directions at once. The destructive myth of faculty members as "triple threats" (Mundy, 1991; Aronoff, 2009) – expected to be exemplary clinicians, outstanding researchers, and superb teachers – casts faculty into impossible situations of role overload. In a survey conducted at one US medical school, 42% of faculty reported they were "seriously considering leaving academic medicine in the next five years" (Lowenstein *et al.*, 2007: 3). Faculty members are increasingly finding themselves stretched thin and forced to set priorities. Too often it is time for teaching that is cut back, since there are fewer institutional rewards for these activities than for research or clinical care. Teaching the patient-centered approach may be time-consuming considering that teachers would want to observe student-patient interactions, to provide constructive feedback and to adequately explore students' personal issues that may be evoked by the discussion. Community preceptors are also expected to be exemplary role models and see enough patients to earn a living. They often provide learning opportunities for undergraduate and postgraduate students and many serve on professional organizations that depend on their involvement. As a result, they too experience role strain.

To avoid replicating their teachers' lifestyle and to prevent burnout, students may impose inappropriate limitations on the responsibilities they will assume. One outcome of the establishment of rigid boundaries between their personal and professional lives is lost opportunities for learning and growth. Examples of such behavior in primary care include working in settings where the hours of work are limited, interactions are superficial, and complex problems are referred; limiting hours of practice or range of services provided (e.g., refusal to provide home visits, hospital visits, intrapartum care, or palliative care). Specialists may reduce their responsibilities by shortening their office hours or by limiting their scope of practice.

While more effective time management will ease some of the competing demands on teachers, the answer is not that simple. Each teacher must discover how to balance patients' needs, students' needs, and personal and family needs. Thus it is important for teachers to strike a balance for themselves to be effective role models for their students. However, there is a limit on what individual teachers can do to remedy their working conditions; schools of medicine must also make changes. There needs to be a better match between what faculty members are asked to do and academic promotion guidelines. In particular, teaching needs to be as recognized and rewarded by promotion as research. "Faculty development programs, which emphasize mentoring, career planning, performance feedback, establishing colleague networks and connectedness and acculturation to one's school and university, are effective interventions that improve faculty satisfaction, productivity, institutional loyalty and retention" (Lowenstein *et al.*, 2007: 37).

TEACHER OVERPROTECTIVENESS

Including students in patient care changes the patient-doctor relationship and creates several challenges for teachers. Clinical teaching makes the doctor's job more complicated – the teacher, in this context, is responsible not only for the quality of patient care but also for the quality of the student's learning experience. Sometimes the two responsibilities seem to be at odds. Physician discomfort in these situations may interfere with student learning. Doctors may be more hesitant to allow students to practice on their patients than the patients are themselves (Weston, 1989). For example, physicians may falsely assume that their patients would not want to discuss their feelings about their illness with a student. This may be a reflection more of the physician's discomfort than the patient's uneasiness. Most patients are willing to allow medical students to participate in their care, provided the students are appropriately supervised and not trying to do something for which they are ill-prepared (Thurman *et al.*, 2006; Shann & Wilson, 2006; Marwan, 2012). It is essential that teachers not undermine the student's position with patients. Whenever possible, teachers should function as consultant to the student and emphasize their agreement with his or her approach. However, if the student has made an error, the facts need to be addressed honestly. One approach is for the teacher and student to excuse themselves from the examining room to allow for frank discussion. When they both return, the student discusses with the patient the error and the new plans for treatment. With postgraduate students in an ambulatory setting, the patient may have already gone home before the error is noted. In this situation, it is essential that the patient be contacted to correct the mistake as quickly as possible. Not everyone will be comfortable with such candor in this age of litigation, even though openness reduces medicolegal risks. Such honesty reassures patients that the monitoring system works, and that a teaching practice offers the advantage of at least two opinions on their problems. In addition, this provides an important opportunity for residents to learn the skills of honest disclosure of error (O'Connell *et al.*, 2003; Disclosure Working Group, 2011).

TEACHERS AS ROLE MODELS

The most important teaching method used by clinical teachers is role modeling. Daniel Tosteson (1979), former dean of Harvard Medical School, emphasized this central responsibility of teachers: "We must acknowledge . . . that the most important, indeed the only, thing we have to offer our students is ourselves. Everything else they can read in a book" (1979: 690). Whether they are aware of it or not, medical school teachers act as models of the profession for students and house staff – either as good examples to emulate or bad examples to avoid (Wear *et al.*, 2011). Teachers must recognize that they are being role models at all times, not just when they are teaching but also in social situations (e.g., making a derogatory comment about a patient in an elevator). Whatever is taught in the preclinical years of medical school is either accepted or rejected by students depending on whether they see "real doctors" doing it. For example, exhortations to "listen to the patient" will be scoffed if most clinicians routinely conduct disease-centered interviews and cut off patients' attempts to express their concerns.

In a case-control study of the attributes of excellent attending-physician role models in internal medicine, conducted in four teaching hospitals in Montreal and Baltimore, Wright and colleagues (1998) found five attributes independently associated with being named as an excellent role model: (1) spending more than 25% of one's time teaching (odds ratio 5.12); (2) spending 25 or more hours a week teaching and conducting rounds when serving as an attending physician (odds ratio 2.48); (3) stressing the importance of the patient-doctor relationship in one's teaching (odds ratio 2.58); (4) teaching the psychosocial aspects of medicine (odds ratio 2.31); and (5) having served as a chief resident (odds ratio 2.07). In addition, excellent attending physicians were more likely to engage in activities that build relationships with residents such as organizing an end-of-month dinner with residents, sharing personal experiences, talking about their personal lives, and trying to learn about the lives of the housestaff (Wright *et al.*, 1998).

In an accompanying editorial, Skeff and Mutha (1998: 2016) point out: "Teachers, even those who are motivated and highly skilled, cannot accomplish these goals without institutional support." In order to develop and nurture excellent teachers, the institution must reward those who spend time with students and residents as well as time in workshops and faculty development activities honing their own skills. Cruess and colleagues describe the profound influence of the hidden curriculum on role modeling:

> For example, an institutional culture that promotes overwork, leaving insufficient time for harried clinical teachers to promote the type of reflective practice needed to demonstrate best practices among students, is detrimental to effective role modelling. Similarly, a culture that tolerates inadequate clinical care or poor interpersonal relationships inhibits positive modelling, as do administrative decisions that fail to show appreciation and support, both financial and non-financial, of those who are trying to be exemplary. (Cruess *et al.*, 2008: 719)

In a seminal study of clinical teachers in three medical schools in Quebec, Beaudoin and colleagues (1998) surveyed all senior clerks and second-year residents about their perceptions of the qualities of their teachers. Almost half of the clerks and one-third of the residents perceived that most of their teachers did not display humanistic characteristics in their role as caregivers and teachers (e.g., valuing contact with patients as an important part of patient care, concern about the overall well-being of patients and not just their presenting complaints, spending time educating patients about their health problems); 75% of clerks agreed that their teachers seemed unconcerned about how their patients adapted psychologically to their illnesses; 78% felt their teachers did not try to understand students' difficulties; and 77% felt their teachers did not try to support students who were having difficulties. Residents were somewhat less critical suggesting that perhaps they were being socialized to accept these deficiencies in patient care and teaching. The authors speculate: "Perhaps their perceptions show how difficult it becomes to attain high standards of humanistic care when health care personnel must deal with increasing strains, constraints and uncertainties. Under these circumstances, perhaps there are limits to one's caring" (Beaudoin *et al.*, 1998: 769).

Wright and Carrese (2002) conducted in-depth interviews with 29 highly regarded role models at two large teaching hospitals and analysed the interview transcripts for major themes. Strong clinical skills were considered essential but insufficient for effective role modeling. Consistency of good behavior was indispensable and truly distinguished role models stepped up their performance in difficult and demanding situations. They sought out opportunities to model particular skills and to teach aspects of medicine that tend to be neglected such as professionalism. Personal qualities were mentioned by all of the role models, particularly interpersonal skills, positive outlook, and commitment to excellence and growth. Teaching skills were also mentioned by all, especially establishing rapport with learners, developing specific teaching philosophies and methods, and being committed to the growth of learners.

A number of barriers to role modeling were mentioned – being impatient and overly opinionated, being quiet, and being overextended.

Students can have mixed experiences in learning the patient-centered clinical method as opportunities for learning from their role models may vary. In focus group interviews with clinical clerks at Western University, students described their observations of their role models and the conflict they experienced in the transition from theory to practice. As one student said, "I think we have been trained well but putting it into practice is another story."

The following comments highlight students' awareness that the patient-centered clinical method is applicable to all physicians and not just family doctors.

> I think that any specialist can be just as patient-centered as the family doctor. It's just how you approach it.

Furthermore, a paucity of role models in the specialities was a concern.

> We don't have the role models in the specialities to reinforce it. I think that time is just an excuse. In an extra minute you can do so much more. Being patient-centered affects everything from helping you with your diagnosis to helping with your treatment plan and management.

As one student observed:

> it's hard to be optimistic about the way we're going to practice patient-centered medicine when we have no role models.

The following comment illustrates the negative effect a role model can have on students when they are attempting to apply patient-centered concepts to clinical practice:

> If you're laughed at by physicians for using this, and they say, "Don't bother with those questions," you stop doing it. Your residents will be directing a lot of your learning along the next two years and when they say, "You don't want to piss off your Attending. He hates those patient-centered questions." So you're not going to ask patients, "What are your ideas about your illness?"

When role modeling was effective, it provided a powerful and memorable learning experience.

One Orthopaedic surgeon I had for clinical methods, I still remember this, I was FIFEing the patient and I found out that the patient had diabetes and was worried about their upcoming surgery, and possible complications. When I told the surgeon that, he didn't laugh at me; he didn't think it was ridiculous. He then went in to see the patient and said, "So do you have any concerns about the upcoming surgery?" And they talked about it. It only took a few minutes.

Learning from role models is both a conscious and unconscious process (Steinert, 2009). At an unconscious level, learners will "catch" the values, attitudes, and behaviors of their teachers by observing their actions and the consequences of their actions (Bandura, 1986). They may be pleasantly surprised (or perhaps horrified) when others comment on how much they have become like their teachers. The literature on apprenticeship describes how a novice learns complex skills and concepts from a master (Gamble, 2001). Often these skills are so complex that they cannot be put into words. Reber (1993: 5) describes this as implicit learning – "the acquisition of knowledge that takes place largely independently of conscious attempts to learn and largely in the absence of explicit knowledge about what was acquired." Students can learn the particulars of good patient-physician communication (e.g., using open-ended questions or reflective listening) in a formal setting with simulated patients. Their teachers can give them descriptions and examples of how to use these skills in talking with patients and provide specific, focused feedback on how they are doing. However, putting these skills together with all the other skills needed for an effective dialogue with a real patient is a much more complex task. This is where role modeling is most effective. Their teachers may be able to demonstrate the skills even though they are at a loss for words to describe exactly how to do it. Polanyi (1969) likened this to how we are able to recognize the faces of acquaintances without being able to describe how we identify them. Such tacit skills "can be communicated only by example not by precept" (Polanyi, 1966: 54).

However, even though it is difficult, and sometimes impossible, to articulate some of the skills students and residents must learn, it is important to make an effort to describe them as best we can. Cruess et al. (2008) emphasize the importance of protecting time for dialogue, reflection, and debriefing for making the implicit explicit so that students will recognize the important lessons they are learning from their role models. This will deepen their learning and reduce the risk of misinterpreting their observations of their teachers – for example, observing how their teacher calmed an angry, anxious patient and established common ground might look like magic until they have a chance to discuss this encounter with their teacher and, together, identify the specific strategies used. By elaborating on their observations, they are more likely to apply these skills when confronted with a similar situation. Egnew and Wilson (2011) conducted focus groups and long interviews with students and faculty to explore the characteristics of exemplary role models. One key finding was the opinion that effective role models needed "role modeling consciousness." "Role models who made the implicit explicit by articulating the relational qualities they were attempting to portray and the interpersonal struggles they experienced were highly valued by our respondents" (2011: 103).

TEACHING AND LEARNING TEAMWORK

An important feature of modern medical practice is teamwork (Chakraborti *et al.*, 2008; Reeves *et al.*, 2010), as discussed in Chapter 13. Primary care has become too complex for an individual clinician to work as a "lone ranger"; addressing the broad determinants of health requires the specialized skills of professionals from several different disciplines. In the past, a diverse group of health professionals working together for patient care was considered a team. However, without highly honed teamwork skills, they are only a group of people working beside one another and not a team. In an extensive needs assessment of interprofessional teams in Atlantic Canada, nine focus groups with a total of 61 participants were analyzed to identify themes. They concluded that: "Effective collaborative health care teams share common goals, understand each other's roles, demonstrate respect for each other, use clear communication, resolve conflict effectively, and are flexible (Sargeant *et al.*, 2008: 229). Effective primary health care teams also demonstrate a common understanding of primary health care, recognize that teamwork requires work, and have the practical "know-how" for sharing patient care. Communication was highlighted as "'the big thing,' 'the sine qua non,' the glue that holds a team together and enables collaborative work" (Sargeant *et al.*, 2008: 232). Sharing a common language about primary health care teams and having regular formal meetings and opportunities for informal corridor consultations were considered critical. Participants emphasized the importance of really listening to one another but also speaking up when they disagree.

However, team communication is complex and often poorly done. Numerous reports on medical error for over 30 years have identified faulty communication as one of its commonest causes (Abramson *et al.*, 1980; Brennan *et al.*, 1991; Kohn *et al.*, 2000; Greenberg *et al.*, 2007). In a study using semi-structured interviews of a random sample of residents in a 600-bed

US teaching hospital concerning 70 mishap incidents, Sutcliffe *et al.* (2004) describe how communication failure is much more complex than simply poor exchange of information. They suggest that relationships between dyads are at the root of much communication failure. For example, residents tended to withhold information from their supervisors that might make them look incompetent and they were hesitant to contact an Attending in the middle of the night. Also, when patients were transferred, too little information was passed on to the resident who will be responsible for their care. When a resident was convinced that the Attending's orders placed the patient at unnecessary risk they were reluctant to speak up for fear of being criticized. Communication gaps were also identified between general internal medicine residents and residents from other specialties and between residents and nurses. In the Silence Kills study involving 1700 nurses, physicians, clinical care staff, and administrators (Maxfield *et al.*, 2005; Moss & Maxfield, 2007)

> half the nurses and four-fifths of the physicians surveyed in this study witness colleagues break rules, make mistakes, fail to offer support, or appear critically incompetent . . . despite the common occurrence of these disturbing observations, less than 1 in 10 healthcare professionals speak up and surface the concern with their coworker. (2005: 53)

One of the challenges to effective interprofessional collaboration is what Whitehead (2007) terms "the doctor dilemma." Among the barriers to collaboration are the physician's "specific powers, status, professional socialisation and decision-making responsibility. These can make it difficult for doctors to work with other health care professionals in ways that involve sharing responsibility" (2007: 1010). Medical education socializes medical students to accept a major responsibility for decision making and to see themselves as team leaders. Their dominant status is reinforced by the tough competition to get into medical school and their rigorous and lengthy training compared with other health professions. In addition, government health care usually covers the cost of physicians' services but not the services of other health professionals, and legal responsibility focuses on the role of physicians. Although this "medical chauvinism" is anachronistic and counterproductive, physicians do not easily give up their privileged status in the health care system. Similarly, the training of other health care professionals promotes the development of separate silos:

> Each profession has struggled to define its identity, values, sphere of practice and role in patient care. This has led to each health care profession working

within its own silo to ensure its members (its professionals) have common experiences, values, approaches to problem-solving and language for professional tools. It is not only the educational experiences, but also the socialization process which occurs simultaneously during the training period that serves to solidify the professional's unique world view. At the completion of their professional education, each student will have mastered not only the skills and values of his/her profession, but will also be able to assume the occupational identity. (Hall, 2005: 190)

One of the ways in which professional education molds the unique character of its graduates is through a discipline-specific approach to teaching – the "signature pedagogy" of each profession (Shulman, 2005a, 2005b). Special to medicine is the ritual of teaching rounds where a student, caring for a patient, presents a synopsis of the clinical findings and outlines a plan for investigation and management with justification for his or her opinions, followed by questions, sometimes "pimping" (Detsky, 2009) from the Attending to explore the patient's problem and the student's understanding. This, in turn, may be followed by a brief teaching session. For law, the signature pedagogy is the case method (Miller & Garretson, 2009) as depicted in the film *The Paper Chase* from 1973, in which Professor Kingsfield grills members of the class on points of law, using a quasi-Socratic technique, to teach them how to think like a lawyer, just as teaching rounds in medicine teaches students how to think like a doctor.

> Signature pedagogies are important precisely because they are pervasive. They implicitly define what counts as knowledge in a field and how things become known. They define how knowledge is analyzed, criticized, accepted, or discarded. They define the functions of expertise in a field, the locus of authority, and the privileges of rank and standing. (Shulman, 2005a: 54)

Although the signature pedagogies of each profession are important for the knowledge and skill development as well as identity formation of each clinician, if professional education remains constrained by separate silos, it will continue to be difficult to teach clinicians how to think like members of an interprofessional team. Students need opportunities to work in effective intra- and interprofessional teams where they can learn with, from, and about one another. They need to learn how to be effective team members and team leaders. Young health care professionals in training have an opportunity to complement their traditional education by learning from teachers in other health disciplines. Team teaching is a powerful method for faculty members to model collaborative teaching and learning. Another valuable way in which students learn about the roles and functions of other professionals is by sharing learning experiences with students from other health care disciplines. Three specific skill sets are particularly valuable to prepare clinicians for teamwork: using checklists and participating in team huddles and team meetings.

Checklists have been demonstrated to improve patient safety, especially on surgical teams (Pronovost & Freischlag, 2010; Gawande, 2010). The Rourke Baby Record is a good example of a checklist in primary care (Rourke *et al.*, 2010). Medicine has become so complex that it exceeds the reliance on expertise and memory alone. Gawande (2010: 48) points out that

> checklists seem able to defend anyone, even the experienced, against failure in many more tasks than we realized. They provide a kind of cognitive net. They catch mental flaws inherent in all of us – flaws of memory and attention and thoroughness. And because they do, they raise wide, unexpected possibilities.

Checklists and training in team communication go hand in hand – for example, the SBAR acronym/checklist for communicating among team members improves handover and referral.

- Situation: "Dr Preston, I'm calling about Mr. Lakewood, who's having trouble breathing."
- Background: "He's a 54 year old man with chronic lung disease who has been sliding downhill, and now he's acutely worse."
- Assessment "I don't hear any breath sounds in his right chest. I think he has a pneumothorax."
- Recommendation "I need you to see him right now. I think he needs a chest tube." (Leonard *et al.*, 2004: i86)

The team huddle is "a brief, frequent form of structured communication among members of the health care team to plan for daily tasks and roles, and to review any barriers or facilitators of the day's work" (Fogarty & Schultz, 2010: 158). Typically, a huddle will be scheduled for a few minutes at the start of each half-day office session – a 5-minute "heads up" for the whole team. Participants in a huddle can include everyone who has contact with patients (e.g., physicians, nurses, social workers, pharmacists, patient educators, receptionists, and learners). Topics can include the following.

- Which patients are most appropriate for a student or resident to see? Does anyone have any quick tips to help the learner avoid pitfalls or important background information about these patients that would affect care?

- Which patients might benefit from seeing the pharmacist for a medication review, or a health educator to help them understand their complex treatment plan?
- Check for patients who may need more time and assistance because of age or disability and decide who can help.
- Will any patients need an interpreter?
- If there are patients booked for a procedure, what equipment will be needed?
- Who needs an update on their immunization?
- Are there any lab results that need to be tracked down?
- Does anyone on the team have new important information about any of the patients?

To be practical, have everyone stand, and limit the huddle to 5–7 minutes (Stewart & Johnson, 2007). For more on huddles, search "huddles" on the Institute for Healthcare Improvement's website (www.iHI.org).

Clinical team meetings are longer and less frequent than huddles, typically occurring once a week for an hour. They provide occasions for all members of a team to discuss patient care, often focusing on complex patients with multimorbidity who require the care of several members of the team. It is an opportunity to brainstorm and to provide support for team members dealing with situations that are desperate, discouraging, or frustrating. Regular meetings improve collaboration and communication on teams, which, in turn, leads to better patient outcomes (Molyneux, 2001; Xyrichis & Lowton, 2008; Brown *et al.*, 2009). The electronic health record enhances team communication through the common messaging system by providing minute-to-minute patient information among health care providers – for example, a social worker, seeing a patient with increasing symptoms of depression, contacts the family physician through the messaging system, requesting a quick consultation about the patient's medication (Denomme *et al.*, 2011). As team members learn from their experiences of patient care and from one another, an effective interprofessional team becomes more than the sum of its parts. Lave and Wenger's (Lave & Wenger, 1991; Wenger, 1998) concept of "situated learning" describes how practitioners learn more from their social relationships in work settings rather than in classrooms. Describing their manuscript as an attempt to "rescue the idea of apprenticeship" (Lave & Wenger, 1991: 29), they explain how learning is situated in specific contexts such as the clinical setting. They suggest a different way of thinking about learning. Instead of focusing on the accumulation of knowledge in the minds of individual learners, situated learning addresses the evolving roles and responsibilities of learners within communities of practice – "groups of people who share a concern, a set of problems, or a passion about a topic, and who deepen their understanding and knowledge in this area by interacting on an ongoing basis" (Wenger *et al.*, 2002: 4). The novices begin their journey as *newcomers* with the responsibility of *legitimate peripheral participation* – they are involved with care of patients but do not yet have full responsibility for management. "In contrast with learning as internalization, learning as increasing participation in communities of practice concerns the whole person acting in the world" (Lave & Wenger, 1991: 49). Over time, the newcomer is given increased responsibilities for more complex problems and, eventually, becomes an "old-timer" ready to pass on the learnings, traditions, and rituals of the community of practice to the next generation of newcomers. "Learning thus implies becoming a different person with respect to the possibilities enabled by these systems of relations. To ignore this aspect of learning is to overlook the fact that learning involves the construction of identities" (1991: 53).

The concept of "shared mind" (Leung *et al.*, 2012; Epstein, 2013) or "distributed cognition" (Lingard, 2012) may help to explain how the members of an effective team share their thoughts, feelings, and hunches to arrive at an understanding that no single team member could discover alone. Such teams share an understanding of one another's roles and the overarching goals of the team, and, through their interactions and struggles to find a way to help each patient, new and deeper understandings of their mission emerge. Learners at all levels should be invited to participate actively in huddles and team meetings; senior learners in all professional fields should have opportunities to participate as leaders in both venues with feedback on their performance from their supervisors and other team members.

Case Example

Allison Tsui, a first-year resident in internal medicine, was consistently an hour late at the end of her outpatient clinics. Patients and staff were complaining and the Chief Resident, Russ Johar, arranged to meet with her to discuss these mounting concerns. Dr Tsui attributed the problem to overbooking. She felt that she was expected to see too many patients in the time allotted – they all had many complex medical problems and many of them also had personal problems that were very time-consuming. She felt overwhelmed. Dr Johar wondered how he would address his junior colleague's difficulty. He decided to approach Dr Tsui as an adult learner and asked what she thought they could do together to address these issues. He offered to meet with her in one of the clinics to review the bookings and to observe her with a few patients. He discovered that she was doing complete assessments on many of the patients and that she was spending a lot of time in patient education and counseling rather than referring patients to the nurse educator, social worker, or other appropriate staff. Her prior experience had not prepared her to work collaboratively with other team members and, as a junior she did not feel she could ask other team members, who all seemed so busy, to assist with her patients. Dr Johar realized that he had failed to provide Dr Tsui with an adequate orientation to the role and function of the interprofessional team in the outpatient clinic. He apologized to Dr Tsui for this oversight and, in doing so, role modeled open and direct communication as an important aspect of good teamwork.

CONCLUSION

In this chapter we have described some of the challenges experienced by both teachers and learners as they endeavor to learn, teach, and practice the patient-centered clinical method. These challenges include personal, professional, and systemic aspects. Each one affects the others. Thus solutions are not simple and must include tackling the educational challenges in concert. It is particularly important to acknowledge the unrecognized complexity of patient-practitioner communication and the powerful influence of role models on the socialization of students in the health professions. Learning to be patient-centered cannot happen in isolation but must be respected and reinforced at all levels of professional education.

11 Teaching the Patient-Centered Clinical Method: Practical Tips

W Wayne Weston and Judith Belle Brown

> The setting for learning in a medical school is moulded by many things, but the major artisan is the teacher whose work penetrates to unnumbered patients who profit or suffer from encounters with his students. This responsibility is too heavy for tradition, inertia, or ennui to be allowed to dictate his actions – as a scientist he can do no less than prepare himself for this responsibility as carefully as he prepares to be a physician or investigator. The means are at hand. All he need do is use them. (Miller *et al.*, 1961: 296)

In previous chapters we addressed a number of theoretical issues and explored general principles of teaching clinical and communication skills; in this chapter we concentrate on the practical application of these principles to the day-to-day challenges of teaching patient-centered medicine in a clinical setting.

Fitting students into an already hectic schedule is challenging. Some research has indicated that the presence of a learner in a community practice increases the workload by 52 minutes per day and decreases the number of patients seen by 0.6 per hour (Vinson *et al.*, 1996). However, it depends on the office setup and the level and skill of the learner. Studies by Walters (Walters *et al.*, 2008; Walters, 2012) and by Tran *et al.* (2012) demonstrate that general practitioner preceptors had no reduction in the number of patients seen each day with a parallel consulting schedule. While the preceptor was seeing patients, third-year medical students were seeing patients on their own for 30 minutes before being joined by the preceptor for an additional 15 minutes. Also, patients reported a small increase in the quality of the consultation compared to having students sit in on the preceptor's consultation. Postgraduate students may even increase the number of patients the practice can see each day. In a study of precepting in a community-based family medicine residency program, Lillich *et al.* (2005) demonstrated that the 4-point POwER model of precepting, including the use of team huddles to plan and assign patients, the microskills approach to teaching, a more active role for preceptors in coordinating workflow, and a debrief with the team at the end of the session improved time management and decreased patient wait time.

Preceptors include students and residents in their community practices in a number of ways. Some schedule fewer patients on days with students – for example, leaving a few blank spots during the day for catch-up time and teaching. Others schedule more spots for walk-in acute problems. These patients are often more interesting and appropriate for students. Sharing the teaching with colleagues allows preceptors to catch up on days when they do not have a student and provides students a view of different styles of community practice. Students with little previous clinical experience will benefit from sitting in on their teacher's consultations initially but should soon be given more responsibility. Even preclinical students can be involved in speaking with patients on their own about their concerns. In fact, being freed of the expectation of making a diagnosis, allows them to explore patients' health and illness experiences thus making a significant contribution to their care and providing insights into the impact of illness on patients' lives.

Sometimes new clinical teachers wonder if they have anything worthwhile to teach students and residents – these young people seem to know so much and may be more up to date than they are. However, students often have trouble applying all that "book learning" to real patients who often have multiple

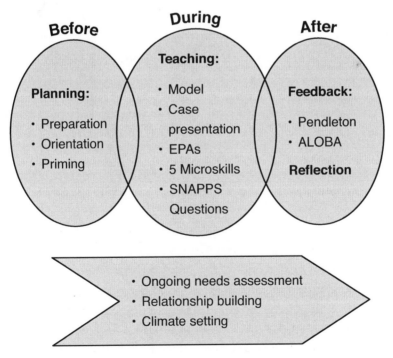

FIGURE 11.1 Framework for clinical teaching (based on Irby, 1992; Irby & Bowen, 2004)

medical problems as well as social and psychological difficulties. Students, and even residents, may feel lost in the uncertainties and complexities of practice. They greatly appreciate learning the practical tips their teachers have acquired from years of working in "the trenches."

It may help preceptors to remind themselves what it is like as a clerk or new resident constantly changing rotations – for example, just as they get comfortable working up patients on internal medicine, they are moved to obstetrics or surgery. They are constantly trying to sort out what is expected – it is like starting a new job every month. Being greeted in a friendly manner and welcomed onto a new clinical team goes a long way in reducing the anxiety of starting out in another new setting.

Based on structured interviews, a think-aloud exercise with a written case, and week-long observations of teaching rounds by six distinguished teachers in general internal medicine, Irby (1992: 630) developed "a model of instructional reasoning and action." He noted that these teachers all spent a considerable amount of time planning before rounds and reflecting after rounds. We have adapted this model for use in ambulatory settings, although the general principles apply in a hospital setting as well. In the rest of this chapter we will elaborate on this framework as shown in Figure 11.1.

BEFORE

Before students arrive, it is important to learn about the expectations of the learner's home institution, inform the clinic staff about the roles and responsibilities of students, and let patients know about the possible involvement of students in their care. Soon after students arrive they should be oriented to the clinic and their initial learning needs should be determined. Patients should be selected for student involvement, with patient permission, based on the student's learning needs. Students should initially be primed before seeing each patient to enhance their learning experience and the quality of care they provide.

Learn about Program Expectations

It is important to be aware of the objectives or competencies expected by the student's home institution, and methods and format of assessment required. Knowing the overall plan of the curriculum, and how his or her block fits in, will assist teachers to tailor the educational experiences to match the student's needs.

Prepare the Practice

The clinic staff need to be aware of the involvement of the practice in training young physicians and the level of student responsibility for patient care so that they can help prepare patients to see a student or resident and answer any questions about this process. It may help to coach staff on how to present a learner to patients. It is essential to educate the receptionist about the role of students and how to schedule patients for them. Patients also need to be informed that students may participate in their care. It may be helpful to post a sign in the waiting room about the involvement of the practice with the medical school. Posting the name of the student or resident in the waiting room near the reception area may remind patients of their name and make it more likely that they will follow up with the same learner.

Orientation: Mutual Sharing of Expectations

It may be useful to contact the student or resident before he or she arrives to provide information about the practice and community. Ask the learner to describe his or her background, especially about what he or she has done so far in the clerkship or residency. When the student or resident first arrives, find out about his or her previous clinical experiences and his or her special interests. What does the student or resident hope to learn? What areas of medicine does he or she find difficult or confusing? What skills does he or she want to practice (e.g., using the ophthalmoscope, doing pelvic exams, doing procedures)? Students are often reluctant to admit any area of weakness until they feel more comfortable with their teacher and trust that this information will not be used against them in their evaluation. A brief orientation to the office or hospital and introductions to the staff will help them feel welcomed. Let them know about the system of assessment. Make sure they understand what is expected of them (e.g., responsibility for patient care, punctuality, dress code). Making these issues clear at the start can prevent problems later on. Tell them about the community and the special attractions they might enjoy during their time off. Find out if they will be absent for holidays, conferences, or other approved activities. It may be helpful to have a checklist or handout for the student or resident outlining the key points in the orientation.

Some Suggestions for Orientation in a Busy Clinic

- The staff can assist with the orientation (e.g., tour of the clinic, overview of the community, and dress code).
- Do not try to cover everything on the first day – it may be overwhelming.

The important thing is for the new learner to feel welcome and have a clear idea of how they will fit in on the clinical team.

- Orient the learner to the electronic health record if used in the practice. A short manual on the electronic health record can be invaluable.
- If teachers have students or residents regularly, it will save time to develop a brief handout about the office and community, their approach to teaching and supervision, and their expectations of learners. Then teachers can spend time responding to questions after the student has reviewed the handout. A good orientation will save a lot of time in the long run. One study showed that it took students up to 2 weeks to figure out how to focus their workups, write up charts, and present cases (Kurth *et al.*, 1997).
- Provide a copy of the core learning objectives of the rotation and have the student highlight his or her priorities and consider adding a few personal objectives. It may take a few days before the student has a clear idea about the available learning opportunities. After observing the student for a few days, the preceptor will be in a better position to recommend any changes in the student's priorities if the student had been unaware of some of his or her learning needs. Then circulate the list for everyone who will be teaching the student. Over time additional learning needs may be recognized and a revised list should be distributed.

Selection of Patients and Priming Students

A team "huddle" at the start of each clinical session is often helpful – the physician, nurse, and student gather around the patient list to identify which patients a student will see and to briefly outline their reasons for visit. If the student has time, he or she could quickly look up information about the patients' problems in order to be better prepared. Identifying patients and their problems the night before would give students a better chance to prepare. Preceptors might also want to take some time before the clinic to update their knowledge of conditions they are less familiar with. The "huddle" is also an opportunity to clarify the nurse's role with each patient and whether or not additional equipment might be needed for particular visits. Often the nurse or other team member has had contact with patients between visits and this is an opportunity to share new information with the team.

While most patients are suitable for involvement with students, there are some issues worth considering. First, some patients may prefer not to see a learner: they may have a very difficult personal issue to discuss; they may have seen students several times before and need a break from teaching; they may be in a rush and not have the extra time required to be seen by a student. Next, the student's ability needs to be considered. An inexperienced student at the start of clerkship may be overwhelmed by a patient with several complex problems and may not be able to deal with some patients who are abrasive or uncooperative. It may be best to start these students with more straightforward cases – for example, friendly patients with typical examples of one or two problems.

Priming, also referred to as *briefing* (Miflin *et al.*, 1997), involves spending a minute or two preparing students just before each patient encounter – quickly checking with the student what hunches he or she has about the patient based on the student's chart review and the stated reason for visit. The student should be able to describe the features of the history and physical exam he or she will focus on, what differential the student is considering or what approach he or she thinks will be most helpful, recognizing that he or she may need to change his or her approach once the student listens carefully to the patient's story. The student needs to be clear about what questions he or she needs to be able to answer at the end of his or her assessment (e.g., what is the differential diagnosis, or what investigation or treatment is indicated?). Clear expectations need to be provided regarding how much time the student should spend doing the workup and what he or she should focus on. For example:

- take 10 minutes to find out all the issues the patient wishes to discuss, or
- determine the patient's priorities and explore the top two, or
- take a detailed history of these two issues and conduct a targeted physical exam, or
- come up with a differential diagnosis and a plan for investigation and management.

Once the student has been primed several times, this process becomes much quicker. Experienced students and residents will soon be able to prime themselves by reviewing the chart before seeing the patient. It is particularly helpful to review the patient's problem list, medication list, last visit note, and any recent lab investigations.

Ongoing Needs Assessment

This is one of the most important teaching tasks and one that is often neglected. It simply means finding out what the student is good at and what they need more help with – this is important so that the teacher can concentrate on teaching what the student needs rather than what they would like to teach whether the student needs it or not. Teachers can guess at the student's needs based on other students they have taught at the same level but student variability is so great that it is essential to assess each student individually.

Teachers can begin the needs assessment during the initial orientation of the student using questionnaires or interviews but, because they are based on self-assessment, they may miss the student's blind spots. Therefore, the needs assessment must be ongoing – teachers will continue to learn about their student's needs every time they observe the student with patients and during every case presentation, chart review, and discussion with the student. Grant (2002: 157) cautions us to avoid being overly prescriptive: "Exclusive reliance on formal needs assessment in educational planning could render education an instrumental and narrow process rather than a creative, professional one. This is especially so in a profession where there is inherent unpredictability and uncertainty." The needs assessment should address not only the gaps in the student's knowledge of the core requirements of the educational program but also his or her personal goals for learning.

DURING

Irby (1992) highlights the complexity of clinical teaching – the teacher must determine that the patient's medical problem has been properly diagnosed and treated, determine the student's learning needs, and provide instruction to learners at many levels, often sleep-deprived, in a setting characterized by inter-ruptions and multiple urgent demands. He cites an example of the thoughts of a clinical Attending during hospital teaching rounds:

> I'm asking myself, does the intern have a good understanding of what is going on? I'm evaluating the person's competence in regard to this specific problem. First you listen for a level of confidence, facility with words, a certain smooth-ness that causes a favorable impression and that builds confidence. And then the proper use of jargon and surrounding content. In almost all cases I will ask a few key questions. And the way the person answers the questions, both in terms of what they say and how they justify what they say, tells me whether a person has a good knowledge and understanding of the problem. (1992: 634)

In this section we will address several features of clinical supervision important for student learning and patient safety:
- some common effective and less effective teaching methods
- a compendium of teaching strategies
- variations of the triadic relationship among teacher, student, and patient
- deciding how much responsibility to grant to a learner based on entrustable professional activities

- case presentation and discussion
- two popular models of clinical teaching – the "One-Minute Preceptor" and the "SNAPPS" method
- asking questions that encourage thinking.

Common Effective and Less Effective Teaching Methods

There are several commonly used teaching methods – some are very effective but others can interfere with student learning (*see* Table 11.1). Great teachers over the ages have used parables – stories with a message – to instruct and inspire their students. "War stories" may be entertaining and even instructive, but often they are told to enhance the reputation of the teller. A crucial distinction rests in the purpose of the narrative – whether to brag or teach. A common distortion of the Socratic method is "Guess what I'm thinking!" Rather than probing and questioning learners to help them deepen their own understanding, the teacher asks leading questions or gives hints to help students guess the "right" answer. One hazard of this approach is that students stop thinking for themselves and, instead, start second-guessing the teacher. Some teachers think that being Socratic means never answering students' questions. Often teachers like this will turn every question back on the student: "What do you think about that?" or "Why don't you look that up tonight and tell me tomorrow what you learned?" Used appropriately, these techniques are invaluable but sometimes students are so confused or overwhelmed that they need more help. Frequently the answers they seek are not in the books; sometimes, especially in an ambulatory care setting, the student needs immediate advice to help a waiting patient. When teachers never answer students' questions, they begin to think they do not know any of the answers and their credibility and effectiveness as teachers are lost. On the other hand, answering students' questions

TABLE 11.1 Comparing Common Clinical Teaching Methods

Less Effective	More Effective
"War stories"	Parables and narrative approaches
Mini-lectures	Dialogue
"Guess what I'm thinking!"	Guided discovery
"Put down"	Critique the behavior, not the person
Never answering the question	Helping the learner answer the question or providing the answer when appropriate
Grilling	Challenging
Dictating	Coaching

too often may foster dependence and might convey the message that students are not capable of learning for themselves.

One of the most destructive acts a teacher can commit is to "put down" a student; students rarely forgive such behavior and they will not respect a teacher who does not show respect for them. Students may learn facts from teachers they do not like but they will not heed the teacher's principles or values. It is especially dangerous for teachers to put down one student in front of others; they then lose the respect and credibility of the whole group of students.

While drill may be appropriate for memorizing the dosages of emergency drugs, grilling – putting a student "on the hot seat" – is usually inappropriate. Those who advocate its use argue that it helps toughen up students and prepares them to keep cool in the stressful situations of clinical practice where they must think and act quickly. In its typical form, grilling involves repeated questioning of one student until he or she gives a wrong answer or "gives up" by confessing that he or she does not know the answer. The teacher moves on to other students and continues the process until all have been shown inferior to the teacher. This approach is said to motivate students to try harder but usually ends up in "pimping" (Brancati, 1989; Detsky, 2009) – a game of clinical one-upmanship and the focus is often on esoteric or trivial information. This approach reinforces teachers' power because they control the questions and know the answers. It may encourage competition rather than teamwork, teaches that not knowing is "bad" and may leave students feeling put down. It is difficult for students to develop comfortable relationships with teachers who utilize this approach excessively. The vast majority of students in medicine are motivated to work hard. Excessive pressure from the teacher is not only unnecessary but also may be counterproductive. An overanxious student does not learn well. In a supportive environment where teachers demonstrate a genuine interest in the people they teach, students generally blossom and put forth their best efforts. In such a setting, teachers can challenge students' conclusions or even their basic assumptions without provoking so much defensiveness that they cannot learn. An effective challenge preserves, and may even enhance, the learner's self-esteem. Detsky (2009) suggests a positive view of pimping as a strategy to increase retention by being provocative:

> finding the right balance between humiliating the student who gives incorrect answers, and boring the audience by simply providing the answers is a real skill. The lesson is to not take pimping too seriously and remember that often more can be learned from incorrect answers than from correct ones. (Detsky 2009: 1381)

Another important teaching strategy is coaching. The teacher, as coach, works with students to identify skills to be learned and, together, they decide on how best to learn them. For example, consider a student who has difficulty finding common ground with diabetic patients who seem uneasy taking responsibility for self-care. The student has already discovered that providing lots of advice and cajoling patients is ineffective and is looking for more effective strategies. The teacher might jump in too quickly and direct the student to try specific interviewing methods thus replicating the ineffective strategies the student had tried with patients. Alternatively, the teacher can collaborate as a coach. The coach will assist the student to clarify his or her learning needs and identify specific skills to practice either by using role-play or observing the student with real patients and providing constructive feedback. While teachers who act as directors dictate the learning agenda, coaches support and encourage self-directed learning.

Each of these teaching methods illustrates the distinction between teacher-directed and learner-centered approaches to education, as described in Chapter 9. Of the more effective methods shown in Table 11.1, all focus on the needs of the learner more than the interests of the teacher and are rooted in a fundamental respect for the learner.

A Compendium of Teaching Strategies

There are a great many ways to help students learn the patient-centered clinical method at all levels of education. Many of these learning methods involve practice followed by feedback. In the structured environment of the preclinical curriculum, it is relatively easy to teach the basic skills of patient-centered care (e.g., in clinical skills courses). However, in the hurly-burly of clinical education, these skills may be easily ignored. Table 11.2 outlines several practical methods to incorporate the teaching of patient-centered medicine into day-to-day clinical education.

TABLE 11.2 A Compendium of Teaching Strategies

Method	Indications	How
Demonstrations of skills by faculty	To help a novice learner understand what he or she is trying to learn To demonstrate to an experienced learner that there is still more to be learned	Prepare the learner for the observation – discuss with him or her what to watch for in the demonstration A "debriefing" afterward is helpful to consolidate the learning and to respond to questions
Impromptu role-plays	To provide an opportunity to "try out" a new skill in a safe situation and receive immediate feedback about how to improve before using the skill on a real patient	Teachers need to be aware of the common "first time" skills of students at different stages in their learning and have examples of role-plays to practice (e.g., breaking the news of a new diagnosis of a serious chronic disease)
Simulated patient interviews	To practice more complex skills that are difficult for faculty to role-play (e.g., an angry or depressed patient) To reduce risk to real patients	Lay out the "ground rules" carefully first Allow "time out" if the student-doctor is stuck Provide constructive feedback allowing the "student doctor" to go first Some simulated patients are trained to provide constructive feedback
Patients playing themselves (e.g., a recovered alcoholic playing the role of an alcoholic in denial)	To practice complex skills with a real patient and get feedback from the patient All of these role-playing approaches can be used to provide experiences with important but uncommon situations that the student might otherwise not experience	These patients are carefully prepared in the same way as simulated patients, but they are playing "themselves" at an earlier phase in their illness when they were still having problems coming to terms with their diagnosis Because of their personal experiences they are able to create more depth to the role and provide invaluable insights about the impact of interviewing methods on patients with similar problems
Extended discussions with patients – this could be conducted in the patient's home	To help students understand the impact of illness on the lives of patients and their families and how their context influences their illness	Set aside 45–60 minutes for the student to have an extended conversation with a patient (or group of patients with the same problem) The focus should not be on the diagnosis but on the patient's unique illness experience Seeing more than one patient with the same disease will highlight the distinct impact of the same disease on different individuals
The student presents the patient by role-playing the patient	To help the student "enter the patient's world" and his or her illness experience and to give the other team members an opportunity to practice interacting with the patient's "proxy"	The student is instructed to interview the patient in sufficient detail and depth to be able to role-play the patient for the team Other team members interview the student who is in the role of the patient The focus can be on the interview or on the diagnosis or both (Information about physical examination and lab findings can be provided when requested)

Method	Indications	How
Present a short video clip of an interview with a patient	To provide feedback on patient-centered skills and to demonstrate them to the other members of the team It is helpful if the faculty members also show segments of their own interviews	This requires a setting in which video cameras are mounted on the wall of the interviewing room Students are encouraged to view the tape themselves first and to select a short segment or segments to show to the team The segments can be as short as 1 or 2 minutes to illustrate a particular skill or can be 20–30 minutes long if there is time The other team members provide constructive feedback
Use the "Patient-Centered Case Report" (see Chapter 12)	To practice "seeing" patients in a broad context that includes the humanistic aspects of illness This is a powerful way to reinforce the other teaching strategies listed here	This approach adds to the traditional case presentation of the disease It incorporates a description of the patient's experience of illness and the family and community context Developmental and relationship issues and finding common ground about treatment are also included
Screening exercise with real patients	To provide practice using screening methods with real patients	Assign the student to approach several patients on the ward or in the office and screen them for a common health issue (e.g., alcohol problems, depression, or immunization status) Ask the student to describe the screening technique used and the results obtained Ask how the student might apply what he or she learned to other patients Option: the interviews could be audiotaped and constructive feedback provided
Observed interviews with real patients followed by constructive feedback	"Real" patients are often more challenging and unpredictable than simulated patients It is important to consolidate skills learned in simulated situations by using them in the "real" world	Faculty can observe directly or by monitor or later by viewing a video recording After a feedback conversation, it is helpful to observe again to assess any changes in performance
Self-reflection and reading	To enhance self-awareness and to consolidate and integrate learning from reading and experience It is important to begin self-directed learning during medical school in preparation for a lifetime of learning after graduation	Provide time for reading and reflection around patients they provide care for Encourage regular review of core journals, discuss key articles, challenge students with related ideas from nonmedical journals and the humanities Model self-reflection and invite students to attend a journal club

(continued)

Method	Indications	How
Portfolios	To explore and come to terms with the personal effects of becoming a physician	Many programs now require students and residents to keep a portfolio of their reflections on their experiences caring for patients and their relationships with their peers, teachers, and family members Teachers can deepen the students' understanding and clarify their goals by discussing selected portions of their portfolios
Evidence-informed discussion of patient-centered medicine	To help learners realize that patient-centered care is based on robust research and has important measurable outcomes	Discuss key research on the impact of patient-centered approaches to care Apply this research in case discussions and the care of patients
Teaching clinical reasoning	To help students integrate the four components of the patient-centered clinical method	The One-Minute Preceptor and SNAPPS models of teaching stimulate students to be explicit about their clinical reasoning Asking students to describe how they integrate guidelines and patient's preferences and values in finding common ground requires them to bring together their analysis of their patient's medical condition with their understanding of their patient as a whole person

The Roles of Patient, Student, and Teacher

Teaching in the ambulatory setting involves a complex triadic relationship between teacher, learner, and patient. Patients are generally supportive of student participation in their care (Jones *et al.*, 1996; Bentham *et al.*, 1999), as long as they perceive that the student is working at their level of ability. Mavis *et al.* (2006) surveyed patients about factors that would influence their willingness to have medical students involved in their care. They are more willing if the request comes from their physician than from another member of the team. Student attributes (being respectful, polite, caring, gentle, neat and clean, "listens to me," and is easy to talk to) are strongly correlated with patients' willingness. Also, in one study, 93% of patients expected that their consent for involvement would be gained and should not be asked in the presence of the student, so that patients have a chance to decline (Chipp *et al.*, 2004).

Teachers, students, and patients all take on a variety of roles depending on the situation and the educational goals. Traditionally, patients have only been allowed a passive role in medical education as "teaching material," but when patients are acknowledged as experts, as described by Tuckett *et al.* (1985), they can make important contributions to student learning. By describing how interactions with their physician influenced their perceptions of health, experience of illness, and clinical outcomes they help students understand the ways in which physicians can be patient-centered. In addition, patients can play a valuable role in teaching physical examination skills. A literature review of the role of patients as teachers concluded: "If patients are given appropriate support, training, and remuneration, evidence shows that, in specific settings, patients offer unique qualities that can improve the acquisition of physical examination skills and communication, instill confidence, and change attitudes towards patients" (Wykurz & Kelly, 2002: 820). The "Patient Partners" program has patients with rheumatologic conditions trained to provide constructive feedback to students on the physical examination of their joints – focusing on proper technique and tips to minimize patient discomfort. This program has been used in several countries and has been shown to be "at least equal to Consultant Rheumatologists in the teaching of musculoskeletal examination techniques for arthritis" (Hendry et al., 1999: 674). However, another study found that students performed better on an Objective Structured Clinical Examination if they were taught by rheumatology faculty rather than Patient Partners (Humphrey-Murto et al., 2004).

Bleakley et al. (2011) point out that the traditional approach to apprenticeship, where the teacher models a strong relationship with patients, might interfere with students developing their own skills. The teacher's dominant role in the triad of teacher-patient-learner makes it difficult for students to have meaningful autonomy or sense of making any meaningful contribution to the patient's care. If teachers focus more on facilitating a stronger role for students they will learn more from these interactions and patients will feel that they have made a significant contribution to the training of the next generation of physicians. Ashley et al. (2008: 24) describe the benefits of developing a strong relationship between students and patients:

> In the most effective teaching consultations, doctors promoted a level of participation that realized patients' and students' mutual sense of responsibility by orientating them to one another, creating conditions for them to interact, promoting and regulating discourse, helping students to perform practical tasks and debriefing them afterwards.

Students valued teachers who were friendly and approachable, clarified their expectations, and oriented students to patients. Students indicated that it was important for them to know that patients had consented to being seen by a student. They valued the opportunity to interview patients on their own before the preceptor joined them in the examination room.

In the examples given here, we offer a variety of options for the roles of teacher, learner, and patient. For simplicity we have shown only one teacher in the diagrams, who could be any member of the clinical team, but we acknowledge that the teacher could include several members of the team.

Observation ("shadowing"): The teacher acts as a role model while providing the patient care. The student observes. This is especially useful to help clarify objectives by demonstration. New students benefit from this but so also do seasoned learners who are trying to learn from teachers a skill that is difficult to describe in words. 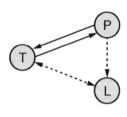 Sometimes, when the patient's problem proves too complex for the student, it is useful for the supervisor to take over and demonstrate how to sort out the problem. Learning is enhanced if teachers use a "think aloud" technique by explaining the thought processes governing their actions and decisions. Patients can be invited to provide insights into their illness experience and the ways in which physicians have been helpful to them.

Partial care. The student provides a portion of patient care (e.g., taking a history and perhaps performing part of the physical examination). This is especially suited to inexperienced students who are unfamiliar with treatment options. It is also a useful format for practicing a newly learned skill. Patients can be asked to provide feedback to 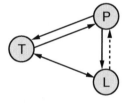 students about their physical examination skills (e.g., how hard to push on their abdomen to palpate their liver by comparing the student's examination with the teacher's).

Collaborative care. Teacher and learner together provide care (e.g., discussing treatment options and finding common ground with a patient). This allows the student to see how it is done and to be actively involved at the same time. The teacher may gradually withdraw and give more responsibility to the student. It is helpful to prepare students in advance to avoid putting them on the spot 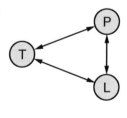 and appearing uncertain about the advice they are giving to the patient. It is important to make sure patients feel comfortable expressing their own ideas and preferences about treatment and not be intimidated by the recommendations of the two physicians in the room.

Supervised care. The teacher provides "backup" and may double-check portions of the history or physical examination on request from the learner, but the student provides the majority of care. This is appropriate for situations where the learner is comfortable assessing the patient's problem and will recognize when they need assistance.

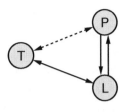

Teachers must see all patients in person and provide close supervision of care provided by an undergraduate medical student to assure patient safety and to comply with medicolegal requirements. The teacher may observe the interaction by sitting in a corner of the examination room or indirectly by a video monitor. Monitoring is done for a variety of reasons – to respond to the learner's questions, to provide feedback to the student, or to reassure the patient about the quality of care. Students benefit from the opportunity to spend some time alone with patients – to participate as a doctor-to-be and feel that they have made a difference by contributing to the care of the patient. For more experienced learners, supervision can be provided indirectly by discussing the case without the supervisor seeing the patient. The patient is in a good position to provide feedback to the learner, as well as the supervisor, about the care they received by completing an anonymous survey (Evans *et al.*, 2007).

Facilitator. The teacher functions as a facilitator of learning; the learner provides full care to the patient. Experienced learners can be entrusted to decide when they need assistance from their teacher. This situation is appropriate when the patient problem is within the competence of the learner. The teacher may observe in order to provide constructive feedback but usually supervision is

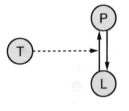

provided by request of the learner or patient or by chart review and end-of-day debriefing. The patient's role is to provide direct feedback to the learner and he or she may be in a position to provide tips on providing patient-centered care (e.g., approaches he or she has seen with more experienced physicians).

Entrustable Professional Activities

New clinical teachers are often unsure how much responsibility to give to their learners. They know that students learn best when they must make their own decisions about patient care rather than simply following the suggestions of their teacher. Granting too much responsibility may overwhelm a resident who is not ready and places patients at risk, but not granting enough responsibility holds residents back and reduces their learning (Cantillon & Mcdermott,

2008). "Carrying out activities that are just at the edge of one's competence can stimulate maximum comprehension and a steep learning curve" (Sterkenburg *et al.*, 2010: 1408). Residents need to learn how to apply their skills when they are facing the stress of being responsible for the well-being and the lives of their patients. However, preceptors also recognize their responsibility to assure patient safety. This balancing act can be challenging. Often, clinicians assume a level of competence in their learners based on their year of training. Although that approach provides a rough estimate of a learner's capabilities, it is often inaccurate.

Recently, Olle ten Cate (2006) has proposed the concept of entrustable professional activities (EPAs) to guide clinical teachers in this important decision. There are three overlapping sets of abilities or traits that need to be considered in granting increased responsibility (*see* Figure 11.2). All EPAs will require appropriate personal qualities and basic clinical skills; specific EPAs will relate primarily to context and content specific abilities. Typically, an EPA will be granted in stages – for example, taking a history, then performing a focused physical examination, then developing a differential diagnosis, and, finally, generating a treatment plan. Different domains of practice will have their own EPAs since they require different specific abilities.

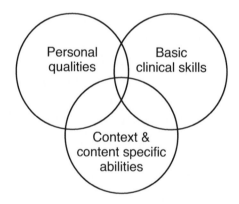

FIGURE 11.2 Factors to consider in granting an entrustable professional activity

Personal Qualities

Three personal qualities are essential to protect patient safety before allowing residents to see patients independently – truthfulness, conscientiousness, and discernment (Kennedy *et al.*, 2008). Most residents are conscientious and most will be truthful, unless their teachers punish them for being honest about their uncertainties and their inability to conduct impossibly complete assessments in the short time available. Most residents are not very accurate in self-assessment

(Eva *et al.*, 2004; Davis *et al.*, 2006) but should be able to sense when they need to slow down, rethink their assessment, or ask for help (Moulton *et al.*, 2007; Epstein *et al.*, 2008). Medical education tends to encourage a "macho" approach of trying to get by without needing any assistance. It is important for preceptors to dispel this false ideal and replace it with the ideal of getting help when needed to assure patient safety.

- *Truthfulness*: trust that what they said or recorded are accurate reflections of what they actually did. They are honest about their confusion or lack of knowledge. They do not modify their presentations simply to impress their teacher.
- *Conscientiousness*: they go the extra mile for patients when necessary and take responsibility for their actions. They do not cut corners in ways that might compromise patient welfare. They do what is right even when no one is looking.
- *Discernment*: they are aware of their limits and when they need help, and will take appropriate steps to get assistance. They are effective at "self-directed assessment seeking" (Eva & Regehr, 2008: 14). Patient welfare is their first concern and is more important than "looking good" in the eyes of their supervisor. They are aware of personal beliefs, attitudes, and emotions that may impair their judgment.

Basic Clinical Skills

Basic clinical skills are essential for adequate assessment of patients' problems and concerns. Effective patient-centered interviewing is important to set patients at ease and involve them in setting the goals for the visit and incorporating their values and preferences in treatment. Unless patients are comfortable with the resident they may not disclose some of their concerns. Also, if they are not involved in decisions about management, they may not follow through on the treatment plan. Skills in history taking, physical examination, and clinical reasoning are obviously essential for safe patient care. Unfortunately, students are not observed enough during medical school so many residents do not all have well-developed skills in these areas. Some studies suggest that teachers need to observe residents 8–16 times to accurately assess these skills (van Thiel *et al.*, 1991; Schechter *et al.*, 1996). The degree of autonomy and independence granted to a resident will be determined by their teacher's assessment of the resident's ability to provide safe care. The following description of competencies outlines the many abilities that teachers look for in their residents but their final decision is more often based on a gut reaction than on a detailed analysis of this long list of competencies.

If clinical supervisors think of their trainees, they would be able to identify those whom they would entrust with a complex medical task because they will either perform well and seek help if necessary or not accept the task if they don't feel confident. Supervisors often know who to pick, even if they can't tell exactly why. This gut feeling does not always match with formally assessed knowledge or skill, but it may be more valid for its purpose. (ten Cate, 2006: 749)

- *Interviewing*: they apply the patient-centered clinical method in all consultations with patients using evidence-based interviewing skills as described in the Calgary-Cambridge Guides (Silverman *et al.*, 2004). They are particularly effective in putting patients at ease, not interrupting the patient's opening monologue, using open-ended inquiry, reflective listening, and empathy. They explore the patient's unique illness narrative to understand the patient's ideas about what might be causing his or her concerns, how the patient feels about them, how they affect the patient's daily function, and what the patient hopes the physician will do to help him or her. They involve patients in setting the goals for the encounter and in decisions regarding investigation and treatment. They use the electronic medical record to enhance collaboration with patients.
- *History-taking skills*: they quickly review the problem list, medication list, and last visit note before seeing the patient. They determine all of the patient's concerns and, together with the patient, decide whether or not they can all be addressed at this visit and then set priorities. They explore each concern appropriately recognizing when it is important to supplement the patient's history with information from family, other physicians, and the past medical record. They recognize which historical features have high predictive value. Their data gathering is guided by their search for a differential diagnosis as well as to clarify treatment issues – for example, simply knowing the diagnosis is not adequate for planning management; treatment will be quite different for a chronic stable condition compared with an acute exacerbation. They are also skilled at exploring patients' narratives and integrating information related to disease with the meanings derived from the narrative.
- *Physical examination skills*: their physical examinations are organized and conducted skillfully. They are able to distinguish normal variants from abnormalities.
- *Clinical reasoning*: they are able to apply both analytic and nonanalytic approaches to clinical reasoning and recognize the inherent risks of error of

each approach (Palaccia *et al.*, 2011). They consider both probability and payoff in developing an appropriate differential diagnosis and recognize red flags. They are able to manage uncertainty appropriately and can recognize when it is appropriate to reassure the patient or use time as a diagnostic tool or when it is important to investigate more intensively, or to act quickly or refer. They are able to prioritize problems. They recognize that patients consult physicians for many reasons, not just disease, and are familiar with McWhinney's taxonomy of illness behavior (McWhinney, 1972) and can modify their approach to address the particular needs of their patients. They are able to make appropriate decisions regarding their patients' predicaments even when they cannot make a definitive diagnosis.

- *Case presentation*: their case presentations are clear, well-organized, and include the key information on which they based their decisions, including important negative findings. Their case presentations also include a summary of the patient's illness experience and how patient preferences are incorporated into the treatment plans.
- *Record keeping*: their medical notes are a concise, well-organized and accurate record of their findings and decision making.

Content- and Context-Specific Abilities

The first two sets of qualities and abilities are somewhat general and apply to a wide range of patients and their problems. However, the third domain is highly content and context specific. For example, residents may be very skilled in the assessment and treatment of patients with asthma but limited in their abilities with patients with diabetes. This is largely a reflection of their prior experience with patients with specific conditions. Because of this, it is important for clinical supervisors to assess their residents' abilities with a range of clinical presentations and not assume that, because they were skilled in managing the last patient with angina, they will be equally skilled with the next patient suffering with dementia. However, once the supervisor has seen a resident perform well in managing several patients with a range of conditions, it is reasonable to assume that they will do well with the next patient. As long as the resident will seek assistance when they feel out of their depth, then patient safety can be assured. The supervisor will take into account a number of factors related to the patient when considering how much independence is appropriate. The seriousness of the patient's condition, complexity of multimorbidities, and challenging behavioral or social factors may all merit more careful supervision and affect the level of responsibility given.

A Competent Resident will Demonstrate the Following Abilities

- They are able to apply disease-specific knowledge in assessment by appropriately modifying their approach to the history and physical examination.
- They are skilled in applying principles of the behavioral sciences appropriate to the patient's presentation.
- They are skilled in applying their competencies in different settings – in a family practice office, in the emergency department, on a hospital ward, or in a patient's home. (Skill in one setting does not necessarily transfer to skill in another.)
- They are skilled in caring for patients across the life cycle and across diverse populations.

Case Presentation and Discussion

Presenting a case in a well-organized manner that includes only the information needed for assessment and treatment is a complex skill that is gradually learned by most students as they progress through the clinical clerkship. One of the challenges for students is the lack of any standard format – every teacher seems to want a different approach. Most teachers like to start with basic demographic information (e.g., "Mary Smith is a 64-year-old married white female . . ."), but there is little agreement about what comes next. Some teachers prefer to have the student present a complete problem list followed by a list of presenting complaints; others want to hear more about the personal situation of the patient (e.g., living situation, job). Some like a problem-oriented format; others, a more traditional outline. It is important to not leave students guessing; let them know the teacher's preferred format for case presentation and provide a short handout. Suggesting to students that their case presentations should include information about the patient's life situation, their ideas about what is wrong with them, and their preferences for treatment gives a strong message about the importance of using a patient-centered approach in their care. (*See* Chapter 12 for a description of the patient-centered case report.)

While listening to the case presentation, teachers may quickly recognize a familiar disease pattern, or they may be developing hypotheses about the patient's diagnoses and considering what should be done next. They may have many questions to explore the differential diagnosis but it is best to save these until after the presentation. From the students' perspective, the ideal presentation is one that is not interrupted too often – interruptions may confuse them and are often seen as criticisms of their presentation (Lingard *et al.*, 2003). Students also tend to downplay uncertainty, considering it a sign of weakness, whereas teachers need to know when the student is uncertain in order to explore these areas in more detail. Interruptions may be valuable to help the student stay on track or get back on track, to explore important areas omitted by the student, and to make a teaching point. Be careful that these "detours" do not sidetrack the presentation, leading to major sections being left out – for example, when a student presents a patient with diabetes, it is tempting to launch into the teacher's favorite teaching script on diabetes. If the case presentation drags on, teachers may be concerned about getting behind in their schedule and proceed to seeing the patient before the student has told them about the patient's other potentially serious problems lower down on the problem list.

It is often valuable to have students present their findings in front of the patient (Rogers *et al.*, 2003). This saves time, patients like it better, it may provide information about the interaction between the student and patient, and it facilitates teaching about clinical skills. It also gives the patient an opportunity to correct any misinformation and reassures the patient that the teacher has heard the whole story. However, students should warn their teacher if the patient has very personal issues or a potentially serious condition. In this case, it may be preferable to discuss the case first away from the patient. Sometimes it is useful to discuss the case separately from the patient to facilitate an exploration of the student's clinical reasoning. Also, some students lack confidence and feel very uncomfortable presenting in front of patients. In this case it is best to let them present privately until they gain confidence.

Students should be able to present cases without reading their clinical notes. However, novice learners may need to use cue cards to keep themselves organized and not leave out important information. It is important for students to learn to present in a manner that "makes the case" for their diagnosis rather than in the same order in which they collected the data. For learners who have trouble providing a concise case presentation, teachers could suggest: "Summarize the patient's situation in three sentences." This can be a great strategy for getting them to hone their skills in case presentation and prepares them for telephone case presentations that often need to be very brief.

Some Tips on Clinical Supervision

- Focus on one aspect of the interview for a day such as the initial determination of all the patient's concerns or focusing on how well the resident explains the treatment plan to patients or how well they find common ground with patients. Focusing on one skill for a whole day fits well with what we know about deliberate practice – concentrating on a very specific task and repeating it over and over again with feedback after each trial until it is mastered (Ericsson, 2008).

- Ask "What else could this be?" when working with strong residents who have a good knowledge base and excellent clinical reasoning skills. Sometimes these residents get so confident that they start taking too many short cuts. Their experience is usually not good enough to be relying solely on pattern recognition.

- Use a monitor to view a resident-patient interaction. This is a good strategy for giving students and residents a greater sense of being on their own and being responsible for patient care decisions. It is particularly valuable for monitoring communication and relationship skills.

- Address issues dealing with uncertainty. It is important to help residents, especially in their senior years, learn how to deal with the discomfort of decision making in conditions of uncertainty. They need to learn how to differentiate uncertainty related to their own learning needs from uncertainty inherent in the patient's condition and they need to recognize when they need help. They need to learn how to evaluate the seriousness of a patient's condition even when they cannot make a diagnosis.

- Use "What if" questions to challenge strong residents – for example, What if this patient with pneumonia had been traveling in California or Arizona recently? What if this was a rural setting? What if the patient was a child, or a senior? What if you were practicing in a remote location?

- Demonstrate aspects of the physical examination on the resident – for example, how hard to push over the sinuses to determine tenderness or over costochondral junctions to diagnose costochondral pain.

- Give residents more independence. They will learn more if they have to take more responsibility for decisions about patient care and not feel too comfortable knowing their teacher will bail them out. Pushing residents to make their own decisions teaches them a lot more than if they had just watched the teacher passively.

- If there is time, consider providing an immediate opportunity for the learner to practice a skill they have just learned – for example, if they have just been assisted by their supervisor to provide instructions to a patient, it will help to consolidate their learning if they have a chance to practice these patient education skills with the teacher playing the role of the patient. This may take only 2–3 minutes but will pay dividends in their learning. Another valuable use of role-play is rehearsal just before the learner sees a patient – for example, they can be instructed on how to ask about treatment

adherence or about how to break bad news and then have an opportunity to try it out with the teacher role-playing the patient.
- Provide a conceptual framework. Decision trees and diagrams are helpful to organize masses of data or to uncover gaps in information. When students are confused or unclear about a patient's problem, it is often useful to depict the situation as shown in Figure 11.3. In these situations it is common to have a large mass of data about the patient's diseases and even some ideas about the patient's illness experience and health concerns. However, often, the sections on "Person" and "Context" are sparse. This visual representation assists the student to recognize the deficiencies in their understanding of the patient and suggests areas for further enquiry. The diagram can also be used to document the accumulating knowledge about the patient.

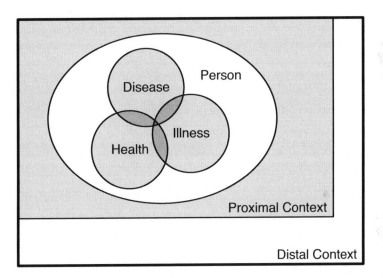

FIGURE 11.3 The whole person

When a student is having difficulty working with a patient, the source of trouble is often related to finding common ground. Box 11.1 illustrates a useful grid for identifying disagreements between patient and physician regarding treatment. In our experience, difficult interactions are reflected by differences of opinion about the nature of the problem, the goals of treatment, and the respective roles of the patient and doctor. Filling in the grid makes the conflict obvious and leads naturally into a discussion about how to deal with their differences.

Box 11.1 Finding common ground

Issue	Patient	Doctor
Problems		
Goals		
Roles		

- When students reach the limits of their knowledge, ask how they are going to seek more understanding of the issues. Schedule a definite time to follow up on what they learn. Students will remember more if they have struggled to find the answers for themselves. Effective teachers get to know their students well enough that they can judge how much challenge is appropriate – too much leaves them overwhelmed, but too little reduces their learning (Ambrose *et al.*, 2010). When the decision cannot wait, you may need to offer a suggestion. If possible, offer options and encourage students to choose from them and to explain their choices. Use questions to clarify what students are saying rather than to probe their ignorance.
- Chart review is particularly helpful for assessing the strength of the evidence for the student's diagnostic conclusions and proposed investigation and treatment. The traditional record needs to be modified to fit the patient-centered clinical method. For example, students should include information about the patient's "illness experience" (feelings, ideas, effects on function, and expectations).
- Video review is valuable for helping students examine their communication skills and reasoning process (Vassilas & Ho, 2000; Nilson & Baerheim, 2005; Kelly, 2012). It has the special advantage of allowing students to monitor their own performance, with, or even without, the teacher acting as a facilitator. It also enables the teaching occasion to be postponed until more time for the analysis of the recording is available. The video stimulates

recall of the student's thought processes during the interview and can be used to explore why they asked certain questions, why they ignored others, and why they did not ask questions that were on their minds. Studies of the use of video recording in teaching interviewing skills show significant advantages. For example, Verby *et al.* (1979) studied the impact of general practitioners providing peer review of their colleagues' videotaped interviews. A control group submitted video recordings that were not discussed. The peer learning group improved in a number of ways (compared with the control group): they picked up more leads; clarified more; used more facilitation; improved their questioning style; ended the interview more smoothly. Maguire and colleagues (1989) found similar results in a series of well-designed and controlled studies. Even 4–6 years later, the students who had received feedback on videotaped interviews were more likely to retain their skills than the control group.

- Learning from role models should not be a passive activity. Students must be prepared, by their teachers, to focus on specific behaviors and then have an opportunity to discuss their observations. Before the teacher and student enter the examining room, it is helpful for the supervisor to explain his or her goals and particular techniques that he or she intends to use. For example, if the student has already seen the patient but been unable to determine the patient's experience of illness, the teacher may remind the student about the four dimensions that need to be explored and briefly outline the kinds of questions that could be asked. Following the encounter, they will discuss the student's observations and the teacher's reasons for certain actions.

The One-Minute Preceptor Model

Teaching in a busy clinical setting must be quick. There is reasonable evidence that the One-Minute Preceptor model (also referred to as the Five Microskills Method) (Neher & Stevens, 2003) is an effective approach (Furney *et al.*, 2001; Aagard *et al.*, 2004). This is a set of basic clinical teaching skills that are effective in many teaching situations. Some or all of these skills can be applied after a student has presented a case to enhance his or her learning. However, they should not be used as a recipe – in some situations, other skills should be used.

- *Get a commitment.* This means getting students to commit themselves to an opinion about the diagnosis or about investigation or treatment. They need to feel comfortable enough with their teacher to be able to "stick their neck out" in making the commitment. By making a commitment, they feel more responsible and are more motivated to learn.
- *Probe for supporting evidence.* Ask students to provide a rationale and

evidence for their commitment – how they came to their conclusions. This provides important insights into their knowledge base, reasoning skills, and learning needs. This is an important part of the ongoing needs assessment of the student. Of course, teachers will also be forming an opinion about the student's strengths and weaknesses during the case presentation and subsequent questioning.

- *Teach general rules.* For example, "When a patient's hypertension is poorly controlled, ask about adherence to medication and alcohol intake," or it may be a recommendation to read up on a particular topic. Even better, ask the learner about their "take home" message from their experience with a particular patient. General rules enhance the likelihood that the student will be able to apply what he or she has learned to another similar case. Sometimes there will be time to provide a mini-lecture – a brief outline of a clinical pearl that may be hard to find in a textbook. Having a file of articles or notes allows teachers to provide handouts to reinforce and amplify what they have taught. It is also helpful to have good websites bookmarked for later reference by the student. Having a small, up-to-date library of core texts is also valuable for reference when clinical questions arise although this is less necessary now that so many online resources are available including whole textbooks through university library systems.
- *Reinforce what was right.*
- *Correct mistakes.* These last two important elements of the One-Minute Preceptor model are further discussed in the section on feedback later in this chapter.

The SNAPPS Framework

The SNAPPS framework (Wolpaw *et al.*, 2003) is particularly useful for a confident student or resident who is ready to take more responsibility for his or her own learning. In this model the learner takes control of the discussion around the case presentation. SNAPPS is an acronym for the following six steps.

1. **S** – Summarize briefly the history and findings (generally no longer than 3 minutes). This should include a description of who the patient is, a full list of the patient's problems, and the patient's current concerns, followed by a brief history, physical examination, and laboratory findings of each active problem. This should be condensed to the key relevant positive and negative findings.
2. **N** – Narrow the diagnosis or treatment of each active problem to two or three relevant possibilities. This is analogous to "make a commitment" in the One-Minute Preceptor model.

3. **A** – Analyze the reasoning by reviewing the findings or examining the evidence – compare and contrast the possibilities. In this step, the learner presents his or her thinking in ruling in or ruling out each diagnostic possibility.
4. **P** – Probe the preceptor by asking questions about uncertainties or by asking for help in reviewing part of the physical examination.
5. **P** – Plan treatment: this is often done in collaboration with the teacher.
6. **S** – Select a case-related issue for self-directed learning.

Some teachers would add another **S** – Solicit feedback.

There are many similarities with the One-Minute Preceptor model – except in this approach, the learner leads the process and the teacher may be relatively silent until probed about the learner's uncertainties. However, the teacher may be quite actively involved in the conversation if the learner is struggling – for example, in guiding the learner to consider other possible diagnoses or treatment options or in correcting any errors. The teacher may need to coach the learner initially but he or she should quickly encourage the learner to take over the lead role. The teacher's main role is to act as a guide. Both the One-Minute Preceptor and SNAPPS models focus on diagnosis and treatment and tend to ignore issues related to communication, relationships, and development.

Addressing this gap is narrative-based supervision, an approach developed by Launer and others (Launer & Lindsey, 1997; Halpern & Morrison, 2012). Using this approach, the learner brings an issue or concern to the supervisor, whose role it is to help the learner explore the issue by asking a series of short, open-ended questions. The goal is to help the student reflect on the story the student is telling him- or herself about the issue so that he or she can consider alternative stories. Their conversation is a form of shared narrative leading to a new way of thinking about the issue or concern. "The supervisor accepts the supervisee's story and does not offer any interpretations or advice, but allows the supervisee to come up with his own solution" (Halpern & Morrison, 2012: 51). This approach is consistent with the learner-centered approach described in Chapter 9 and can address important questions related to the student's development as a clinician.

Questions: A Fundamental Teaching Tool

Questions are the teachers' primary tool for stimulating thinking in the learner. It is helpful to ask questions from a low to a high level of complexity and to start with the most junior member of the team. Avoid asking a junior to answer a question a senior has been unable to answer – it can be humiliating for the senior. Create a comfortable environment in which anyone can say, "I don't know," even the teacher (Lake *et al.*, 2005). Inform learners that often more is learned from an incorrect answer than a correct one – it may point out a common misunderstanding that needs clarification. This may encourage learners to take their best guess at an answer rather than remaining silent. Sometimes follow up a correct answer with another question to check how they arrived at the answer – students may get the right answer for the wrong reason. Make sure to involve everyone on rounds when asking questions. Some of the most useful questions the teacher can ask are the following:

- "What do you think is going on with this patient?"
- "How did you reach that conclusion?" or "What is the evidence for that conclusion?"
- "What else could it be?"
- "What do you think we should do next?"
- "How would you explain that to the patient?"
- "What are the patient's ideas or concerns?"
- "What are you feeling right now about this patient?" "What is it about the patient that makes you feel this way?"
- "In what ways can you be helpful and comforting to the patient?"

Common Errors in Asking Questions

- Asking questions that require memory but not thought – for example, "What is the starting dose of pravastatin?" This is a rather trivial question that can easily be looked up. On the other hand, it is important to know the correct dose of medications needed in an emergency when delay could be harmful to the patient.
- Not waiting long enough for an answer. Waiting only a few seconds longer will increase the likelihood of students answering and will result in better answers (Rowe, 1986). If the question is met with silence, wait at least 10 seconds before rephrasing the question or providing additional information.
- Avoid leading questions – questions that imply a particular answer. For example, "Don't you think that he is more likely to have heart failure, given his chest findings and gallop rhythm?"
- Putting students down for not knowing the answer. When this happens the teacher loses the students' respect and students become fearful and learn less. Even a wrong answer may be partially correct. Teachers can respond in this way: "You are partly right, but there is another aspect that we need to consider . . ."

AFTER

In this section we provide a detailed analysis of feedback with examples of effective and less effective methods, and address its emotional impact, the learner's role in feedback conversations, and two popular models of feedback – Pendleton's rules and ALOBA (Agenda-Led, Outcome-Based Analysis). We conclude with a discussion of reflection for learners as well as teachers.

Feedback Conversations in Clinical Teaching and Learning

Feedback is "information communicated to the learner that is intended to modify his or her thinking or behavior to improve learning" (Shute, 2008: 153). Feedback can come from observing the consequences of one's actions, from personal reflection, from peers, from patients, and from teachers. In the not too distant past, when teacher-centered approaches dominated thinking about medical education, feedback consisted of the authoritative pronouncements by teachers about their students' performance – what they did right and what they did wrong. It was often an unpleasant and sometimes humiliating experience. The learners' role in receiving feedback was passive – they were expected to accept their teachers' opinions without question and change their behavior accordingly.

More recently, learner-centered approaches to medical education have become prominent (Ludmerer, 2004). Feedback, in this approach, is a collaborative enterprise in which teachers and learners together explore a student's performance seeking to understand better how it went – what went well and what could be done even better. The following definition of feedback reflects this approach: "Constructive feedback is the art of holding conversations with learners about their performance" (Mohanna *et al.*, 2004). In the same vein, Jenny King (1999: S4) comments: "Giving feedback is not just to provide a judgment or evaluation. It is to provide insight. Without insight into their own strengths and limitations (trainees) cannot progress or resolve difficulties." For example, a deeper understanding of what went well enables the learner to achieve the same ends at will in future occasions. An effective feedback conversation answers three questions:

1. Where am I going (what are the goals)?
2. How am I doing (what progress is being made toward the goal)?
3. Where to next (what activities need to be undertaken to make better progress) (Hattie & Timperley, 2007)?

Feedback is essential for learning (Cantillon & Sargeant, 2008). Without feedback, the learner can practice over and over again but may never know if he or she is doing it right. Research on effect size shows that feedback is one of the most powerful influences on learning (Hattie & Timperley, 2007; Norcini, 2010). "Indeed, in an educational context it is now argued that learning is the key purpose of assessment" (Norcini & Burch, 2007: 855). However, some research has shown that students and residents are not observed frequently enough and the feedback they do receive is often vague and unhelpful (Day *et al.*, 1990; Bing-You & Trowbridge, 2009; Perera *et al.*, 2008). Assessment is important during all phases of education: during orientation (needs assessment); throughout the educational program (ongoing feedback); and at the completion of the program (summative assessment to certify competence). Summative assessment is important periodically to assure that students are on track for successful completion of the program and to identify faltering or failing students or residents who need additional or modified educational opportunities or other interventions to address their individual needs.

Regular assessment of students and residents is important to assure patient safety. On a busy clinical service, teachers may assume that a senior student or resident will be capable of working up patients without direct supervision. They may observe a learner a few times and, being satisfied with their performance, assume that they can carry on with minimal supervision. Supervisors need to observe samples of behavior for many different topics in different settings to get an overall sense of competence. If the sample is too small, they may be lulled into a false conclusion. Learners can help supervisors gain a more accurate assessment of their abilities by openly disclosing their areas of weakness or difficulty and by regularly asking for feedback.

How Students can Contribute to the Feedback Conversation

Supervisors should recognize that student and resident self-assessment is inevitably inaccurate (Davis *et al.*, 2006). In their seminal paper "'I'll Never Play Professional Football' and Other Fallacies of Self-Assessment," Eva and Regehr (2008) suggest that programs should not attempt to improve the quality of self-assessment (which they regard as impossible) but, rather, focus instead on *self-directed assessment seeking*. Others have argued that a habit of feedback seeking is essential for lifelong learning (Duffy & Holmboe, 2006). In a study by Milan *et al.* (2011), clinical clerks were given a 90-minute workshop on how to elicit feedback from their supervisors and residents. Students "were encouraged to present an attitude of emotional readiness to learn from their mistakes and to assist their instructors in feedback formulation by presenting them with specific questions" (2011: 905). Before the workshop, 39% of students indicated that they never asked for feedback but only 3.5% never asked for feedback after the workshop. Eighty-four percent stated that the feedback helped to improve their clinical skills.

Students and residents can assist their teachers to provide helpful feedback in several ways (Rudland *et al.*, 2013). Teachers can offer the following list of suggestions to their learners.

- Ask your supervisor to observe you performing a particular task (e.g., examination of the knee, breaking bad news, or explaining a treatment plan to a patient) and ask for feedback on particular aspects of your performance. It helps if you can provide specific comments on how you thought you did to begin a dialogue about your strengths and areas to work on. At its best, feedback is a conversation with your teacher focused on trying to understand at a deep level what went well, what you did to make it go well, and what you might do to make it even better.

- If the feedback is vague or general, even if it is positive, ask for suggestions on how to improve – for example, "I'm wondering if you can help me think of ways I could have done that even better." Or you can ask for comments about specific aspects of an interaction with a patient – for example, "I thought the history was going well until I started asking about his relationship with his wife. At that point he started giving me one-word answers and seemed to not want to talk about it. I couldn't think of a way to get back on track. What do you do in those situations?"

- If you receive negative feedback, pause and think before responding. The initial pain of negative feedback will fade. Resist the powerful urge to explain yourself. "Well the reason that I did that was because . . .," "That was because I . . ." Explanations cut off further feedback, they are interpreted as statements that you are not ready to hear more. Students with a learning orientation use feedback as a tool to help them improve; students with a performance orientation are more focused on demonstrating competence to others. Research shows that those with a learning orientation are less likely to give up and are more willing to tackle difficult or challenging tasks where success is less likely (Archer, 2010).

- Indicate verbally and nonverbally that you value the feedback, even if you disagree with it. Remember that teachers usually feel uncomfortable providing negative feedback and that it takes courage to tell you about their concerns. Use facial gestures and nodding of your head to acknowledge the feedback. Ask questions for understanding. Summarize and reflect what you hear to show that you are really listening. Ask for it to be repeated if you did not fully understand it.

- Try to suspend judgment; work to accept the feedback as possibly correct.

However, don't take negative feedback personally or blow it out of proportion and assume everything you do is bad. Use the 1% rule (assume that all of the feedback is at least partially true – at least 1%). Assume it is constructive until proven otherwise. Often others can see us better than we can see ourselves. Accept it positively (for consideration) rather than dismissively (for self-protection).

- Show appreciation to the person providing the feedback.
- Take time after the feedback to reflect on the information and consider specific areas for improvement. Use feedback to clarify your goals and to track progress on your goals.

Feedback and Emotions (Molloy *et al.*, 2013)

Although feedback is "the cornerstone of effective clinical teaching" (Cantillon & Sargeant, 2008), providing feedback is challenging because of the multiple needs it must satisfy – the fundamental need to protect patient safety, the need to assure that feedback is honest and accurate, and the need to protect the self-esteem of the learner. "Students' emotions greatly influence the way in which they are able to receive and process feedback, and sometimes the value of such feedback may be 'eclipsed by learners' reactions' to it" (Värlander, 2008: 146). When feedback, critical of a performance, is experienced as a judgment about the person, the remarks may be magnified with damage to self-esteem and confidence. It is more helpful to offer feedback about deficiencies as suggestions for improvement rather than as a list of weaknesses. Positive feedback tends to produce feelings of well-being and energy in students, but negative feedback arouses feelings of anxiety and depression. Students receiving negative feedback may discount it as useless, burdensome, critical, or controlling (Baron, 1988). Providing positive feedback first makes negative feedback more tolerable and believable. Involving students in discussion about the feedback makes it less threatening and more effective. Peer feedback is less intimidating because it is reassuring to learn that others share the same difficulties. When students feel a lack of power and recognition from their teacher they may experience fear, anxiety, and low self-esteem.

Another important paper, by Mann *et al.* (2011), describes some of the tensions that interfere with the feedback process. For example, students may want feedback yet fear disconfirming information. They may want to be able to question others and learn from feedback, yet not want to look incompetent or share areas of deficiency. The studies of feedback highlight the importance of developing a relationship between teacher and learner that is supportive and in which they feel safe to disclose their struggles. If learners do not trust the positive intent of their teachers they are likely to discount any negative feedback their supervisor provides and will not learn from it. When medical education is structured so that feedback is provided by a series of supervisors, often from different clinical rotations, it may be ineffective. It is important for learners to have an ongoing relationship with a small number of supervisors who they respect and trust. The "culture of assessment" needs to change from one in which any learning need is seen as a deficiency to be criticized, to one in which feedback is experienced as a gift to enhance learning. Reframing the supervisor as a coach rather than a judge might be a step in the right direction. A coach's role is to pinpoint areas that the learner performed well and identify approaches he or she could use to perform even better, and then, together with the learner, develop a plan to acquire and practice the new skills.

Frameworks for Feedback

Having a framework for providing feedback is helpful. The following two frameworks are used for teaching communication skills. Pendleton *et al.* (2003) developed a popular framework, dubbed "Pendleton's rules" that were "designed to create a safe environment in which learners could respond more positively to recommendations, avoiding defensiveness. This would be an environment in which learners could take risks in their development and experiment without fear" (2003: 77). Prior to or at the beginning of a feedback session, teacher and learner should clarify the process: the timeframe for the discussion, the learner's agenda, the teacher's agenda, and the roles and responsibilities of each. It is important to have a clearly established focus for the feedback conversation. It is not fair to raise concerns about an issue that had not been on the agenda unless there is mutual agreement to add it. The feedback session itself is framed by four rules or principles that should be applied flexibly depending on the circumstances:

1. Briefly clarify any matters of fact (but no rhetorical questions please!)
2. Encourage the learner to go first
3. Consider what has been done well first
4. Make recommendations rather than state weaknesses. (Pendleton *et al.*, 2003: 77)

Positive feedback preserves or enhances the learner's self-respect, whereas negative feedback may damage self-respect and provoke defensiveness or resistance to change.

The ALOBA shares many similarities with the Pendleton approach but is more elaborate (Kurtz *et al.*, 2005). It is often used with a small group of learners. The first step is to organize the feedback process.

- Start with the learner's agenda – the problem(s) they would like help with.
- Look at the outcomes the learner and patient are trying to achieve – this encourages a problem-solving approach.
- Encourage self-assessment and self-problem solving first.
- Involve the whole group in problem solving – to help the learner and also to help themselves in similar situations.

Then give feedback to one another.

- Use descriptive language to encourage a nonjudgmental approach – be as specific as possible to avoid vague generalizations.
- Provide balanced feedback – learning from what went well and what didn't work so well.
- Make offers and suggestions; generate alternatives rather than making prescriptive comments – they should be offered in the spirit of ideas for consideration.
- Show respect and be sensitive to one another.

Then consolidate the learning.

- Rehearse suggestions – all members of the group try out alternative phrasing by role-playing.
- Value the interview as a gift of raw material for the group to learn from.
- Introduce theory, research evidence, and wider discussion as appropriate and if time permits.
- Structure and summarize learning so that a constructive end point is reached.

Additional Tips on Providing Feedback

- Making notes, when observing a learner, helps teachers recall the points they wish to make – this helps them to be more specific. For example, "When the patient said . . . you changed the subject and later the patient brought it up again. Then you picked up nicely on his question and expressed empathy when you said . . ." By recording exactly what was said you are able to remind the resident about the interaction. Sometimes they are surprised by the words they used.
- Comment favorably on what was done right. Students may not realize how good it was. Reinforcing this behavior makes it more likely they will keep doing it.

- Describe the observed behavior, not the person. It is usually best to avoid making assumptions about motives – just describe what was observed. In describing their behavior, be as specific as possible. Don't "beat around the bush" in an attempt to sugarcoat areas needing improvement – the risk is that they will not understand the comments and not realize they had made a mistake, or they may know by the teacher's tone of voice or facial expression that they did something wrong but not know what it was.
- End the feedback with a discussion about what the learner can do to improve any deficiencies. Start by asking the student what ideas he or she has for further learning.
- Follow up with positive feedback and praise when improvements are noted.
- Sometimes it helps to be explicit about providing feedback because learners often underestimate the amount of feedback they actually receive, thinking it was just a discussion. You could say, "Let's discuss how that last interaction went. I will give you some feedback about what I think, but I'd like to work together with you and find out first what you think."

TABLE 11.3 Examples of Feedback

Quality	Good Example	Poor Example
It is descriptive not evaluative	"I notice you didn't make eye contact with the last patient during the interview."	"You are not interested in patient care."
It is specific rather than general	"You were able to convey empathy and understanding during the interview. For example, when he looked upset discussing his recent divorce, you . . ."	"You did a good job."
It is focused on issues the learner can control	"When taking the history, it would help to speak slower and check for understanding."	"My patients cannot understand you because of your accent."
It is well timed	Provided regularly throughout the learning experience, and as close as possible to the events stimulating the feedback	Provided only at the end of the rotation
It is limited in amount	Focused on a single, important message	Learner overwhelmed with information
It addresses learner goals	Addresses learning goals identified by the learner at the beginning of the rotation	Learner's goals are ignored

What To Do if the Student or Resident is Not Doing Well

The teacher's first responsibility is to discuss their concerns with the student or resident to try to figure out the nature of the problem. Learners struggle for many reasons and often have little insight into their problems. In addition to assessing the learner's contribution to their poor performance, it is important to sort out the role of the teacher and the system (Leung, 2012). Does the teacher have unrealistic expectations, or ineffective teaching methods; is there adequate ongoing feedback? All three sources of difficulty must be addressed to help faltering or failing students. If dealing with problems in the teaching and the system do not resolve the learner's difficulties, it is essential to make sure the learner is aware of the seriousness of their deficiencies. Tell the student: "I am concerned that you are not doing well *and that you might fail this rotation* if your performance does not improve." It is natural for teachers to feel uncomfortable discussing such concerns and they tend to put it off hoping the student is "just having a bad day" or similar excuse to avoid confronting them. The sooner the teacher talks to the student the better. Don't avoid the "f" word with vague comments such as: "You aren't doing as well as I hoped" or "You need to work harder." These comments do not convey the seriousness of the problem.

It may be helpful to ask colleagues who have also been teaching the student for their opinions. Does the student have poor study habits; is the student overwhelmed by the vastness and uncertainties of clinical medicine; does the student have problems with unprofessional behavior; does the student have a physical or mental illness; does the student have personal problems? He or she may need to be referred to a faculty member with special skills in working with students in difficulty. Finally, provide clear and specific advice to the student about what he or she needs to do to improve.

This should be tailored to the student's particular learning needs – for example, if the student's problem is poor clinical reasoning, he or she needs to read up on the cases he or she is seeing by reading about two or three common related problems. If the student saw a patient with shortness of breath, he or she should read about congestive heart failure, chronic obstructive pulmonary disease, and asthma and focus on the similarities and differences in the presentations of each so that he or she will be able to assess patients with shortness of breath more effectively. If the student's problem is poor interviewing skills, it would be helpful to observe several short segments of the student's interviews and provide specific feedback on how he or she could improve. Role-playing with the teacher playing the role of a patient is another helpful strategy. If the student's problem is related to professional behavior (e.g., frequent lateness or arrogant behavior with allied staff), teachers tend to become more uncomfortable, but the principles are the same. Teachers need to discuss their concerns as soon as they notice the problem. Ask the student how he or she thinks he or she can remedy the problem and follow this up in a few days.

As soon as the teacher recognizes a student who is not doing well, it is important to consult the appropriate departmental or program coordinator for advice. They need to know about students who are struggling in order to provide additional help if needed and to address the student's problems in the context of the whole clerkship or residency program. It is important to provide clear and direct feedback to students about their deficiencies as soon as possible to give them a fair chance to correct the problems before the end of that rotation.

Lacasse and colleagues (Lacasse, 2009; Lacasse *et al.*, 2012a,b) provide a comprehensive approach to assessing and managing challenging learning situations. Rubenstein and Talbot (2013) offer a valuable list of common difficulties experienced by learners and outline strategies for determining the causes of the problems and suggestions for treatment.

Time for Reflection

While it is important for students to be actively involved in patient care during their clinical training, it is equally important for them to have time for reflection and reading in order to consolidate what they are learning, to relate it to what they have already learned, and to "make it their own." Without such reflection, there is the risk that they simply learn "recipes" for care, without a deeper understanding of the rationale for the approach and without knowledge of the evidence supporting it. Teachers should be clear that they expect students to read around the cases they see. Periodically ask them to review a topic and provide a summary the next day.

In addition, they need time to reflect on their emotional responses to their experiences with patients. Clerkship is a time when they may first encounter death and the terrible unrelenting suffering that some patients endure and they need time to come to terms with the intense feelings these experiences may stimulate. Otherwise, in self-defense, they may close off their emotional reactions. It is important to be sensitive to student's reactions to patients, especially dying patients and "difficult" patients. If teachers are open about their own reactions it may make it easier for students to discuss their feelings. Becoming a physician is a profound life-changing process that can be challenging and frightening for some students.

Some preceptors like to spend 15–20 minutes at the end of the day reviewing the most challenging cases or picking up on one key topic that came up during the day. Teachers could ask, "Who was the most interesting patient this afternoon?" or "Did anything surprise you today?" or "How is your experience different from what you expected?" You might end the day discussing learning objectives with the student. Ask them what they would like to learn about that evening – they need to be specific and realistic and should outline what resources they will use (journal articles, course notes, texts, the Internet). However, make sure they also have some time off for recreation each week.

Rachel Remen (1999: 44) encourages regular reflection by students and physicians:

> I suggest they spend a few minutes each evening with a special bound journal just for this purpose, and ask themselves three questions about their day. The three questions are: What surprised me today? What moved me or touched me today? What inspired me today? The answers need not be long. What is important is to review the experience of the day for a brief time, looking at it in a new and different way.

Teachers also benefit from reflection on their teaching. At the end of the day identify a teaching interaction that was particularly effective or ineffective in helping the learner enhance his or her competence or develop insight about his or her growth as a physician. Then ask two questions:
1. Why was this approach effective or ineffective?
2. What, if anything, would I do differently next time and why? (Ferenchick, 1997).

When teachers try out new teaching methods it may feel awkward at first and they will be tempted to stick with what they are used to. However, if they stick with it for about 5 weeks, the new approach becomes more comfortable and maybe even second nature. It is best to try out one new thing at a time until it feels natural; then another new technique can be added.

CONCLUSION

In this chapter we have highlighted a number of practical guidelines for teaching the patient-centered clinical method based on the "Before-During-After" framework first described by Irby (1992). Effective clinical teachers take time to plan before learners arrive by familiarizing themselves with the program expectations and preparing their staff and patients. They provide an orientation for new learners on their arrival, conduct a needs assessment, and prime students before they see each patient. During their supervision of learners they use a variety of teaching strategies, including the One-Minute Preceptor, the SNAPPS method, and narrative-based supervision and modify the roles of preceptor, learner, and patient to match the student's stage of development.

They consider the student's personal qualities – truthfulness, conscientiousness, and discernment – along with his or her basic clinical skills and the unique content and context of each patient's problems to decide how much responsibility to entrust to each learner. They engage learners in feedback conversations where together they explore the student's strengths and identify areas needing more study and practice. They recognize faltering or failing students early and develop strategies to address their specific learning and personal needs. Finally, they encourage students to reflect on their experiences of becoming clinicians and reflect on their own experiences as teachers always striving to discover more effective approaches to enhance their students' learning.

12 The Case Report as a Teaching Tool for Patient-Centered Care

Thomas R Freeman

Case reports have frequently been criticized as representing anecdotal experience and, therefore, very low in the prevailing hierarchy of medical evidence (Sackett *et al.*, 1996). In the late nineteenth century, medical journals largely consisted of case reports, but by the late twentieth century case reports had all but disappeared from the most influential journals.

Nevertheless, case reports and presentations remain a mainstay in the wards of teaching hospitals and wherever medical education takes place. "As a fundamental ritual of academic medicine, the narrative act of case presentation is at the center of medical education and, indeed, at the center of all medical communication about patients" (Hunter, 1991: 51). As described by Weston elsewhere, the case method is a "signature pedagogy" in medicine and is very difficult to change. Nevertheless, there has been increased interest in the how these activities, essential to transmission of knowledge, may be improved. They are recognized as useful in teaching clinical reasoning skills (Bannister *et al.*, 2011).

This chapter describes a format for formal case presentations that is organized on the principles of the patient-centered clinical method.

REVIEW OF CASE PRESENTATION APPROACHES

The traditional format of the case presentation that evolved during the time of Sir William Osler was recognized very early as a valuable tool in the teaching of medicine (Cannon, 1990). It generally begins with a brief description of the patient, followed by the history of the present illness. Next comes past history, family history, patient profile, and examination findings. Investigative results such as laboratory work, X-rays, pathology reports, a problem list, and a management plan usually round out the presentation. This form of presentation accurately reflects the conventional clinical method, which is based on the biomedical model (McWhinney, 1988).

The written medical record was greatly improved by the method described by Weed (1969), and his Problem-Oriented Medical Record has been widely accepted. This method made problems the organizing principle of the record and separated subjective and objective elements. This form of written record has had a great influence on the format of oral case presentations as well. The increased use of the electronic health record has introduced new dimensions into record keeping (Lown & Rodriguez, 2012).

The bio-psychosocial model proposed by Engel (1977) was an attempt to apply systems theory to clinical problems. This model, along with the recognition that psychological and social factors play a role in illness events, has led to the inclusion of these topics in many case presentations.

The conventional case history or report has been criticized for being heavily dependent on scientific language, which, although seemingly precise, leaves much of reality aside (Schwartz & Wiggins, 1985). Abstract scientific language excludes the human, lived experience of patients and obscures the fact that where illnesses are unique, disease labels are classificatory terms only (McCullough, 1989). This problem is as true of chronic illness as it is of acute illness (Gerhardt, 1990). By minimizing the importance of the patient's story and subjective experience, the conventional case history separates biological processes from the person (depersonalization) and minimizes the physician's role in producing findings or observations (Donnelly, 1986). This form of presentation is primarily doctor- and disease-centered. "The message is clear, disease counts; the human experience of illness does not" (1986: 88). Recently described expectations of general internal medicine consultants regarding the content of oral case presentations continue to neglect this issue (Green *et al.*, 2009, 2011).

Hawkins (1986) advocates a method she calls the clinical biography, in which the scientific and humanistic are complementary, each representing different attitudes to the human experience. She points out that case history and biography are similar, in that they involve a lot of interpretation and are to be understood in the "context" of the narrative.

From a phenomenological perspective, the clinical encounter can be viewed as a hermeneutical exercise involving the interpretation of multiple "texts." These consist of the "experiential text" of illness as lived by the patient, the "narrative text" arising from history taking, the "physical text" of the patient's body as objectively examined, and the "instrumental text" constructed by diagnostic technologies. Such a hermeneutic model poses a number of questions, the most important being: "How can the ill person, both as text and cointerpreter, be restored to centrality in the clinical encounter?" (Leder, 1990). In the traditional case presentation, the patient's perspective is, to some extent, represented under the heading "subjective." The symptoms described therein have been described as an important source of medical knowledge (Malterud, 2000).

Efforts to change the focus of case histories to include more accurate descriptions of patients as person, range from the elegant literary work of Luria (Hawkins, 1986) and Sacks (1986) to the innovative and pragmatic teaching methods of Donnelly (1989), Charon (1986, 2004) and Cassell (2013).

Donnelly (1989) suggests that the human aspects of medicine can be addressed by teaching stories (which pay attention to what has happened in the interior world) instead of chronicles (which stick simply to a recitation of events). He asked house staff to include, in the history, one or two sentences about what the patient's understanding of the illness was and how it affects his or her life, in an effort to help the physician empathize more accurately.

Charon (1986, 2004) states that the physician's effectiveness increases with empathy and the physician teaches the "empathic stance" by asking medical students to write stories about their patients. These stories are considered as adjuncts to the hospital chart and do not replace the traditional case writeups. Charon has suggested that the students are molded into the kind of doctor their teachers want by becoming the kind of writer their teachers want (Charon, 1989).

Cassell (2013: 248) advises medical trainees that writing succinct summaries of patients is a skill that must be developed:

> Include a brief personality description. Follow with a description in succinct terms of the patient's background, education and employment, current family (married or single, children) or other significant relationship. Following that there should be a brief description of the patient's physical appearance. Start with the patient's appearance prior to undressing. If there are distinguishing features of speech or presentation of self they should be mentioned. Then focus on the unclothed appearance-body habitus, general development, musculature, and prominent distinguishing features such as major birthmarks, scars, or deformities. The whole description is usually not more than a paragraph.

Narrative medicine has developed a literature in its own right (Charon, 2001, 2004; Greenhalgh & Hurwitz, 1998; Greenhalgh, 1999), and has helped inform our understanding of how we seek meaning in the events of our lives. Evaluation of the impact of narrative medicine workshops for faculty are in the early stages (Liben *et al.*, 2012). For the most part, however, the narrative format lacks the structure desirable in transmitting important knowledge quickly in clinical settings. There remains the need for a bridge between the thin description of the traditional case presentation and the thick description of the narrative approach, especially in the teaching of students and house staff. Basic changes have to occur in the way that medicine is taught. Combining narrative in the standard case report and placing the history of present illness at the end has been advocated (Bayoumi & Kopplin, 2004).

Anspach (1988) points out that the presentation of case histories is an important part of the medical training of students, interns, and residents. Usually presented before an audience of peers and senior medical people, these presentations are important for both their content and as part of the socialization process. They are a powerful way of teaching and reinforcing a particular worldview. Such exercises are important in the development of professional identity (Jarvis-Selinger, 2011). They are a method for communicating standards of practice (Spafford et al., 2004) and can serve to teach management of uncertainty in clinical decision making (Holmes & Ponte, 2011) as well as ethical values (Charon & Montello, 2002). Learning to balance the use of evidence with the particulars of a case serves to foster in the learner the development of practical knowledge.

The absence of clear instructions on how case presentations should be done may result in acquisition of unintended professional values and delayed development of effective communication skills. "Teaching and learning of oral presentation skills may be improved by emphasizing that context determines content and by making explicit the tacit rules of presentation" (Haber & Lingard, 2001).

With the evolution of the clinical method, it is an appropriate time for a change in the way that case histories are presented, to more accurately reflect and reinforce the patient-centered clinical method and the worldview on which it is based.

DESCRIPTION OF THE PATIENT-CENTERED CASE PRESENTATION

The following is a description of a full case report method to be carried out at special end-of-rotation teaching sessions or Grand Rounds.

In a sharp departure from the conventional case report, which focuses on the organic pathology of the patient, the patient-centered case presentation (PCCP) gives primacy to the patient and the total experience of the illness and associated pathology. Unlike the conventional method, in which "the objective truths of medicine are recorded in the 'language of abstraction'" and are not "related to the existence of the individual patient" (Wulff et al., 1986: 132), the PCCP regards objective truth as of less interest when it is not related to the individual.

The PCCP focuses on an "acquaintance with particulars" (McWhinney, 1989a). It begins with a description of the particulars of the case under study and then proceeds to a discussion of the general – that is, other cases or studies that may share similar features. There may be a discussion of a single case or several cases that seem to express a common theme.

The PCCP, by going from the particular to the general and from the subjective to objective and back again, performs a cycle that ultimately informs the presenter with a greater understanding of the patient.

Table 12.1 compares the conventional case presentation and the PCCP and highlights how the items of information of the conventional approach are incorporated into the PCCP.

1. *The Patient's Chief Concern or Request.* This consists of a brief statement of the symptomatology as well as the illness behavior (McWhinney, 1972) that brought the patient to the encounter. It should address the patient's actual reason for coming.

2. *The Patient's Health and Illness Experience.* A description of the experience of the illness should include some quotations from the patient that particularly illustrate the subjective quality of the illness. For example, when discussing an individual for whom pain is a predominant feature, it would be appropriate to include the pain descriptors that the patient used in communicating the discomfort. Metaphors are particularly helpful here, as they are linguistic structures that bear epistemological weight (Carter, 1989; Donnelly, 1989). Knowing the metaphors that patients use to describe their illness gives the clinician greater insight, understanding, and empathy. The language for the metaphoric landscape is "not found in traditional textbooks of medicine, but in articulate memoirs of illness, insightful fiction, poetry, drama, and the examined experience of our own illnesses and those of our family and friends" (Donnelly, 1989: 134–5). As in the patient-centered clinical method, the patient's feelings, ideas, effects on function, and expectations are mentioned here, including the significance of the symptoms to the patient. A statement of the patient's meaning of health and how the patient's illness affects his or her ability to achieve a state consistent with his or her particular aspirations in this regard is appropriate here (corresponding to the Health and Illness Experience portions of Figure 1.2 in Chapter 1).

3. *Observations.* The observation portion of the presentation involves the Disease, Person, and Context dimensions shown in the diagram (Figure 1.2

TABLE 12.1 Comparison of the Conventional and Patient-Centered Case Presentations

Conventional Case Presentation	Patient-Centered Case Presentation
1. Chief Complaint	1. Patient's Chief Concern or Request
2. History of Present Illness	2. Patient's Health and Illness Experience Quotes from the patient: meaning of health and aspirations, feelings, ideas, effects on function, expectations

3. Past Medical History
  • Medications
  • Allergies
  • Observations
	3. Disease
	  • History of Present Illness
	  • Past Medical History
	  • Review of Systems
	  • Physical Exam
	  • Laboratory, etc.

4. Family History	4. Person
	  • Patient Profile
	  • Individual Life Cycle Phase

5. Patient Profile	5. Context
	  • Proximal (for example:
	    — Family History
	    — Genogram)
	  • Distal (for example:
	    — Culture
	    — Ecosystem)

6. Review of Systems	6. Patient-Doctor Relationship (the Clinical Encounter)
	  • The Dyad Itself
	  • Transference/Countertransference Issues
	  • Finding Common Ground
	    — Problems
	    — Goals
	    — Roles

7. Physical Exam	7. Assessment (Problem List)

8. Laboratory Database	8. General Discussion
	  • Illness Experience – Literature (pathographies, poetry)
	  • Medical Literature (Clinical Epidemiology, Pathophysiology, other case reports, medical anthropology)

9. Problem List	9. Proposed Management Plan
10. General Assessment	
11. Proposed Plan	

in Chapter 1). This section is subdivided into observations about the disease, including the standard elements of the medical history (history of present illness, past medical history, review of systems, physical exam, and relevant laboratory work), issues related to the person (patient profile, life cycle phase)', and context, both proximal (e.g. family, employment) and distal (e.g. culture, ecosystem).

4. *The Patient-Clinician Relationship (The Clinical Encounter)*. This involves a discussion of not only the technical management issues (e.g. drug and nondrug therapies) but also a discussion of how the patient-clinician dyad can be developed into a healing relationship (Cassell, 1985, 2013). Issues of self-awareness, feelings about the patient, and struggles to make effective connections are appropriate, as are any issues related to finding common ground between the doctor and the patient. *See* Chapter 6 for a detailed description of finding common ground and Chapter 7 for more on enhancing the relationship.

5. *Assessment (Problem List)*. This section summarizes the issues that need further assessment or intervention in any of the five areas of health, disease, illness, person, or context.

6. *General Discussion*. Having discussed the particulars of the case, the presentation then turns to the general issues raised by the case. The issues selected for discussion are chosen by the presenter from elements of the case which he or she found most interesting or puzzling. In this way the case helps to instruct the presenter. General issues can be subdivided into those that relate to the experience of the illness and those issues related to pathophysiology, epidemiology, sociology, and medical anthropology.

First-person accounts of the experience of illnesses have become common. Literature and poetry provide many examples of individuals who have written in a lucid and illuminating way of their personal experience of an illness (Styron, 1990; Mukand, 1990; Cousins, 1979; Broyard, 1992; Frank, 1991; Heshusius, 2009; Carel, 2008; Stein, 2007; Atkins, 2010; Hadas, 2011). In addition, the movie industry has focused on this area and occasionally a short video can very effectively communicate the trials of a particular sickness (Alexander *et al.*, 2012). Illness blogs are common on the Internet (Hilnan, 2003) and work has begun on content analysis of cancer blogs (Kim, 2009). Indeed, this type of writing has recently undergone a resurgence and an acquaintance with it will provide the presenter with improved insights into the patient's experience of the illness. It will be necessary for faculty to accumulate a usable bibliography of such material, as it appears not only in journals but also in newspapers, magazines, and books (Baker, 1985).

This section of the PCCP includes a discussion of any relevant medical literature pertaining to the case. It should incorporate the current understanding of any pathology or clinical epidemiology (i.e., prevalence, natural history, the sensitivity and specificity and predictive value of any tests, effects of intervention).

This section also demonstrates knowledge of the published scientific literature concerning the disturbed psychological and social functions that have been observed in other individuals with similar problems.

7. *Proposed Management Plan.* This is an opportunity to use the information gleaned from the discussion of the general issues and to integrate this knowledge into a management plan.

Case Example

The following is a case illustrating the level of detail to be encouraged by learners at the undergraduate or postgraduate level. This case takes place in Singapore.

Margaret L: Case Illustrating a Patient-Centered Case Report

Gerald Choon-Huat Koh

1. Patient's Chief Concerns

Margaret had four main concerns when I visited her, which was slowly revealed as the consultation progressed.

a. Copious saliva production for months
b. Right knee pain for months
c. Bilateral ankle swelling
d. Left eye cataract

Current Medications

● Metformin 425 mg bd
● Glipizide 5 mg om
● Aspirin 100 mg om
● Famotidine 20 mg bd
● Diltiazem 100 mg om
● Simvastatin 10 mg eon
● Paracetamol 1 g tds
● Tramadol 50 mg bd prn
● Glucosamine 500 mg om

2. Patient's Illness Experience

She complained of thick saliva production in the recent months. "I keep spitting out saliva, even when I am not talking . . . and need to keep a tissue paper in my hand to soak it up," shared Margaret. "Is there any way it can stop?" she asked.

Margaret also highlighted that she has had pain in her right knee for the past few months. She's had osteoarthritis in her knees for years and has previously received intra-articular hyaluronic acid injections in her knee joints. However, her right knee pain has been getting worse recently. "It's been acting up again, Doctor, and I'm finding it hard to walk recently. I need to use the walking frame more and my maid to help me get around."

Margaret also mentioned that her right ankle (and sometimes the other ankle as well) would become swollen in the evenings but the swelling would subside by the next morning. "It's not really painful. It's just worrying because you know what people say, ankle swelling could be signs of problems with the heart or kidney or liver, so I'm worried," explained Margaret.

Lastly, she expressed a desire to have her left eye cataract to be operated upon. She previously had a right eye cataract operation with good results at a local hospital but her residual left eye cataract made binocular vision impossible. "Although I can now see with my right eye, I can't judge distances well because I can't see anything with my left eye," she shared. "And with my stroke, you know, I'm not steady on my feet and I'm afraid I might fall if I misjudge the depth of uneven floors or steps. Could you refer me to the eye surgeon again to have the left cataract removed like the last time with my right eye?"

3. Observations

Disease

History of Present Illness

Margaret is an 85-year-old Chinese lady who had a stroke in March 1997, when she presented with cognitive impairment and dysphasia. She was found to have a middle cerebral artery infarct and residual functional impairment and dysphagia. She was reviewed by a swallowing therapist who assessed her as safe to eat orally with modification of food consistency and use of thickeners for fluids. Currently, she drinks only three to four glasses of water a day because she does not like the texture of the fluids when she uses the thickener and she wets diapers only twice a day. This suggests that she is not drinking enough fluids and this is causing her saliva to be thick.

Margaret also has had osteoarthritis of both knees for 10 years. She was seen by an orthopedic surgeon 5 years ago and was given three rounds of intra-articular hyaluronic acid injections in the ensuing few years. She found that the intra-articular hyaluronic acid injections were no longer helpful after

Greenfield Medical Library - Issue Receipt

Customer name: Byrne, Rachel Bridget

Title: Patient-centered medicine : a human
experience / David H. Rosen, Uyen B. Hoang.
ID: 1007816600
Due: 24/04/2018 23:59

Title: Patient-centered medicine : transforming
the clinical method / Moira Stewart ... [et al.].
ID: 1006967674
Due: 24/04/2018 23:59

Total items: 2
27/02/2018 12:48

All items must be returned before the due date
and time.
The Loan period may be shortened if the item is
requested.

www.nottingham.ac.uk/library

her second round. She had also received physiotherapy but had found it too strenuous so she stopped a year ago. She was counseled about the options of total knee replacement or arthroscopic debridment but she was not keen for surgery as she felt her operative risk was too high, a concern validated by her orthopedic surgeon. She reported that her pain is controlled by paracetamol and only takes her nonsteroidal anti-inflammatory drugs occasionally. This is important because nonsteroidal anti-inflammatory drugs can cause kidney and stomach toxicity in the elderly and should be used sparingly in this age group.

Margaret has a history of ischemic heart disease but has never been diagnosed with congestive heart failure. Her bilateral pedal edema was not associated with shortness of breath, exertional dyspnoea, paroxysmal nocturnal dysponoea, and chest pains. On physical examination, her blood pressure was normal, her jugular venous pulse was not raised, her lungs were clear, and she had no pallor, jaundice, or signs of uremia. All this suggests that her pedal edema was not due to any new onset of heart, kidney, or liver failure. Moreover, her annual blood investigations were also not suggestive of any renal or liver disease. As she was on diltiazem (her antihypertensive medication), which is associated with nonserious pedal edema, she was diagnosed to have mild pedal edema from diltiazem use.

Margaret has an intra-ocular lens in her right eye, inserted 10 years ago. This operation went well and she has positive memories of it. Although she can see with her right eye, she is unable to judge distances well because she does not have binocular vision. Given that she has functional impairment from her old stroke, she is at risk of falls, especially with uneven floors or stairs. As she is keen for a cataract operation for her left eye now, I was keen to refer her.

Past Medical History

Margaret has a past history of diabetes mellitus for more than 20 years, hypertension for 10 years, and hyperlipidemia for the past 5 years. She also has a history of ischemic heart disease but is functionally unimpaired now that she does not have symptoms of anginal chest pains any more.

Review of Systems

Functional Status

- Ambulation: furniture walker but independent without aid.
- Activities of daily living: independent in all activities of daily living.

Fall History

No recent history of any previous falls.

Cognition

Margaret is partially cognitively impaired. Her Abbreviated Mental Test score is borderline abnormal (6 out of a maximum score of 10) but she is still able to hold a conversation and retains decision-making capacity.

Speech

She has word finding difficulty and hence her speech is slow. However, given time, she is able to express herself and her needs.

Psychological Assessment

Margaret does not have any symptoms of depression, a condition I am wary of, as her husband passed away a year ago. She was very cheerful and very forthcoming with history. No anxiety or psychotic symptoms were elicited during mental state examination and from history.

Urination

Margaret is currently on diapers, as she often cannot make it to the toilet on time and does not want any accidents.

Defecation

Margaret defecates once every 1–2 days. Her stools are normal in consistency and have no visible blood. She is occasionally constipated and this is probably related to her self-imposed fluid restriction.

Sleep History

Although Margaret sleeps during the day, she is also able to sleep well at night.

Appetite and Nutrition

There has been no recent change in her appetite and it remains adequate.

Physical Exam

- General condition well
- Blood pressure = 105/55 mmHg (sitting), heart rate = 72 beats per minute, respiratory rate = 16 breaths per minute
- No pallor or cyanosis; no pedal edema; no raised jugular venous pulse

- Visual acuity (with glasses): right eye – reads print; left eye – perceives light only; right intra-ocular lens seen from previous cataract; left cataract seen but red reflex still present
- Hearing: bilaterally normal
- No pallor or jaundice
- No enlarged cervical lymph nodes; jugular venous pulse is not raised
- Heart: S1, S2, no murmur
- Lungs: clear
- Abdomen: soft, non-tender, no palpable masses organomegaly, bladder non-palpable, bowel sounds active; rectal examination normal
- Musculoskeletal system:
  — both knees – crepitus felt on full range of movement; osteophytes seen with bilateral lateral ligament involvement; significant muscle wasting of both quadriceps observed; patient unable to stand up from a squatting position and has difficulty rising from a low chair
  — both hands – osteoarthritis of proximal and distal interphalangeal joints also seen
- Neurological system: cranial nerves grossly normal; power 4+/5 on all four limbs. Reflexes: normal; plantar reflexes down-going bilaterally; no parkinsonism or cerebellar signs
- Feet: mild pedal edema bilaterally; skin normal; sensation decreased in stocking distribution; pulses diminished but still palpable

Laboratory Investigations

- Pre-lunch capillary blood glucose = 7.3 mmol/L
- Annual blood and urine tests (including HbA$_{1c}$), which are done by Margaret's daughter-in-law (who is a doctor): normal.

4. Person

Patient Profile

Margaret is an 85-year-old Chinese lady who was a homemaker all her life. Margaret came from a poor family and suffered in her youth during the Japanese occupation of Singapore during World War II, where many of her relatives perished. Fortunately, her parents survived the war, but, as they were uneducated, her family had to work hard to rebuild their lives after the war. Margaret married her husband, a civil servant, and gave birth to two sons. Being a firm believer in the value of education, Margaret sold traditional snacks and cakes rooted in Nonya (a unique culture that is derived from persons with both

Malay and Chinese heritage) to earn money to send her children to university. It is no wonder that she was very proud that one of her sons became a doctor. She was living with her husband after their children moved out a decade ago, but when her husband died a year ago from dementia and aspiration pneumonia, Margaret has since moved into her first son's home. Although Margaret's first son has four children (two teenage boys and two girls in their early twenties), both girls are living abroad at the moment and only the boys (Margaret's grandsons) are living in the same house. Margaret also has a full-time caregiver, who looks after her needs and sleeps next to her room at night.

Individual Life Cycle Phase

Margaret is at her last stage of the life cycle but she still has a zest for life and looks forward to each day.

5. Context

Proximal

Family History

Margaret is widowed (her husband passed away in 2008) and she currently stays with her older son and his family (wife and two sons). She is a nonsmoker and nondrinker. Margaret has very good social support from her two sons, nieces and nephews, and many grandchildren, all of whom visit her weekly. She also has a full-time helper who helps her in her activities of daily living.

Genogram

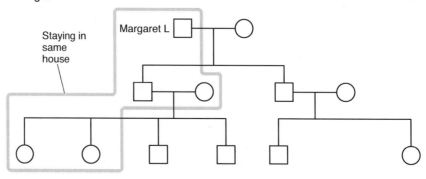

Home Environment

The son's house in which Margaret is staying is a single-story apartment with an outdoor garden on the same level. Unfortunately, to get to the house, Margaret needs to climb about 20 steps, as the house is perched along the slope of a low hill. However, once inside the home, there are no longer any steps for her to maneuver. She has a room for herself and her helper sleeps within calling distance. Her toilet and shower room both have sufficient space for a wheelchair to maneuver. There are grab bars installed in both her toilet and the shower room. There are a few stray wires and lighting is adequate throughout the house during the day and night. Margaret currently uses a walking frame to ambulate inside the home and a wheelchair to ambulate outside the home.

Distal

In Singapore's Asian culture, filial piety is still very much alive and it is not uncommon for parents to live with their children, especially when they become disabled. In the local context, spitting thick saliva is considered very rude, unhygienic, and associated with lung disease, which explains why Margaret was so uncomfortable with her thick saliva. This association probably originates from the early days of Singapore when tuberculosis was rampant and anyone with thick oral discharge was considered to be infectious with tuberculosis and avoided. In the same way, bilateral leg swelling is also associated with serious disease and impending death. This fear probably originates from the early days of Singapore when malaria and malnutrition was rampant and pedal swelling occurred with "blackwater fever" in late stages of malaria and kwashiorkor with protein-calorie deficiency, two conditions associated with certain death.

4. Patient-Doctor Relationship (the Clinical Encounter)

The Dyad Itself

Margaret's eldest son is a colleague. I felt a little pressure, to be seeing a colleague's mother. Margaret was happy for me to be her attending family physician and was comfortable with me from the first time I saw her. Margaret's first son was happy that she finally encountered a family physician she liked and trusted. He would often ask me to reiterate a specific advice to his mother when she refused to listen to him. For example, he once told me, "Can you please tell my mother to use the thickener? She won't listen to anyone except you."!

Transference/Countertransference

Personally, I found caring for Margaret to be a complete joy. She is a very warm and pleasant lady who always makes me comfortable when I visit her. In turn, I think she is very pleased that I am her family physician and is always cooperative and open.

Finding Common Ground

I advised Margaret to drink more water to make her saliva less thick and reinforced the need to use the thickener. She was reluctant at first but then I highlighted to her that the thickener could be added to her favorite drink (i.e., Chinese jasmine and herbal teas) and soup (Margaret, like most Chinese, likes soups because they are associated with beneficial qualities and goodness). She agreed to use it more often.

Problems, Goals, Roles

When I explained to Margaret that I felt that her bilateral pedal edema was just due to her antihypertensive diltiazem and reassured her that she was unlikely to have any serious illness such as heart, liver, or kidney failure, she was very relieved. I offered to change her antihypertensive to another one that is less likely to cause pedal edema. However, Margaret replied that she was happy with diltiazem and just needed to know that there was nothing serious.

When I told Margaret that the only definitive treatment to relieve her chronic knee pains was surgery, she reiterated that she was not keen. I suggested that she continue to use her paracetamol as her main analgesic and nonsteroidal anti-inflammatory drugs for breakthrough pain. I was very concerned that Margaret would get gastritis or renal toxicity with use of nonsteroidal anti-inflammatory drugs and I was prepared to add a third analgesic (an opioid) for her. However, an opioid would increase the risk of falls, as it also has sedating effects. I explained the risks to Margaret carefully and she decided to stay with paracetamol as her main analgesic and nonsteroidal anti-inflammatory drugs for breakthrough pain. She too was concerned about falling and sustaining a hip fracture, because she had a friend who recently fractured her hip and needed an operation to fix it. She also reassured me that with the current regimen, her pain will be adequately controlled. I suspect that with education of the alternative solutions to her pain and their possible adverse effects, Margaret was able to better tolerate her knee pain with her current analgesic regimen.

Margaret was also pleased when I offered to refer her to an ophthalmologist who was an expert in cataract surgery, especially in elderly with multiple medical problems.

5. Assessment (Problem List)

- Diabetes mellitus (controlled)
- Hypertension (controlled)
- Hyperlipidemia (controlled)

- Ischemic heart disease (controlled)
- Old stroke with functional, swallowing, and speech impairment (stable)
- Thick saliva from self-imposed fluid restriction
- Osteoarthritis of both knees
- Mild bilateral pedal edema from nifedipine use
- Left cataract impairing binocular vision
- Risk of falls because of visual impairment, osteoarthritis of the knees, and numbness of her feet.

6. General Discussion

Illness experience

I found it instructive to reflect upon how older persons in Singapore view certain symptoms. Singapore evolved from a developing country to a developed country within a short span of 30 years. This has resulted in the eradication of many diseases that were once endemic, such as malaria and malnutrition, and the control of tuberculosis. However, many of the memories of these devastating illnesses still persist in the minds of older Singaporeans, diseases that I myself have never seen in Singapore since I started in medical school. So I have learned to apply the historical context of my elderly patients to their ideas, concerns, and expectations to better appreciate their personal life perspectives.

Literature (Pathographies, Poetry)

Treating the elderly is challenging, but I enjoy it because they are repositories of a lifetime of experiences and they are fascinating people if you slow down to find out who they are, the lives they have lived, and the lessons they can share with us. During my work with older persons, I encountered a particular poem on what it is like to be an elderly patient and it helped open my eyes to their frailty, humanity, and history. It was written by an old man who died in the geriatric ward of a small hospital near Tampa, Florida. After his death, when his nurses were going through his meager possessions, they found this poem. Its quality and content so impressed the staff that copies were made and distributed to every nurse in the hospital. The old man's sole bequest to posterity has since appeared in the various venues including the Christmas edition of the *News Magazine* of the St. Louis Association for Mental Health and I reproduce it here.

Crabby Old Man

What do you see nurses? ....What do you see?

What are you thinking......when you're looking at me?

A crabby old man,..........not very wise,
Uncertain of habit ....with faraway eyes?
Who dribbles his food............and makes no reply.
When you say in a loud voice ...."I do wish you'd try!"
Who seems not to notice ....the things that you do.
And forever is losing .... A sock or shoe?
Who, resisting or not............lets you do as you will,
With bathing and feeding ...... The long day to fill?
Is that what you're thinking?.......Is that what you see?
Then open your eyes, nurse......you're not looking at me.
I'll tell you who I am .... As I sit here so still,
As I do at your bidding,......as I eat at your will.
I'm a small child of Ten.......with a father and mother,
Brothers and sisters ....who love one another
A young boy of Sixteen ......with wings on his feet
Dreaming that soon now..........a lover he'll meet.
A groom soon at Twenty ......my heart gives a leap.
Remembering, the vows.........that I promised to keep.
At Twenty-Five, now .... I have young of my own.
Who need me to guide ......And a secure happy home.
A man of Thirty .... My young now grown fast,
Bound to each other .... With ties that should last.
At Forty, my young sons ....have grown and are gone,
But my woman's beside me.......to see I don't mourn.
At Fifty, once more, ... Babies play 'round my knee,
Again, we know children .... My loved one and me.
Dark days are upon me .... My wife is now dead.
I look at the future ....I shudder with dread.
For my young are all rearing......young of their own.
And I think of the years....... And the love that I've known.
I'm now an old man............and nature is cruel.
'Tis jest to make old age ......look like a fool.
The body, it crumbles..........grace and vigor, depart.
There is now a stone......... where I once had a heart.
But inside this old carcass ...... A young guy still dwells,
And now and again ....my battered heart swells.
I remember the joys.............. I remember the pain.
And I'm loving and living............life over again.

> I think of the years …all too few……gone too fast.
> And accept the stark fact……….that nothing can last.
> So open your eyes, people ………open and see.
> Not a crabby old man…….Look closer….see………ME!!

Remember this poem when you next meet an older person who you might brush aside without looking at the young soul within . . . we will all, one day, be there, too!

Medical Literature (Clinical Epidemiology, Pathophysiology, Other Case Reports, etc.)

The association between use of calcium channel blockers and pedal edema is well documented in medical literature and it is believed to be secondary to a local vasodilator phenomenon (Williams *et al.*, 1989; Van Hamersvelt *et al.*, 1996). Some doctors treat calcium channel blocker–induced pedal edema with diuretics instead of cessation of the drug, but research has shown that diuretics are not effective in reducing this condition (Van der Heijden *et al.*, 2004).

7. Proposed Management Plan

My final proposed management plan for Margaret was as follows:

- Copious saliva production for months – increase hydration through greater use of thickener in her favorite drinks and soups.
- Right knee pain for months – to continue using paracetamol as her main analgesic and nonsteroidal anti-inflammatory drugs for breakthrough pain.
- Bilateral nifedipine-induced ankle swelling – to leave alone.
- Left eye cataract – to refer to eye surgeon for left cataract operation.

SHORT FORM OF THE PATIENT-CENTERED CASE PRESENTATION

In day-to-day clinical work in the office or ward, it is necessary to use a shortened form of case presentation while continuing to emphasize the values of patient-centered medicine. In these settings learners should be instructed to describe the patient's chief concern or request; the patient's health and illness experience; brief summary of proximal context assessment; and suggested plan. When learners lapse into a truncated and impersonal case description (e.g., "I have a 54-year-old woman with pain and weakness in her shoulders and hips"), they must be gently, but firmly instructed in "re-humanizing" their report by beginning with the patient's name, followed by the elements of the shortened PCCP.

ADVANTAGES OF THE PATIENT-CENTERED CASE PRESENTATION

Case presentations can be viewed as "highly conventionalized linguistic rituals" that serve to socialize physicians in training to a particular worldview (Anspach, 1988). The PCCP, by placing the patient at the core of the presentation, reinforces the primacy of the person rather than the disease, without excluding the process of clinical decision making. In this way it can serve to inculcate a more humane form of medicine and reinforce the basic values inherent in the patient-centered clinical method. It does this without sacrificing the more conventional type of information found in the standard case presentation.

In increasing numbers of medical schools there has been a shift away from passive learning (i.e., lectures) to a less structured format in which learners take greater responsibility for setting learning goals. This is more effective at developing "lifelong learners." Nevertheless, it is not an unusual experience, after starting into practice, to feel somewhat at a loss as to how to continue to be well informed. The rapid expansion of medical knowledge makes it impossible for any individual to always be completely up to date. Therefore, it is necessary that the practicing physician have a method for continuing medical education that takes into account one's individual learning needs. Most experienced physicians acknowledge that their most demanding teachers are ultimately their patients. The PCCP, when a part of medical education, develops a useful framework for later use by practicing physicians when considering their challenging cases. It recognizes the role of the patient in teaching us what we most need to know.

The usual reasons for making a written case report are (a) a unique case, (b) a case of unexpected association, and (c) a case of unexpected events (Morris, 1991). The philosophy of the PCCP is that every case is unique and may – indeed, often – will involve the unexpected. The only necessary motivation for undertaking a PCCP is a desire to come to a deeper understanding of the patient.

CONCLUSION

The patient-centered case presentation suggests a way of presenting case material in medicine that is consistent with new clinical methods. It recognizes that case presentations are an important part of the socialization of training physicians as well as other health care professionals. By giving primacy to the subjective aspects of illness, this form of presentation reinforces an attitude of "patient-centeredness."

ACKNOWLEDGMENTS

Parts of this chapter have been previously published in *Family Practice: An International Journal* (Vol. 11, No. 2, 1994).

The text has benefited from careful review and suggestions by Dr Wayne Weston.

PART FOUR

The Health Care Context and Patient-Centered Care

Introduction

Moira Stewart

This part of the book presents aspects of the health care context within which patient-centered care occurs.

The first and most immediate context is the health care team. The implications of team care may be positive for patient-centered care if team members all agree on and aim to provide patient-centered care. If, however, there are competing definitions of the goals of care and members of the team are pulling in different directions, then patient-centered care may be threatened.

In an effort to reinforce the four components of patient-centered care (in rather the same parallel way as we reinforced them in the framework of learner-centered teaching presented in Chapter 9), we propose in this part a method for creating and sustaining a team. This method presents the four components adapted for use early in a team's formation, and later for subsequent regular efforts to sustain positive teamwork in health care.

The second context is the health care policy environment within which we work in the era leading up to 2020. This policy environment has many facets but one key facet is the shrinking budgets for health care and health care organizations. In such an environment, it is important for us to learn about the implications of patient-centered care for efficiency in the health care system (and about effectiveness, which is covered in Part Five). Here in Part Four, we present one chapter on patient-centered care and costs. This chapter, which focuses on Canada, complements and supplements similar work in the United States by Epstein *et al.* (2005b). The Canadian chapter and the US papers have found, in fact, that patient-centered care is associated with *lower* costs of overall care, leading to a conclusion that patient-centered care is good for the system.

Also, highly policy-relevant is the finding that patient-centered care is effective across all levels on the socioeconomic spectrum (Jani *et al.*, 2012). The policy implications are that resources needed to ensure patient-centered care should be available at all socioeconomic levels. This would require policies that overcome the inverse care law, which holds that resources for excellent health care vary inversely with population need (Hart, 1971). Policies supporting enough time with each patient and supporting continuity of care must be enacted vigorously, especially in deprived regions.

Part Four of this book aspires to heighten awareness of two contexts: the team and the policy.

13 Team-Centered Approach: How to Build and Sustain a Team

Moira Stewart, Judith Belle Brown, Thomas R Freeman, Carol L McWilliam, Joan Mitchell, Lynn Brown, Lynn Shaw, and Vera Henderson

Acknowledging that health care often takes place in the context of teams rather than single practitioners, we ask the following questions: Does patient-centered care enhance team care or not? And does team care embellish or impede patient-centered care? Is it possible for these to be mutually reinforcing and if so, how?

Our past experience in articulating the parallels between patient-centered care and learner-centered education, led us to consider whether a similar parallel process might be helpful in thinking through positive attributes and processes to enhance team function. Knowing that modeling a behavior or relationship is one effective way to educate a group of trainees or improve

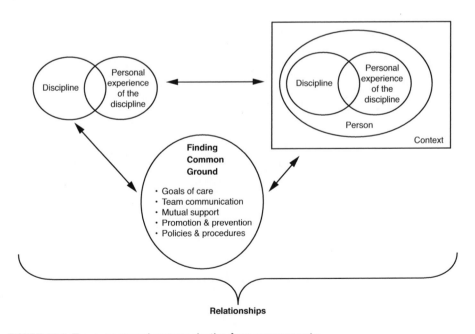

FIGURE 13.1 Team-centered approach: the four components

care in a health care organization, we propose a process of team development that mirrors the patient-centered clinical method, potentially enhancing both.

We present a parallel process of a team-centered approach based on the four components of patient-centered care. The team-centered approach is presented as a diagram in Figure 13.1 and outlined more fully in Box 13.1. The first two components – Component 1, exploring both the disciplines and the members' personal experiences of their discipline, and Component 2, understanding the whole person of the team member – focus on the individual team members, asking them to reflect on and share their own discipline and some of their life history and personal context. Components 3 and 4 consider the team itself and the attributes that characterize the team.

The *first* component encourages each team member to be ready to share and to learn about others regarding each member discipline's formal scope of practice as described by their respective licensing body. The implication of this component is that each team member becomes prepared to explain his or her legal and sanctioned role of practice in relation to other health professionals. It is somewhat surprising how common it is that these roles are implicit, unlearned, and out of date. This first step toward seamless team care firmly grounds the team in the realities of their current policy context.

Simply knowing the official scope of practice of the other disciplines may not be enough. Another important feature of this component is for health care team members to share and learn about all members' personal experiences of their discipline – for example, their unique professional history and ways of thinking about health care. This sharing may open everyone's eyes to the myriad of ways formal roles can be enacted and may bring the formal roles to life. Also, they may learn what they like about their role and what aspects they find challenging. Additionally, this exchange is especially important for teams who are at the beginning of their journey together. Knowledge of one another's formal discipline and experience within the discipline is an interprofessional competency outlined by the Canadian National Interprofessional Competency Framework (Bainbridge *et al.*, 2010). Further, we contend that the mutual process of learning about each other's discipline promotes mutual respect and enables a more trusting interprofessional practice.

The *second* component stresses the need for understanding the whole person of each team member. The reflection, necessary for a team member in preparation for sharing their own story, may help prepare the health professional for the experience of being on a new team. Each member will be encouraged to share relevant aspects of his or her life history, personal context, and his or her perceived ability to respond to change and manage conflict. As well,

Box 13.1 Team-Centered Approach: How to Start and Sustain a Team

1. Exploring both the disciplines and the members' personal experiences of their discipline:
   - the discipline as described by the licensing body, scope of practice
   - the member's personal experiences of their discipline.
2. Understanding the whole person of each team member:
   - the "person" (life history, and personal context, perceived ability to respond to change and manage conflict)
   - the context (opportunities and constraints of the team environment, time available for each individual).
3. Finding common ground – toward the shared language, culture, and philosophy of the team care:
   - underlying goals of care
   - formal and informal team communication (meetings, electronic medical record)
   - supporting one another's strengths, knowledge, and skills
   - promotion of team health and prevention of team dissonance, leadership issues
   - policies and procedures including regarding conflict resolution.
4. Enhancing ongoing team relationships:
   - sharing power
   - trust
   - empathy, respect, genuineness
   - individual professionals' commitment to the team
   - self-awareness, awareness of others.

sharing one anothers' understanding of the team's current context, in terms of each member's perceptions of the opportunities and constraints of the team environment, may assist in getting the team started and, ultimately, sustain the team. Such sharing fosters mutual understanding of team members as individuals, thereby enabling each to relate to the others in ways that promote effective team functioning. Also, studies show how social activities and opportunities for sharing life events are created and maintained by teams as they develop their unique routines and rituals. Social activities and sharing life events foster relationships and team cohesion (Brown *et al.*, 2010). Also, social relationships in the workplace can contribute to both personal fulfillment and pride and to the maintenance of effective teams (Hodson, 2004).

The *third* component, Finding Common Ground, represents the shift, from the focus on the individual team member sharing his or her history and experiences, to all team members co-creating the new team environment, moving toward a shared language, culture, and philosophy (Marra & Angouri, 2011). Components 1 and 2 have provided some of the necessary building blocks of information and experiences from the past.

One element of the *third* component, Finding Common Ground as a team, is to outline the underlying broad principles and goals of care. Some of this work may be explicitly shared early in the team's development; some of it may also become revealed as the team functions in its first weeks and months. A mechanism to encourage finding common ground as a team is to specify the formal and informal communication strategies of the team. For example, will team meetings occur and, if so, what is their agenda? Would team huddles as described in Chapter 10 suffice? Will the main communication strategy among the health professionals be the patient chart, these days usually an electronic medical record? If so, the approach to recording the clinical notes should be discussed and agreed upon. Regularly scheduled team meetings may be a vital mechanism for communication on the team. The need for meetings builds on findings reported in prior studies (Apker *et al.*, 2006; Higgins & Routhieaux, 1999; Craigie & Hobbs, 2004; Ruddy & Rhee, 2005; Brown *et al.*, 2009). Craigie and Hobbs (2004) have described team meetings as a safe place to raise issues and to participate in a problem-solving process that is both respectful and collaborative. These opportunities can both serve to build team cohesion and develop creative strategies for sustainment when teams are confronted by stress or conflict (Ruddy & Rhee, 2005). As meetings themselves can be a source of stress if inadequate time and remuneration become an issue (Petrini & Thomas, 1995), and the location and timing of meetings can create tension on the team, particularly when certain agenda items are viewed by some members as mundane or not relevant to their role function (Freeth, 2001). Thus clinical and administrative meetings may need to be held at separate times (Payne, 2000). When this is not feasible it is important to create distinct agendas for each component of the meeting, including identification of the leadership or chair of designated agenda items. Teams must collectively agree upon required mandatory attendance by all members versus those meetings that are pertinent to specific disciplines only (Payne, 2000). These issues need to be addressed in order for optimal communication to occur.

Informal communication is an important part of the daily interactions of the team members as they work together. Communication about patient care issues needs to be immediate. Ellingson (2003) has described this as "backstage communication," which occurs outside of formal team meetings and is essential in the provision of patient care. Hallway consultations may remain the preferred means of communication for clinical as well as business matters that are time sensitive. As teams grow in size the hallway consultation may not be an effective communication strategy for administrative or organizational matters, but it may remain critical for core team communication regarding patient care. Hence, the accessibility and physical proximity of team members is essential. Approachability is also key.

Another element of finding common ground in a team is supporting each other's strengths, knowledge, and skills. The extent to which this is done becomes one of the shared philosophies of the team. The team learns about these individual team members' attributes through successfully exploring the disciplines and members' personal experiences (Component 1) and understanding the other team members' personal and professional context (Component 2), but also by observing the contributions over time as part of finding common ground (Component 3).

Another element moving the team toward a shared language, culture, and philosophy may be the ways in which the team promotes team health and prevents team dissonance. Inherent in this element will be mutual agreement on policies and procedures through mutual discussion and efforts to test out approaches. For example, timely follow-up of patients discharged from hospital to primary health care requires an organized approach, as various team members address different aspects of the community-based care. Further, such policies need to attend explicitly to conflict resolution processes that can be followed early and equitably.

Role boundary issues, scope of practice, and accountability have been persistently identified as sources of team conflict in the literature (Bailey *et al.*, 2006). Even though there is extensive documentation of these conflictual issues in the literature, accompanied by helpful suggestions on how to address them, they continue to disable team functioning in hospitals (Grunfeld *et al.*, 2000; Laschinger *et al.*, 2001) and in the community (Brown *et al.*, 2011). An important team strategy in addressing conflict in larger teams may be the development and active use of conflict resolution protocols (Porter-O'Grady, 2004). It is important to recognize that conflict is normal and inevitable in any group of individuals. Attempts to avoid it lead to misunderstandings and may contribute to errors in patient care. In effective teams, all members take responsibility for clarifying disagreements and misunderstandings and hold one another accountable for following through on commitments. Smaller teams may benefit from learning to use frameworks when discussions are particularly important. These processes can help teams to find a common voice and can assist in broadening and strengthening the team's ability to succeed.

The *fourth* component of a team-centered approach is enhancing the ongoing team relationships. As clinical care transpires and team members gain experience with one another and with the cadre of shared patients, the ongoing relationships mature. One element of the team approach to relationships stems directly from the development of a common philosophy, one that encompasses sharing power. This is a requirement of a patient-centered approach and it is equally germane to the team approach. Each professional needs to reframe his or her notion of particular aspects of care as belonging to his or her discipline – instead, recognizing that other disciplines have skills and interests in that domain too. Team structures that place individuals in less powerful positions could be a barrier to team functioning. Prior work has focused primarily on the hierarchical relationship between doctors and nurses and the inherent conflict in this dyad (Bailey *et al.*, 2006; Zwarenstein & Reeves, 2002). More widespread recognition of nursing as a professional discipline has contributed to an increase in the status of nurses within the health care system. While nurses may have achieved more equality in the team environment, other team members with less status remain vulnerable (Brown *et al.*, 2011). A literature review by Mickan and Rodger (2000) on characteristics of effective teamwork suggests that team functioning is impeded when the concerns and views of team members are devalued or dismissed.

Another element, crucial in responsible clinical practice, is trust. Members must trust their team's processes if they are to provide superb communication and high-level clinical care. When trust is broken, the processes outlined in finding common ground such as conflict resolution must be implemented to restore trust among team members.

Aligned with trust are the three bedrocks of ongoing counseling relationships: empathy, respect, and genuineness. Studies suggest the importance of openness, willingness to find solutions, and respect (Craigie & Hobbs, 2004; Freeth, 2001; Lemieux-Charles & McGuire, 2006; Mickan & Rodger, 2000). Research has also suggested that humility is the foundation on which respect is enacted (Brown *et al.*, 2011).

Another element of ongoing team relationships is the commitment of each individual professional to a shared approach. The degree to which the commitment is wholehearted and steady, in contrast to partial and inconsistent, will affect the team's potential; the potential will vary depending on how narrow or broad is the vision of interprofessional practice, and the commitment of participating members to this approach.

All of these elements of enhancing ongoing team relationships depend to some extent on the ability of each team member to nurture self-awareness and gently encourage it in others. The self-knowledge that one feels threatened by some aspects of sharing clinical roles or that one responds (positively or negatively) to some types of individuals, goes a long way to smoothing out rough patches in the early and continuing evolution of teams.

Box 13.2 Team Members' Perspectives of Health Issues, Goals, and Roles

	Health Issues	Goals	Roles
Patient and patient's family			
Dietician			
Nurse practitioner			
Family practice nurse			
Family physician			
Social worker			
Other health practitioner, such as pharmacist; psychologist; physiotherapist; occupational therapist			

As in all patient-centered care, the patient is the focus. Therefore, the patient is considered a member of a health care team. We propose using the grid shown in Box 13.2 as one way of helping a team that is stumbling in its effort to provide patient-centered clinical care. This may be one of the tools to decrease conflict, because it explicitly offers each player, including the patient, the opportunity to clarify his or her health issues, goals of care, and roles he or she would propose to take on.

The following case is used to illustrate the grid as shown in Box 13.3.

Case Example

Forty-two-year-old Martina Morgan had denied the symptoms she had been experiencing over the last several months including weight loss, frequent urination, and occasional blurred vision. When she finally went to her family doctor she declared, "I have diabetes." Mrs Morgan was in fact very familiar with diabetes, as her mother had been diagnosed with diabetes over 30 years previously and had suffered from numerous related complications.

Box 13.3 Team Members' Perspectives Regarding Martina Morgan

	Health Issues	Goals	Roles
Patient	Difficulty accepting the diagnosis Experience of mother's diabetes Fears Overwhelmed "diabetes was final blow"	Reluctant to follow plan, frozen Felt need to regain control	Not willing or able to assume a role in her care yet
Nurse	Serious diabetes Potential for sequelae	Education about foot care	Health education Advocate for patient Go at patient's pace Try to find achievable plan
Family physician	Serious diabetes	Begin insulin injections Refer to specialist	Coordinator To achieve blood sugar control Try to find achievable plan
Social worker	Mother's diabetes Father's abandonment Diabetes as final blow	Explore strengths in the family Explore husband's fears	Communicate fears and family issues Advocate for patient Try to find achievable plan
Dietician	Serious diabetes Poor diet	Tight control of diet	Diet education Try to find an achievable plan

However, Mrs Morgan refused to accept the doctor's recommendation that she begin insulin injections to control her very high blood sugars. Furthermore, Mrs Morgan adamantly declined a referral to an endocrinologist because, from her perspective, interventions from such specialists had hastened her mother's deterioration. In response, the family doctor, serving in the role of coordinator, invited several other health care professionals including the dietician, a family practice nurse, the social worker, and the nurse practitioner to assist in addressing Mrs Morgan's serious health problems. The doctor led the first meeting of the team of the five health professionals; the patient was not asked to attend. Because the team's focus was primarily on getting Mrs Morgan's diabetes under control, efforts to coordinate care leaned toward the medical model, such as modifying her lifestyle by attending to tight diet control, providing education about proper foot care, and exploring options for financial aid to assist with her financial difficulties. In spite of each individual team member's best intentions, over the next 4 months, Mrs Morgan remained reluctant to follow their recommendations and attempts at coordinating services faltered.

The more she didn't adhere, the more the primary health care team intensified their efforts to educate Mrs Morgan. Also, each team member was focused solely on achieving his or her own professional goals, specific to his or her discipline. While they were not engaging in turf wars there was neither a shared language nor a shared vision for Mrs Morgan's overall care plan. What the team, collectively, had failed to ascertain was Mrs Morgan's meaning of health, life aspirations, experience of illness, and her current context.

A second meeting of the five health care professionals was convened at the request of the nurse practitioner. A plan was made for all health professionals openly to ask Mrs Morgan about her past experiences with diabetes, her beliefs, and her goals for care. The social worker planned a visit to the home to include other family members. It was only after some members of the team began to question and then listen to Mrs Morgan's other issues, not only her medical problems, that change began to occur.

Mrs Morgan had been raised in a very dysfunctional family. Her father had often been out of work and he would frequently "disappear for months" leaving the family destitute. When Mrs Morgan was 16 years old her mother had a below-knee amputation due to complications of diabetes. Her progressively deteriorating eyesight meant she could no longer administer her insulin injections and this responsibility fell on Mrs Morgan. Even though administering the injections into her mother's stumped limb repulsed her,

Mrs Morgan dutifully assumed this task. The entire experience had been very difficult for her.

Thus the diagnosis of diabetes was overwhelming for Mrs Morgan. She was afraid and uncertain about her future. She had witnessed the effects of diabetes on her mother and was terrified that she would suffer the same long-term consequences of the disease. The only way she could handle her fear was to avoid even thinking about her diabetes. For Mrs Morgan, this was the "final blow" from her family of origin.

In meeting with Mrs Morgan's husband, the social worker learned that although Mr Morgan was supportive and understanding, he was struggling to cope. Further exploration by the social worker revealed that Mr Morgan was worried that his wife was going to have a hypoglycaemic reaction in her sleep and die in bed next to him. Consequently, he was often awake in the night. He found it difficult to talk to his wife about his fears and was reluctant to reveal his terror that she might die.

In her work with Mrs Morgan on diabetic self-care issues, the nurse practitioner learned that Mrs Morgan desperately needed to regain some control over her life. The nurse practitioner began to appreciate the strong link between Mrs Morgan's struggles with her own diabetes and her past family relationships. She was immobilized by what she perceived the future would bring. Her past experiences had propelled her to future possibilities and her ability to exercise current options was frozen. The nurse practitioner's task, along with other members of the team, was to help weave the past, present, and future together into an acceptable and achievable care plan for Mrs Morgan. They had to connect with her by acknowledging her story, empathizing with her terror, and, together with the patient, discovering some small steps she could tolerate as a beginning in reducing the harm caused by her diabetes.

Eventually, the social worker, visiting nurse, Mrs Morgan, and her husband began to move toward a more collaborative and interdisciplinary team approach regarding Mrs Morgan's care. They now understood the multiple reasons for Mrs Morgan's nonadherence but it was still a hard sell to the rest of the team. A third meeting, including the five health professionals and Mrs and Mr Morgan, moved the whole team from coordinated care to a more powerful position of sharing the patient's complex story, of adjusting goals to those the patient can accept and deal with, and working at the patient's pace. The team members could begin to find ways to interact with Mrs Morgan that were empathetic to her context, compatible with her capacity, and which opened new doors to caring.

One recognizes that using a grid such as those shown in Boxes 13.2 and 13.3, may be useful for teams early on but may not be necessary for teams after they have gelled and the role blurring makes the boxes less relevant. We suggest that treating other team members with the same principles as one treats patients, in a patient-centered or team-centered manner, could enhance both team functioning and patient-centered care, each reinforcing the other.

In the next case, the story of Francine, every team member held her story. The story and its updates were developed at team meetings and carried from the team meetings to the visits with the individual professionals and back again. The synergy between narrative in health care and patient-centered care has been presented already in this book in Chapter 3. Narrative was the way the professionals on this team encapsulated the information about Francine. Narrative was how Francine understood her life. The narrative was created at two levels: (1) between the patient and each professional where the story was built together and verified repeatedly and (2) among the professionals on the team where the story was twice removed and co-created with team members. When the team functioned well and worked at sufficient depth, the story was rich and true. However, teams can harden around a story and, to guard against such inflexibility, each team member may want to reflect, or verify with the patient and report nuances back to the team. During weekly training seminars, a mixed group of doctors, nurses, social workers, and others

> wrote about their attachment to patients, their emotional responses to patients and families, and their attempts to imagine clinical situations from the perspectives of patients and family members; participants then read aloud their narratives to one another during a facilitated discussion. (Sands *et al.*, 2008: 307)

In focus groups, participants reported the value of the training for team building and getting to know one another as people and their perspectives about care. They also reported that the experience "spilled over" into the team's function as a unit. In Francine's care, the team consciously held a healing narrative in mind, one of hope, in explicit contrast to the struggles she faced. As you will read, the team helped Francine identify unique health outcomes as sparkling events, opening up the possibility of a positive future.

The Team was the Container for Her Story: Case Illustrating a Team-Centered Approach

Lynn Brown

Francine was a petite woman of 41 who had experienced trauma throughout her life including witnessing the homicide of a parent, abuse in her family, and exploitation in adolescent and adult relationships. Born in a different language tradition and with little support to attend school she found reading difficult and direction-finding overwhelming. She usually required someone to assist her in order to attend appointments.

The family lived in dense, subsidized social housing that was not safe. She described events in which she was exploited and directly threatened. These events triggered past trauma and despair. She was unable to earn her way out of this situation because of symptoms of post-traumatic stress disorder, pain, and educational limits. Physical injury to her back during a domestic assault had resulted in chronic pain, for which she had become reliant on opiates. This was an ongoing concern to her family physician. She was receiving the most basic and insecure social assistance income, frequently having to prove her inability to work and unable to manage the letters of instruction. This also triggered intense fear and despair.

Social supports were limited to one main friend who drove her to appointments. Her three adolescent children were her chief source of pride and hope for the future. She was committed to their having a better life and would rally repeatedly to perform the routines she knew they needed. Religious faith at times offered a perspective beyond her surroundings and through her art and painting she could express both suffering and hope.

Francine's family physician was her anchor. She trusted him as he had been a reliable professional in a life where trustworthiness was rare. He created a team for Francine consisting of himself, the social worker, and the nurses. Contacts with all team members were both planned and episodic, with numerous crises.

Francine was not ready to accept referrals for treatment programs. She believed she required the medications for her pain. Her ideas about her health focused on the medication, with some moments when she could consider building into a different future. Her functioning when in despair was severely limited; at those times phone calls and even housework were not possible. When feeling better, her expectations of the team were that they would be interested in her childrens' accomplishments and that some suggestions or hope would be proffered. The team was her major source of support.

The nurses on the team would often assist by repeating information concerning appointments and at times rescheduling appointments that had been missed because of direction and transportation problems. They dealt with medication requests, at times desperate in nature, and provided an enthusiastic audience for the stories of her children. The family physician and the nurses offered some hope when she had lost hers.

The social worker spent many hours with her, sometimes at her home but mainly at the clinic, listening to her horrific story. It was clear that Francine could not participate in trauma therapy, as her life was so unsafe in the present. They began working together to find a more secure foundation for her and her family. It required hours to help her complete an application for a disability pension, which would be more secure and would provide somewhat more income. With each question on the application form, she would offer more of the details of her trauma, although this was not being directly asked. Intense, keening grief would follow. Some sessions were focused on her present despair based on her pain, both emotional and physical intertwined. Months after this, she gained the more established income of a disability pension. During the wait she would call to report the dangers in the housing environment and the social worker began to work toward finding safer housing with crisis calls and concerns about her children intermingled. Finally a move to a safer neighborhood was accomplished after appeals, letters, and efforts to sustain her hope.

The team's presence was crucial to the social worker as she struggled to grasp what was trauma and what was medication related. The team members supported one another in understanding the story of this unique woman, and the challenges of her care were strengthening to all. It appeared that Francine's alliance with her family physician became a form of institutional transference in which all team members were seen as meriting trust. The team shared in monitoring her safety. During dark times she would call and seemed to expect there would be some helpful and knowing response from one of the team. Because she let the team know her, they became her enthusiastic audience in the times of victory. The team members were more able to respond because they knew the meaning of a positive development in a story of frequent sacrifice and turmoil. Although some services offered to her and her family were discipline-specific, all members of the team contributed to providing a container in which her story, the victories, and sadness could be held.

14 Health Care Costs and Patient-Centered Care*

Moira Stewart, Bridget L Ryan, and Christina Bodea

A recent report of the Health Council of Canada (2010) concludes that family physicians' decision making about diagnostic tests is complex. One of several drivers of decisions that the report identifies is patient-centered care, which the authors imply is related to higher costs. Our research draws the opposite conclusion.

Patient-centered care is a high priority in Canada's health care system (CHSRF 2008; MOHLTC 2009). There is considerable Canadian and international evidence that patient-centered care has positive benefits for patient satisfaction (Krupat *et al.*, 2000; Fossum and Arborelius, 2004; Stewart *et al.*, 1999), patient adherence (Stewart *et al.*, 1999; Golin *et al.*, 1996), patient health outcomes such as reduction of concern (Stewart *et al.*, 2000), better self-reported health (Stewart *et al.*, 2000, 2007b) and improved physiological status (e.g., blood pressure and HbA_{1c}) (Krupat *et al.*, 2000; Stewart *et al.*, 1999; Golin *et al.*, 1996; Kaplan *et al.*, 1989a, b; Greenfield *et al.*, 1988; Griffin *et al.*, 2004; Rao *et al.*, 2007). However, there are no comparable Canadian data to support the hypothesis that patient-centered care saves money, whereas there are US data (Epstein *et al.*, 2005b).

The Patient-Centered Outcomes Study (Stewart *et al.*, 2000) found that patient-centered care was associated with not only improved health outcomes but also fewer diagnostic tests. This finding implied a potential for cost savings. The present-day context that both prioritizes patient-centered care and clearly requires cost constraint led us to re-analyze the Patient-Centered Outcomes Study data. We rigorously costed the medical resources associated with diagnostic tests used by the participating family physicians and patients.

There were 311 patients from the Patient-Centered Outcomes Study included in this costing analysis. The perspective for the costing was that of the provincial government's health costs. Other societal costs were not calculated. Costs of diagnostic investigations were determined for each person. First, the

---

* This paper was first published as "Is Patient-Centred Care Associated with Lower Diagnostic Costs?" (Stewart, 2011). This revised version is reprinted with permission.

quantities of diagnostic tests were obtained from a chart review. The quantities were restricted to those diagnostic tests that were related to an index visit (and the associated main reason for that visit) and which occurred from the date of the index visit to 2 months after the index visit. Second, the price per unit of each diagnostic test was determined using Ontario Health Insurance Plan costing schedules from Ontario's Ministry of Health and Long-Term Care. Third, diagnostic costs were determined by multiplying the quantities by the prices per unit. We used the Patient Perception of Patient-Centeredness questionnaire (Stewart *et al.*, 2004) of 14 items on the extent to which the physician attended to the patient's illness experience, attended to the context of the patient and found common ground with the patient concerning problem definition and treatment. The analysis categorized the patient-centered scores into quartiles and determined the mean costs for each quartile.

Table 14.1 provides the mean diagnostic costs by the four quartiles of patient-centered care scores over the 2-month follow-up period of the study. While the mean diagnostic costs for the first three quartiles were fairly similar, those for the fourth quartile were much higher, suggesting a threshold below which costs are implicated. Two possible explanations come to mind: (1) a potential statistical reason is that the fourth quartile consists of visits with a wider range of scores than the other quartiles, including some very low scores on patient-centeredness, and (2) a potential clinical communication reason is that perhaps both patients and family physicians lost confidence; thus, the patient assigned low scores on the patient-centered questionnaire and the physician ordered many high-cost tests in the hope of clarifying some confusion or conflict. It should be noted that these results did not allow determination of the appropriateness of the tests ordered.

TABLE 14.1 Mean Diagnostic Costs during the Subsequent 2 months Following the Family Physician Index Visit, by Quartiles of Patient-Centered Scores (n = 311)*

Quartile of Patient-Centered Score	Mean Diagnostic Cost
First quartile (high patient-centered scores)	$11.46
Second quartile	$13.07
Third quartile	$14.04
Fourth quartile (low patient-centered scores)	$29.48

Note: *The table reveals the clinical significance of this finding. The statistical significance (p = 0.004) was assessed using a multiple regression of the dependent continuous outcome of diagnostic cost with patient-centered scores as the continuous independent variable, controlling for the variables found significant in the bivariate analysis (patient's main presenting problem and marital status).

The costs in Table 14.1 were then projected onto the current Canadian and

Ontario populations (Statistics Canada, 2010) to provide a sense of the magnitude of potential cost savings as a result of patient-centered care. One-fifth of the population visits a family physician each month (Green *et al.*, 2001). One-third of these present new symptoms for which a diagnostic test may be ordered (Stewart & Maddocks, 2013). Dividing the resulting 1/15th of the population into four quartiles and calculating the diagnostic costs based on Table 14.1, we found that in a month overall $14 million would be spent in Ontario and $38 million in Canada. However, if all family physicians were patient-centered at the level of the highest quartile, potentially one-third of these costs would be saved.

The costing for this study was conducted on data from an older study, limiting our ability to draw direct comparisons with the current primary health care context. However, it is likely that the distribution of patient-centered scores is similar today to those found in the original; for example, a recent study using the same measure found comparable mean scores (Clayton *et al.*, 2008). Whether family physicians' actual ordering behavior for particular diagnostic tests might be different today than it was during the original study is more difficult to determine. However, we do know that in Canada, there was an increase between 1993/94 and 2003/04 in the number of CT tests performed (300%) and the number of MRI tests performed (600%) (You *et al.*, 2007). This finding suggests that the potential diagnostic cost savings today may be even greater than in the earlier study.

Other Canadian research has demonstrated that it is possible to provide better primary care that is associated with lower costs (Hollander *et al.*, 2009). Our intention in reporting these results is to encourage further dialogue and future research on the association between patient-centered primary care and costs in today's health care context.

These results lead to several modest recommendations. First, future studies could evaluate the costs as one of the potential benefits of a patient-centered approach. Second, associations of family practice could strengthen their emphases on the education and evaluation of patient-centered care given that training for patient-centered care has been shown to be effective (Stewart *et al.*, 2007b). Third, one could study whether incentives given to family physicians could improve their patient-centered care. Fourth, patients in primary care could be surveyed to assess their perceptions of patient-centered care to provide feedback to family physicians (Reinders *et al.*, 2010). These four recommendations imply future directions for research, education, policy, and practice in improving patient-centered care. Patient-centered care has a role to play in delivering not only effective but also efficient health care services.

PART FIVE

Research on Patient-Centered Care

Introduction

Moira Stewart

The following part summarizes the research relevant to the patient-centered clinical method. Researchers from a variety of research backgrounds have asked questions about the nature and impact of the kind of medical practice that we call patient-centered.

This part will first summarize the evidence from qualitative studies which illuminate patient-centered principles in practice and next turn to a summary of evidence from the epidemiologic tradition on the impact of patient-centered communication on a variety of important outcomes. Our hope is that these two current reviews will help clinicians learn about the distinctive contributions from both of these traditions, enhancing their ability to create an integrated understanding of quality patient-centered practice.

Finally, this part presents updates on the two research measures that we have developed and tested. These measures have both been used in a large number of countries and settings.

15 Using Qualitative Methodologies to Illuminate Patient-Centered Care

Carol L McWilliam and Judith Belle Brown

Parallels between the patient-centered clinical method and humanistic inquiry invite the application of qualitative methods in investigating patient-centered care. Patient-centered care focuses on the patient's health, disease, and illness, and the patient as a whole person. The patient-centered clinical method is a process of acquiring qualitative knowledge and understanding of a fellow human being. Humanistic inquiry explores the nature and experience of being human, eliciting in-depth descriptions or holistic interpretations to enhance understanding. In humanistic inquiry, the researcher and research participant together strive to capture the needs, motives, and expectations of the participant to construct the interpretation of their experience. As well, the patient-centered components, finding common ground and enhancing the patient-clinician relationship, have similarities to the processes of humanistic inquiry.

The "high context" nature of patient-practitioner communication also invites qualitative research, whether it be undertaken to obtain objective description, subjective or intersubjective interpretation, or to correct social injustices associated with inequities and marginalization. In all patient-practitioner communication, much is influenced by the hidden, invisible dimensions of "external" and "internal" context that might be illuminated by explicit description, interpretive understanding, or moral critique. Changes in contemporary society now, perhaps as never before, challenge practitioners to acquire and apply new understandings of the relevance and purposes of patient-practitioner communication. Advances in the prevention and treatment of acute disease mean that more patients suffer longer with chronic diseases. Thus, the traditional goals of healing and transcendence of suffering have taken on renewed significance. Such goals demand that practitioners are prepared to go beyond the application of intellectual understanding of the sufferer's plight to the development of a therapeutic alliance aimed at eliciting the patient's story and assisting with the development of a healing narrative (Egnew, 2009). The need for "thick description," insights and understanding to inform such patient-centered care is readily apparent.

This chapter presents an overview of the current state of the art in using qualitative methodologies to illuminate and develop the theory and practice of the patient-centered clinical method. Of the three paradigmatic options available to researchers wanting to undertake qualitative research, methods eliciting qualitative description within the post-positivist or Western scientific paradigm continue to be the most common application. However, researchers are increasingly undertaking qualitative investigation in the two less familiar paradigms as well – specifically, the interpretive and critical paradigms.

The relevance of these two paradigms to patient-centered care is clearly underscored by their aims and assumptions. Interpretive research aims to promote understanding of subjective, intuitive, dynamic, interrelated, context-dependent experiences of human life. The patient-clinician encounter constitutes one such experience. Researchers have used a diversity of interpretive research methodologies to elicit particulars about human nature and experience, extracting meaning and understanding from words, behaviors, actions, and practices of people. Given its fit with the patient-centered approach to care, not surprisingly, researchers often have applied narrative inquiry as a method to elicit insights and understanding of patient experiences (Blickem & Priyadharshini, 2007; Haidet *et al.*, 2006; Mosack *et al.*, 2005; Nettleton, *et al.*, 2005; Wheatley *et al.*, 2008) that both inform and confirm the relevance of the first two components of the patient-centered clinical method. Recently, however, researchers also have applied a phenomenological lens (Brown *et al.*, 2008; Woolhouse *et al.*, 2011, 2012; Russell *et al.*, 2005), uncovering understandings that not only enhance understanding of the illness experience (hence, patient-centered care) but also afford insights relevant to other components of the patient-centered clinical method – for example, illuminating potential strategies for enhancing the patient-clinician relationship and developing new approaches to finding common ground. Others (Pottie *et al.*, 2005; Scott *et al.*, 2008) have used grounded theory methods to uncover new understandings that may inform practitioners regarding the specifics of executing various components of the patient-centered clinical method, for example, understanding the whole person (Pottie *et al.*, 2005) and enhancing the patient-clinician relationship (Scott *et al.*, 2008).

Investigation undertaken in the critical paradigm presents researchers with the opportunity to achieve both qualitative understanding and quantified generalizable results about human experiences of social injustices, particularly the unconscious or hidden exercise of power and control contained in social relationships. This paradigm has been used much less, but invites researchers to undertake new work to reveal understandings of the whole person in instances in which social injustices or marginalization may potentially come into play, as well as to explore the potential for power imbalances in the patient-clinician relationship. Critical research can illuminate the importance of patient-centered practice as a means of preventing or overcoming human experience of social injustice in the process of seeking and receiving health care. However, to date, there has been very limited application of this paradigm in research in the field of patient-centered care (Waitzkin, 1984), notwithstanding the powerful syntheses provided by Candib (1995) and Malterud (1994), all seminal works that invite and inspire further work of this nature.

The following sections illustrate how the application of qualitative research advances the theory and practice of the patient-centered clinical method. As well, the examples presented illuminate new directions for qualitative research to further our understanding of patient-centered care.

EXPLORING THE PATIENT'S HEALTH, DISEASE, AND ILLNESS EXPERIENCE

Qualitative methodologies are helpful in gaining a greater understanding of the needs, motives, and expectations of patients. Narrative inquiry in particular has emerged as a methodology useful for making sense of an illness experience, as it gives primacy to the patient's voice, to listening for meaning rather than facts, and to providing a relational context that enables the evolution of a patient's story (Sakalys, 2003). As well, however, basic qualitative descriptive studies have proven helpful in identifying the specific needs of patients whose care may present particular challenges for practitioners. Four examples in the current literature illustrate the utility and applicability of qualitative investigation with these orientations.

Arnold *et al.* (2008) used focus groups and basic content analysis to describe the symptom domains and their impact on the everyday life of women with fibromyalgia from their perspective. Findings revealed that pain, sleep disturbance, fatigue, depression, anxiety, and cognitive impairment disrupted relationships with family and friends, created social isolation, reduced both daily living and leisure activities, and had substantial negative impact on career and educational advancement. Study participants described their struggle to keep feelings of stress under control to prevent disease exacerbation, which only intensified their level of stress, particularly creating frustration for "driven" women who were rendered unable to operate at their previous level. Findings underscore the significance of using patient-centered care to capture the needs, motives, and expectations of people who suffer from this debilitating disease.

Another focus group study elicited insights into pregnant women's needs, motives, and expectations related to maternal serum screening, similarly adding to physicians' understanding of the uniqueness of their experience (Carroll *et al.*, 2000). Researchers uncovered three factors influencing women's motives for undergoing or declining prenatal genetic screening: (1) personal values, attitudes, beliefs, and experiences; (2) social support from family and friends; and (3) the quality of the information provided by their physicians. In addition to the desire for quality information, the expectations of this patient population encompassed the right to make an informed choice, and physician sensitivity to their individual needs. As in the previous example, both the expectation of patient-centered care and what constitutes a patient-centered sensitivity to unique needs, motives, and expectations are readily apparent.

A third example (Nettleton *et al.*, 2005) illustrates how narrative inquiry can be used to illuminate the misunderstanding and frustration experienced by people with undiagnosed persistent puzzling symptoms. Through in-depth interviews and template analysis that applied Frank's (1995) typology of illness narratives, researchers uncovered the chaotic structure of study participants' stories, their concern that their symptoms might be "all in the mind" (Nettleton *et al.*, 2005: 207), and their status as medical orphans. Findings not only enhance all practitioners' understanding of this plight but also make abundantly clear the importance of capturing the needs, motives, and expectations of all patients, particularly those whose symptoms do not readily lead to diagnoses and treatment.

Finally, in another narrative inquiry, Mosack *et al.* (2005) applied grounded theory analysis methods to develop a theoretical framework based on Frank's (2010) typology of illness narratives and ambiguous loss theories (Boss & Couden, 2002). The framework illuminated differing orientations to HIV/AIDS illness experiences, including those reflecting benefit, loss, or status quo. Illness narratives reflecting a benefit orientation included experiences of restoration of health and personal growth. Those reflecting a loss orientation were comprised of symptom awareness and psychological distress, while those reflecting a status quo were characterized by calm resignation. The interpretation provides a framework that may help practitioners to determine the needs, motives, and expectations of patients with HIV/AIDS and to develop patterns of and parameters for communication to achieve their goals for patient-centered care.

Of equal importance to understanding patients' illness experience is exploring their knowledge, beliefs, and attitudes toward health. Health professionals need to have a tremendous depth and breadth of understanding of the patient's stage of readiness and self-efficacy related to promoting health or preventing disease in order to determine the appropriate approach to any intervention. As well, it is essential for the practitioner to know what health and/or the prevention of disease means to the patient so that approaches to incorporating prevention and health promotion can be aligned to his or her needs, motives, and expectations, with a view to optimizing positive outcomes. Qualitative methodologies provide the opportunity to capture in-depth descriptions of the experience of health, indirectly informing health promotion and disease prevention. The following two studies serve as illustrations.

Swift and Dieppe (2004) illustrate how narrative inquiry might uncover insights into patient knowledge that might be used to inform the creation or selection of health education materials useful for health promotion or primary and secondary disease prevention. Concerned about optimizing health as a resource for everyday living with chronic disease – specifically, arthritis – these researchers aimed to illuminate and share personal qualities and resources of patients that might be applied by others to maintain a satisfying and productive life, despite having this chronic condition. To obtain relevant insights, Swift and Dieppe (2004) purposefully selected a sample of seven people with extensive experience in coping with arthritis, and used a semi-structured interview guide to explore their everyday activity, work, leisure and social life, social relationships, and personal approaches to everyday issues and health care experiences. With informed consent, individuals' narratives were constructed and elaborated with editorial comment explaining concepts of patient-expertise and self-help. These personal accounts provided real-life evidence of the ability of people to know what may help them to optimize their health, despite chronic disease. Informal evaluation led to the conclusion that both patients and health professionals found this humanistic educational material both appealing and informative.

Brown *et al.* (2004) used qualitative research to evaluate a point-of-care testing strategy for secondary disease prevention of patients with diabetes. Through in-depth interviews with both health care professionals and patients with diabetes, these researchers identified the many benefits of point-of-care testing, including its potential for offering immediate feedback, informing proactive health education, increasing patient-practitioner communication and collaboration, and improving patient adherence. This qualitative understanding has applicability in creating other relevant linkages between disease monitoring activities and health promotion and disease prevention.

UNDERSTANDING THE PATIENT AS A WHOLE PERSON

Understanding the patient as a whole person invites the application of qualitative research methodologies to elicit a more in-depth picture of the larger life context than is immediately apparent. Insights acquired through qualitative investigations not only add to the practitioner's understanding of the specific individuals who have participated in the study, but also have the potential to be applicable in achieving a richer and deeper understanding of other patients who may share similar life contexts.

Three studies illustrate the applicability of qualitative research for enhancing understanding of the patient as a whole person. Brown *et al.* (2008) applied a phenomenological approach in exploring the lived experience of kidney donors. Using in-depth interviews and an iterative immersion and crystallization analysis strategy, this research team uncovered insights into motives behind the decision to donate an organ, intrapersonal and interpersonal factors that enter into the decision and organ donation experience, and the emotional and life-changing sequelae of this experience. Findings pinpoint the fallacy of assuming that individuals' motives will reflect what is supported by published literature, and expose the previously unidentified experience of loss, grief, and vested interest in their recipient's well-being, as well as renewed appreciation of life following donation. These clinical researchers conclude that organ donors may benefit from psychosocial assessment and ongoing emotional support and intervention. The merit of effort to understand the patient as a whole person and the applicability of these findings for those committed to providing quality, patient-centered care to organ donors is highlighted by this study.

Exposing the consequences of not making an effort to understand the whole person and his or her experience of illness is equally helpful to enhancing the practice of patient-centered care, as qualitative research conducted by Arman *et al.* (2004) reveals. This phenomenological study exposed the meaning of patients' experiences of suffering related to the health care provided. Through a secondary hermeneutic analysis of in-depth interviews of women with breast cancer, these researchers uncovered patients' experiences of not having been seen as unique human beings; not having their suffering acknowledged; not feeling cared for; feeling that they had been treated as bodies, numbers, or diagnoses; and having their experience of cancer ignored, pathologized, or explained away. Such experiences meant uncertainty, insecurity, distraction, and increased rather than alleviated suffering for these patients. Study participants clearly articulated the desire to be seen as whole human beings and to have their existential experience of illness understood, a finding that affirms both the theory and practice of patient-centered care.

A third example illustrates how narrative inquiry might be used to assess patient-centeredness, particularly as it relates to understanding the whole person. Researchers (Wheatley *et al.*, 2008) used secondary analysis of the narratives of primiparous women from low-income African American, Mexican American, Puerto Rican, and white families, extracting data on the content and quality of their prenatal care experiences. Template analysis (using the 2005 US National Healthcare Disparities Report markers of patient-centeredness) revealed that all four ethnic groups experienced not being listened to: white women were more likely than the other three ethnic groups to report having received poor explanations; African women were more negative than positive about being shown respect; and Mexican American women were more negative than the other ethnic groups about the time practitioners spent in providing their care. Overall, there was a preponderance of spontaneously volunteered examples of negative experiences related to patient-centeredness across all of three low-income ethnic groups in the study. The findings of this study suggest the importance of using qualitative research to evaluate patient-centered care, a research purpose of increasing importance in this era of evidence-based practice.

Together, these three examples typify the application of interpretive qualitative approaches in research related to understanding the whole person. While we could find no examples of critical research to investigate understanding of the whole person, these three studies illustrate the opportunities for variety, and invite researchers to creatively apply qualitative methods to understanding the whole person.

Pivotal to understanding the whole person is an awareness and understanding of the patient's proximal and distal contexts, as described in Chapter 5. The following three studies examined challenges in the delivery of patient-centered care from different perspectives of the contexts of care.

Pottie *et al.* (2005) explored Central American men's experience of forced migration, exposing their solitary struggle and sociocultural losses in immigrating to Canada. Findings pinpoint the importance of exploring the patients' larger life and health experience and initiating care strategies such as support groups to promote psychosocial health and prevent anxiety, depression, and/or abusive behaviors.

Phenomenological investigation by Russell *et al.* (2005) of community-based and academic practice-based family physicians' experiences of managing patients within the workers' compensation system revealed the challenges arising from this policy context of care. Despite the generally straightforward nature of most of the medical problems encountered, the family physicians in this study confronted suspicion, isolation, and frustration associated with ill-defined or complex conditions. They frequently became wary when dealing with employers, were suspicious of external influences on clinical decision making, and were especially concerned about patient confidentiality. Overall, they experienced conflict between their commitment to patient and insurer requirements for adherence to guidelines and pathways of care. Ethical issues also arose with regard to patient advocacy and confidentiality. Findings reveal the challenges of implementing patient-centered care in a context in which workers' compensation authorities do not understand the complexities of contemporary family practice and the time and cost barriers associated with workplace liaison.

A qualitative study using focus groups to investigate physicians' experiences of barriers and facilitators to the implementation of clinical practice guidelines for care of lower back pain (Dahan *et al.*, 2007) suggests that such practice guidelines also may impede patient-centered care. Findings reveal that physicians' professional decision making regarding the treatment of lower back pain functions on three levels that transpire simultaneously: decision making premised upon familiarity with and commitment to the implementation of the guidelines; decision making premised on patient-centered care considerations; and decision making premised upon the constraints and demands of the workplace, health care system, and environment for care outcomes. Grappling with these three dimensions of decision making is difficult, but the practitioners found that the patient-doctor interaction determined the outcomes of care, whether or not the direction taken ultimately reflected the clinical practice guidelines. Patient-centered care led to a healing process, while care that was not patient-centered led to a vicious circle of unnecessary service utilization. These findings not only illuminate the challenges that the context of health care places on the practitioner's efforts to be patient-centered, but also underscore the importance of making patient-centered care the priority, despite the health care context.

FINDING COMMON GROUND

Finding common ground with patients presents many challenges and opportunities. Patients' perspectives on participation in all components of the health care process vary greatly in both the extent to which they wish to participate and how they wish to participate (Haidet *et al.*, 2006). Coming to a mutual agreement about diagnoses and treatment plans is critical in achieving patient adherence, but it can readily overtax the time and patience of practitioners, particularly when relationships are new or have had inadequate time to develop. Qualitative research may elicit insights into factors that achieve or impede finding common ground, as well as factors that may facilitate the development of the social interaction processes required.

Two qualitative studies describe key elements of the process of finding common ground, illustrating the potential of these methodologies. In one study, researchers (Scott *et al.*, 2001) used a multimethod comparative case study and basic content analysis with a quasi-statistical approach to identify the nature and incidence of patient pressure tactics that countered physician efforts to find common ground regarding the use of antibiotics to treat acute respiratory tract infections. The study found complex connections between physician prescribing practices and patient expectations, revealing the significance of the nature and content of patient-physician communication. The study also addressed some of the challenges in finding common ground when patients and clinicians may not agree.

In another investigation, researchers applied grounded theory research methods to illuminate how the physician's and the patient's experiences together constitute the elements essential to finding common ground (Tudiver *et al.*, 2001). Using constant comparative analysis, researchers describe how a number of patient factors (i.e., expectations, anxiety) and physician factors (i.e., clinical practice experience, influence of colleagues) interact in the process of finding common ground in making cancer screening decisions. Findings also illustrate how a strong patient-physician relationship is central to finding common ground when cancer screening guidelines are unclear or conflicting.

Research by Woolhouse *et al.* (2011) reveals the creative strategies used by family physicians to find common ground with a marginalized group of patients – homeless women using illicit drugs who are participating in sex trade work. This phenomenological study illuminated the delicate exchange between patient and physician as they, often over many crisis-laden encounters, developed a therapeutic relationship. This is a twofold process: first is engagement of the patient, characterized by a "testing" phase, which is addressed by building trust; second is maintenance of the relationship, which involves providing continuity of care and constantly "meeting people where they're at" (Woolhouse *et al.*, 2011: 246). Only once a relationship is established can finding common ground become a reality. Even then, reaching common ground can be tenuous and threatened by the numerous contextual factors undermining the patient including violence, homelessness, and the street drug culture. In spite of this, the family physician participants in this study express their ongoing commitment to finding common ground and always taking into consideration the importance of understanding the whole person.

Shared decision making is, in part, aligned with finding common ground with patients, as described in Chapter 6. Three recent qualitative studies explicate the value of shared decision making in providing patient-centered care to patients with chronic conditions (Peek *et al.*, 2009; Lown *et al.*, 2009; Teh *et al.*, 2009).

Peek *et al.* (2009) conducted a phenomenological study using both in-depth interviews and focus groups to explore the barriers and facilitators to shared decision making by African American patients seeking care for their diabetes. Patient engagement in the shared decision-making process was enhanced when they experienced their physicians as accessible and available and felt their perspective was acknowledged and validated, hence contributing to a shift in the patient-practitioner power imbalance.

Similarly, in Lown *et al.*'s (2009) qualitative study, consisting of a sample of patients with chronic conditions and primary care physicians, reveals how sharing control and finding common ground regarding treatment is enhanced by shared decision making. This dynamic process includes a relational component illustrated through support and advice offered by the clinician, coupled with opportunities for patients to comfortably express their feelings and preferences as well as engage in discussions about care options.

Finally, Teh *et al.*'s (2009) grounded theory study that examined the experiences of older adults with chronic pain through in-depth interviews, supports the notion of the patient-clinician relationship as pivotal in the process of shared decision making and being patient-centered. These authors place particular emphasis on a patient-clinician relationship characterized by mutual respect. Importantly, they report that not all patients wish to participate in shared decision making and this does not pre-empt finding common ground, but rather is the essence of being patient-centered.

ENHANCING THE PATIENT-CLINICIAN RELATIONSHIP

As described in Chapter 7, the patient-clinician relationship constitutes the bedrock on which all care transpires. For this reason, research that uncovers the essence of the complex interactions that occur between patient and practitioner is foundational to building the theory and practice of patient-centered care. Greater in-depth understanding of the attributes of therapeutic relationships, how power is expressed in patient-clinician relationships, how caring and healing transpire, and ways of being in relationships with patients may do much to enhance the self-awareness and practice expertise of professionals, thereby enhancing patient-centered care.

Studies exemplify how the findings of qualitative investigation may enhance the patient-clinician relationship. One poignant interpretive investigation by Arman *et al.* (2004), explored the meaning of suffering by women with breast cancer, experienced in the process of receiving health care. Through second-ary phenomenological analysis of in-depth interviews with 16 Scandinavian women, researchers uncovered that patient-clinician relationships are experi-enced either as not materialized or as distanced, disease-focused encounters devoid of any human connectedness; these relationships are connected in the patient's mind to suffering. Patient suffering related to patient-clinician relationships served to intensify suffering related to the disease, its treatment, and both real and potential outcomes, leaving patients feeling isolated in their experience of disease, guilt and shame about their own mental and spiritual suffering, undermined self-worth, and neglect, including deprivation of caring, human fellowship, confirmation, and support. These findings reveal the impor-tance of clinicians' ways of being in relationships with patients, illuminating the negative consequences of professionally distanced, non-patient-centered approaches. In exposing these negative consequences, these qualitative findings also afford insights into the importance of practitioners' self-awareness and attention to their relationships with patients to achieve patient-centered care.

Indeed, insights into the important elements of relationship-building in patient-clinician encounters specific to women with breast cancer has been studied using phenomenological methodology (McWilliam *et al.*, 2000). Clearly, both the symptoms and diagnosis associated with breast cancer often trigger challenging feelings, such as vulnerability. The findings of this study revealed that physicians who work at relationship-building along with information-sharing ultimately contribute positively to their patient's experi-ence of control and mastery, and, in turn, their learning to live with cancer. By contrast, when patients experienced physicians to be paternalistic, negative, non-accepting, angry, falsely reassuring, giving poorly timed information and no hope, the patients were left feeling vulnerable and out of control. Patients who failed to have a connection with their physician experienced a continued search for meaningful patient-physician communication. Findings not only underscore the importance of creating a working relationship built upon a patient-centered approach but also illuminate key efforts that might contribute to success in this process.

Another investigation contributes additional insights on enhancing the patient-clinician relationship. Scott *et al.* (2008) used a grounded theory approach applying iterative qualitative methods to explore how healing rela-tionships are developed and maintained. From in-depth interviews designed to elicit stories from a purposeful sample of primary care physicians selected as exemplar healers, researchers constructed case studies describing the nature of the relationship of the patient-clinician dyad, which subsequently were analyzed to identify common themes, from which researchers then developed a model of healing relationships. Findings revealed that healing relationships encompass the clinician's valuing and creation of a nonjudgmental emotional bond, appreciation of clinician power, a conscious effort to manage that power in ways that most benefit the patient, and expressed and enacted commitment to caring for patients over time. These relational actions were found to achieve patient trust, hope, and sense of being known. These researchers concluded that healing relationships lead to patient-centered outcomes.

The phenomenological study by Woolhouse *et al.* (2012) explicates the sometimes overwhelming emotional challenges faced by clinicians in their attempt to care for severely disadvantaged populations, which, in this research, were homeless women using illicit drugs, often supported by sex trade work. Their findings reveal both the joys and the sorrows experienced by the physician participants in the care of this marginalized population. In order to sustain their efforts and commitment to these women, participants describe how they alter their expectations of care and engagement with this specific population and rely heavily on the support of team members. The emotional energy expended in the care of vulnerable populations is important to consider when compassion fatigue can severely affect clinicians, and ultimately the patient-clinician relationship.

TEAM-CENTERED CARE IN PROVIDING PATIENT-CENTERED CARE

The final study described in this chapter is relevant to Chapter 13 on team-centered care, as it reveals the tremendous challenges faced by interdisciplinary teams in the provision of patient-centered care. Ethnographic investigation of the structures, practices, and process of implementing interprofessional care in a multiprofessionally staffed stroke rehabilitation ward also illuminates thought-provoking challenges to patient-centered care (Blickem & Priyadharshini, 2007). Findings reveal how patient-centered care is undermined in this context, in which professionals have differing, sometimes irreconcilable, disciplinary and theoretical perspectives on care, as well as differing ideas of the meaning of patient-centeredness. Miscommunication between professionals is not uncommon, eliciting information about context and care arrangements that could help to build patient-centered care is not a straightforward task, and the patient is often placed in the position of being the conveyor of messages from one professional to the other. The researchers conclude that in order for patient-centered care to transpire in any multiprofessionally staffed work context, both patients and practitioners may need enhanced facility to see care from different perspectives, to cultivate the ability to flexibly move between differing subject perspectives, and to receive education that fosters conscious awareness of and attention to the ways in which professionals and patients are positioned to create or impede patient-centered care.

CONCLUSION

Much progress has been made through the use of qualitative research to investigate patient-centered care. However, many opportunities to further advance the theory and practice of patient-centered care exist. While some of the studies were conceived to address directly patient-centered practice, many were undertaken for other purposes. Nevertheless, by virtue of the nature of qualitative inquiry, these studies too illuminate components of the patient-centered clinical method. These studies are especially important, in as much as they spontaneously document the clinical validity of the patient-centered clinical method. As well, they illustrate the many opportunities for researchers committed to the evolution of the theory and practice of evidence-based patient-centered care.

To date, research primarily has explored either the clinicians' or the patients' perspectives, rather than the perspective of both partners in care on any one experience or component of patient-centeredness. More direct observation and more interpretive analysis of the two-way dyadic communication that transpires to create patient-centered care will be important in the future. As well, the absence of work in the critical paradigm invites initiatives in this area of qualitative research.

16 Evidence on the Impact of Patient-Centered Care

Moira Stewart

Research on patient-centered care and patient-centered communication has matured markedly in the past decade. Before then, there were fewer studies and the summaries of their results indicated a mixed effect of patient-centered care on important patient and practitioner outcomes (Lewin *et al.*, 2001; Stevenson *et al.*, 2004; Griffin *et al.*, 2004; Roter & Hall, 2004; Elwyn *et al.*, 2001; Mead & Bower, 2000). Now, as this chapter will illustrate, there are numerous well-executed systematic reviews and meta-analyses. On the whole, they indicate that patient-centered care has a positive influence on patient outcomes such as patient adherence, patient self-reported health, and physiologic health outcomes. Furthermore, they conclude that interventions to improve patient-centered communication are effective in changing practitioner behavior. All in all, this is a good news story, providing evidence that teaching and practicing patient-centered care is worthwhile. It also brings together evidence-based medicine and patient-centered medicine, in that it confirms that patient-centered care has an evidence-base.

This chapter presents four sections. First are the reviews on research linking interventions with improvements in patient-centered practitioner behavior and the patient-practitioner interaction. The second section will cover reviews about patient-centered care and patient adherence to medication or lifestyle regimens. Third, the chapter will summarize the evidence on patient-centered care in relation to patient health outcomes. Finally, the reviews on measures of patient-centered care will be summarized, indicating the concepts and components covered by the measures.

IMPROVING PATIENT-CENTERED INTERACTIONS

Two key recent systematic reviews have evaluated interventions aimed at improving patient-centeredness of the interactions in relation to the subsequent patient-centered behaviors of the practitioners.

Rao *et al.* (2007) distinguished between interventions directed at practitioners (21) versus patients (18). The 21 interventions for practitioners included multiple elements, usually information about concepts, feedback, modeling, and practice. Nineteen of these 21 studies found a significant difference in favor of the intervention group on at least one of a variety of communication behaviors.

The 18 studies of interventions directed at patients described interventions of several types; most were information in the form of written instructions for the patient, others were examples of questions for patients to ask the provider and others included coaching of patients. Of the 18, 13 found the intervention to have an impact on at least one outcome, practitioner behavior.

The systematic review by Dwamena *et al.* (2012) is exceptionally well done and presents valuable information for the reader. Sixteen studies provided a pooled outcome analysis of the process/communication outcome of practitioner behavior, of which four were dichotomous variables and showed no effect of the interventions. However, the remaining 12 studies used continuous outcomes and their pooled analysis favored the intervention groups at a statistically significant and meaningful level; the standardized mean differences were 0.70. This finding allowed the authors to conclude that there is "fairly strong evidence" in favor of interventions improving the patient-centeredness of the interaction between the practitioner and patient. "Is this sufficient to justify the importance that PCC [patient-centered care] has taken on in training programs in Europe, the UK and North America? The answer is yes" (2012: 26).

The most common practitioner behaviors and interactions that were improved in these studies were: clarifying patients' beliefs and concerns, communicating about treatment options, and the level of empathy and attentiveness.

There are two additional key conclusions. First is that, because there were very few studies of undergraduate trainees (such as medical students), their conclusion may not apply to undergraduate education. Second they conducted a rigorous pooled analysis separately for studies of brief training (less than 10 hours of training) and those of extensive training (greater than 18 hours). Both brief and extensive training demonstrated significant impacts leading to the authors' conclusion in their abstract that "short-term training is as successful as longer training (p. 2)."

Taken together, these two systematic reviews provide convincing evidence that education of practitioners is successful in improving the behavior of practitioners and the process/interaction of patients with their practitioners.

IMPROVING PATIENT ADHERENCE

Stevenson *et al.* (2004) summarized, from a systematic review, the kinds of communication about medicines between patients and a variety of health care professionals: doctors, pharmacists, and nurses. While the studies they reviewed revealed mixed results for interventions seeking to improve patients' communication, the results for interventions aimed at health professionals were consistently positive.

A meta-analysis conducted by Zolnierek and DiMatteo (2009) provided the material for the remainder of this section. The authors included 106 correlational studies relating communication variables to the outcome of patient adherence as well as 21 intervention studies of communication training on the outcome.

The 106 correlational studies found that there was a 19% higher risk of nonadherence in patients whose practitioner was a poor communicator. Another way of expressing this is that nonadherence was 1.47 times greater for patients whose practitioner was a poor communicator, or the odds of a patient adhering were 2.16 times greater when the practitioner was a good communicator.

The 21 intervention studies whose outcome measure was patient adherence were summarized and revealed that there was a 12% higher risk of nonadherence in patients whose practitioners had not received training on communication. The risk of nonadherence was 1.27 times greater for patients whose practitioner was not trained. The odds of a patient adhering were 1.62 times greater if his or her practitioner had been trained in one of the communication interventions studied.

A helpful additional analysis permitted the identification of variables that affect the relationship between communication (and communication interventions) and patient adherence. Three clinically oriented variables moderated the effect of communication on patient adherence. They were seriousness of the disease, such that the stronger impact of the communication interventions occurred for patients whose disease was less serious; practitioner was a pediatrician, such that the stronger impact occurred in pediatrician groups compared with non-pediatrician groups; and practitioner experience, such that residents, fellows, and medical students demonstrated stronger associations between their communication and patient adherence than the associations found for practicing doctors.

Also, four research-oriented variables moderated the effect of communication on patient adherence. They were sample size, such that if the number of patients in the study was less than 182, the association between communication and adherence was stronger; self-report adherence measure, such that if an objective measure was used the association was stronger; number of practitioners, such that if the number of providers was 25 or less the association was stronger; and patient perception measure of communication, such that if communication was not assessed by the patient the association was stronger.

Researchers should take note of the decisions on study design and measurement that may therefore reduce the likelihood of finding an association between communication and patient adherence or in intervention studies, of finding an impact on patient adherence. Potentially, such decisions may be a patient sample size larger than 182, the number of providers greater than 25, a self-report measure of adherence, and patient perception of the communication.

Readers interested in patient adherence are encouraged to read another book in the Patient-Centered Care series, *Patient-Centered Prescribing: Seeking Concordance in Practice*, by Dowell *et al.* (2007).

IMPROVING HEALTH OUTCOMES

Dwamena *et al.* (2012) were more cautious in their concluding statements about improving health outcomes than they had been earlier regarding improving patient-centered interactions. However, their meta-analysis results were unequivocal; the 10 studies providing data necessary for pooled analyses "showed positive effects (*on patient health outcomes*) for both dichotomous measures and continuous outcomes measures" (2012: 17, italics added). However, an important caveat was shown in their Table 2 (Dwamena *et al.*, 2012: 148–9), in which all 26 intervention studies are represented. Here only 46% of all 26 trials favored the intervention; the type of intervention most likely to succeed was the intervention training clinicians on patient-centered care and distributing material for patients as well (95% of such interventions achieved patient health outcomes that favored the intervention).

While an impression was emerging as individual studies were published over the past decade, now that the impression has solidified, the most potent interventions simultaneously to improve patient-centered communication and patient health outcomes are found to be those educating both the clinicians and the patients.

Not included in the systematic review, because it was not an intervention study was Jani *et al.* (2012), whose key finding deserves to be highlighted here. They found that patient-centered care (assessed objectively) was associated with positive mental health outcomes for depressed patients. Furthermore, these positive results held for both affluent areas and deprived areas, indicating that patient-centeredness can be a force for equity.

MEASURES OF PATIENT-CENTERED CARE

Building on previous summaries of concepts and measures of patient-centered communication (Epstein *et al.*, 2005a), a recent systematic review of measurement tools found 26 papers with 13 patient self-administered instruments (Hudon *et al.*, 2011). Using patient-centered models of Stewart *et al.* (2003) and Mead and Bower (2000), the authors carefully ascertained the items within each self-administered tool that aligned with the four important concepts outlined. Therefore, one sees in Table 16.1 the list of 13 instruments and the emphasis of each on one or several of the four conceptual dimensions. One can see that very few instruments are balanced, with two exceptions: the Component of Primary Care Instrument and the Primary Care Assessment Tool – Adult. Three lean heavily on the finding common ground dimension (Patient Perception of Patient-Centeredness, Consultation Care Measure and the Medical Communication Competence Scale). The Primary Care Assessment Survey has the majority of items in the Patient-Clinician Relationship dimension.

TABLE 16.1 Patient-centered care measurements instruments included in the review*

Instrument	Authors	Number of Items Assessing Conceptual Framework Dimension			
		Disease and Illness Experience	Whole Person	Common Ground	Patient-Doctor Relationship
Patient Perception of Patient-Centeredness	Stewart *et al.*, 2000	4	1	9	0
Consultation Care Measure	Little *et al.*, 2001a	6	2	9	1
Patient Reactions Assessment	Galassi *et al.*, 1992	0	0	2	6
Perceived Involvement in Care Scale	Lerman *et al.*, 1990	2	0	3	0
Component of Primary Care Instrument	Flocke, 1997	5	5	3	6
Medical Communication Competence Scale	Cegala *et al.*, 1998	0	0	18	6
Primary Care Assessment Survey	Safran *et al.*, 1998	4	1	4	12

Instrument	Authors	Number of Items Assessing Conceptual Framework Dimension			
		Disease and Illness Experience	Whole Person	Common Ground	Patient-Doctor Relationship
Interpersonal Processes of Care	Stewart et al., 2007a	4	0	8	8
General Practice Assessment Survey	Ramsay et al., 2000	2	1	2	5
Patient Perception of Quality	Haddad et al., 2000	0	1	4	5
Primary Care Assessment Tool – Adult	Shi & Starfield, 2001	4	4	2	2
Consultation and Relational Empathy	Mercer et al., 2004	2	1	2	5
Instrument on Doctor-Patient Communication Skills	Campbell et al., 2007	2	0	10	3

Source: *Adapted from Hudon et al. (2011), Tables 1 and 3, with permission.

This systematic review (Hudon et al., 2011) points out the gaps in measurement that exist in the field of research on patient-centered care, in particular the patients' perception of such care.

SUMMARY

This chapter has covered three key outcomes that patient-centered interventions seek to improve: (1) process of care and practitioner behaviors; (2) patient adherence; and (3) patient health. The measurement of patient-centered care itself has been reviewed and the stage is now set for the next two chapters: one on a specific measure of patient perceptions of patient-centeredness and the second on a specific measure of verbal behavior, both of which have been widely used to assess patient-centeredness.

17 Measuring Patient Perceptions of Patient-Centeredness

Moira Stewart, Leslie Meredith, Bridget L Ryan, and Judith Belle Brown

INTRODUCTION

Measures of patients' perception of patient-centered care have been developed that serve to supplement and complement the behavioral measure (MPCC) described in the next chapter. What more patient-centered research approach could one imagine than asking the patient to describe his or her experience of the visit with the clinician in a formal structured way? The measures, described in this chapter, have been used for research, but as well for education, by providing individual feedback to participating physicians on their patients' perceptions.

Patient perception measures are increasingly used to evaluate health care because of the seminal paper of Rosenthal and Shannon (1997). Standard questionnaires to assess patients' views of themselves or to assess their satisfaction with care (which includes implicit comparisons by patients between their perceptions of care and their expectations of care) are not the topic of this chapter. Rather, this chapter covers patients' reports of a recent experience of care. Other researchers have chosen such a focus to evaluate primary care generally (Starfield, 1998; Haddad, 2000; Greco *et al.*, 2001; Steine *et al.*, 2001; Takemura *et al.*, 2006; Campbell *et al.*, 2007; Makoul *et al.*, 2007). In general, such measures are more sensitive to health care delivery changes than long-term health outcome measures, less expensive and more reliable than clinician review methods, and focused on positive aspects of care (not mistakes), hence very suitable for quality improvement initiatives (Rosenthal & Shannon, 1997). These qualities make patient perception measures an important component of any health care research program.

Other researchers who have applied the patient perception approach to the study of patient-centered care include Little *et al.* (2001b). They developed a 21-item questionnaire that they found to be reliable (Cronbach's alpha ranging from 0.96 to 0.84) and which factored into five factors very similar to the components of the patient-centered clinical method described in this book (*see* Chapter 1). Little *et al.*'s (2001b) questionnaire was used before a visit to assess patient preferences (patients overwhelmingly preferred all facets of a patient-centered approach) and after the visit to assess patient perceptions of their experience.

The current chapter presents the questionnaire measures of patients' perception of the patient-centered clinical method described in this book (*see* Chapters 3–7).

THE MEASURE OF PATIENT PERCEPTION OF PATIENT-CENTEREDNESS

Measure Development

The 17 items developed by our colleagues Carol Buck and Martin Bass for a study of patient outcomes in family practice (Bass *et al.*, 1986), were adapted for a study of communication in family practice (Henbest & Stewart, 1990). The latter study served as a partial validation, in that the items on patients' perceptions of the physicians' ascertainment of the presenting problems were correlated with a patient-centered score of the audiotaped encounter (Spearman rank correlating coefficients ranging from 0.296 to 0.416; p values ranging from 0.006 to 0.001; n = 73; Henbest & Stewart, 1990). Revision of the 1990 version (eliminating four items for poor response or irrelevance to the concepts and adding one relevant item) led to the current 14-item version of the Patient Perception of Patient-Centeredness (PPPC) questionnaire (*see* Table 17.1), which was used in two large studies: one of 39 randomly selected family physicians and 315 patients (Stewart *et al.*, 2000); and a version adapted for cancer care in a second study of 52 family physicians, oncologists, and surgeons (Stewart *et al.*, 2007b).

In the late 1990s, pressure to create a shorter version for easy use in practice, especially for the purpose of continuous quality improvement, led to the selection of eight items that were found to significantly associate with either the objective measure of patient-centeredness (presented in the next chapter, Chapter 18) or a health outcome in the 2000 study, plus one new item thought to be necessary to reflect all the components of the patient-centered clinical method. This nine-item questionnaire has two versions: one for the patient to complete and one for the clinician to complete.

Researchers from across Canada and around the world have requested the working paper that describes these two versions of the PPPC (Stewart *et al.*, 2004). Since publication of the second edition of this book in 2003, over

100 requests have been received from Argentina, Australia, Brazil, Columbia, Germany, Italy, Japan, Korea, the Netherlands, Norway, Russia, Sarajevo, Spain, Switzerland, Taiwan, Turkey, the United Arab Emirates, the United Kingdom, and the United States.

The 14-item PPPC has been used in studies with the general population (Stewart *et al.*, 2000; Reinders *et al.*, 2009) and with specialized populations such as breast cancer survivors (Stewart *et al.*, 2007b; Clayton & Dudley, 2008, 2009), and the elderly (Ishikawa *et al.*, 2005). As well as having been used with real patients, the PPPC has also been used with standardized patients (Fiscella *et al.*, 2007).

Reliability and Validity of the Patient Perception of Patient-Centeredness

Inter-item reliability has been found to be adequate for the 14-item PPPC (Cronbach's alpha = 0.71, n = 315). The internal reliabilities (Cronbach's alpha) for the 14-item PPPC total score in four additional international studies are 0.91 (adapted to 12 items, n = 145, Ishikawa *et al.*, 2005); 0.90 (n = 2907, Fiscella *et al.*, 2007); 0.82 (n = 60, Clayton and Dudley, 2008, 2009); and 0.83 (n = 222, Reinders *et al.*, 2009).

The validity of the 14-item PPPC was established through (1) a significant correlation with the objective measure (*see* Chapter 18) (r = 0.16; p = 0.01; n = 315) and (2) significant correlations with patient health outcomes and with efficiencies in the use of health services (Stewart *et al.*, 2000).

Cronbach's alpha reliability of the nine-item patient questionnaire is 0.80 (n = 85). Similarly, Cronbach's alpha of the nine-item physician questionnaire is 0.79 (n = 117). Validity is based on the origin of the items. Eight items were significantly related to either the objective measure (*see* Chapter 18) or a patient health outcome measure. The remaining item was added to enhance content validity.

The Items

The 14-item PPPC is shown in Table 17.1. There are four items thought by the researchers to be relevant to Component 1: Exploring the Illness Experience; one item for Component 2: Understanding the Whole Person; and nine items for Component 3: Finding Common Ground.

TABLE 17.1 The 14-item Patient Perception of Patient-Centeredness

Patient Perception of Patient-Centeredness

Please CIRCLE the response that best represents your opinion.

1.	To what extent was your main problem(s) discussed today?	Completely	Mostly	A little	Not at all
2.	Would you say that your provider knows that this was one of your reasons for coming in today?	Yes	Probably	Unsure	No
3.	To what extent did the provider understand the importance of your reason for coming in today?	Completely	Mostly	A little	Not at all
4.	How well do you think your provider understood you today?	Very well	Well	Somewhat	Not at all
5.	How satisfied were you with the discussion of your problem?	Very satisfied	Satisfied	Somewhat satisfied	Not satisfied
6.	To what extent did the provider explain this problem to you?	Completely	Mostly	A little	Not at all
7.	To what extent did you agree with the provider's opinion about the problem?	Completely	Mostly	A little	Not at all
8.	How much opportunity did you have to ask your questions?	Very much	A fair amount	A little	Not at all
9.	To what extent did the provider ask about your goals for treatment?	Completely	Mostly	A little	Not at all
10.	To what extent did the provider explain treatment?	Very well	Well	Somewhat	Not at all
11.	To what extent did the provider explore how manageable this (treatment) would be for you? He/she explored this:	Completely	Mostly	A little	Not at all
12.	To what extent did you and the provider discuss your respective roles? (Who is responsible for making decisions and who is responsible for what aspects of your care?)	Completely	Mostly	A little	Not at all
13.	To what extent did the provider encourage you to take the role you wanted in your own care?	Completely	Mostly	A little	Not at all
14.	How much would you say that this provider cares about you as a person?	Very much	A fair amount	A little	Not at all

Three scores can be created from PPPC. The 14-item measure was coded so that low scores meant positive perceptions in keeping with other patient outcomes where fewer problems or low scores means a better outcome. The total score is the sum of all responses divided by 14. The second score is for Component 1, in which responses to items 1, 2, 3, and 4 are summed and divided by 4. (The reader will notice that there is only one item for Component 2, item 14, so there is no computed score.) The third score is for Component 3 in which responses to items 5–13 are summed and divided by 9.

TABLE 17.2 Self-Assessment and Feedback on Communication With Patients: Patient Assessment

Please check (✓) the box that best represents your response.

1.	To what extent was your main problem(s) discussed today?	Completely ❐	Mostly ❐	A little ❐	Not at all ❐
2.	How satisfied were you with the discussion of your problem?	Very satisfied ❐	Satisfied ❐	Somewhat satisfied ❐	Not satisfied ❐
3.	To what extent did the provider listen to what you had to say?	Completely ❐	Mostly ❐	A little ❐	Not at all ❐
4.	To what extent did the provider explain this problem to you?	Completely ❐	Mostly ❐	A little ❐	Not at all ❐
5.	To what extent did you and the provider discuss your respective roles? (Who is responsible for making decisions and who is responsible for what aspects of your care?)	Completely ❐	Mostly ❐	A little ❐	Not discussed ❐
6.	To what extent did the provider explain treatment?	Very well ❐	Well ❐	Somewhat ❐	Not at all ❐
7.	To what extent did the provider explore how manageable this (treatment) would be for you? He/she explored this . . .	Completely ❐	Mostly ❐	A little ❐	Not at all ❐
8.	How well do you think your provider understood you today?	Very well ❐	Well ❐	Somewhat ❐	Not at all ❐
9.	To what extent did the provider discuss personal or family issues that might affect your health?	Completely ❐	Mostly ❐	A little ❐	Not at all ❐

TABLE 17.3 Self-Assessment and Feedback on Communication With Patients: Clinician Assessment

Please check (✓) the box that best represents your response.

1.	To what extent was your patient's main problem(s) discussed today?	Completely ❑	Mostly ❑	A little ❑	Not at all ❑
2.	How satisfied were you with the discussion of your patient's problem?	Very satisfied ❑	Satisfied ❑	Somewhat satisfied ❑	Not satisfied ❑
3.	To what extent did you listen to what your patient had to say?	Completely ❑	Mostly ❑	A little ❑	Not at all ❑
4.	To what extent did you explain the problem to the patient?	Completely ❑	Mostly ❑	A little ❑	Not at all ❑
5.	To what extent did you and the patient discuss your respective roles? (Who is responsible for making decisions and who is responsible for what aspects of your care?)	Completely ❑	Mostly ❑	A little ❑	Not discussed ❑
6.	To what extent did you explain treatment?	Very well ❑	Well ❑	Somewhat ❑	Not at all ❑
7.	To what extent did you and the patient explore how manageable this (treatment) would be for the patient? We explored this . . .	Completely ❑	Mostly ❑	A little ❑	Not at all ❑
8.	How well do you think you understood the patient today?	Very well ❑	Well ❑	Somewhat ❑	Not at all ❑
9.	Regarding today's problem, to what extent did you discuss personal or family issues that might be affecting your patient's health?	Completely ❑	Mostly ❑	A little ❑	Not at all ❑

The nine-item questionnaire has two versions. The patient version is shown in Table 17.2. The physician version is shown in Table 17.3. A total score of the patient version is the sum of responses to all items divided by 9 and ranges from 1 to 4. The nine-item questionnaires were coded so that a high score meant positive perceptions in order to enhance the ease of interpretation of the feedback to physicians, with high scores intuitively meaning better performance. For formative feedback to the physician, two displays were provided. First, the proportion of patients of the doctor who responded with the most positive rating was shown for each item in a bar graph, allowing each physician to see what aspect of patient-centered care he or she was better at or worse at. Second, the level of agreement between the patient and physician rating was shown for each item in a bar graph.

Descriptive Results

TABLE 17.4 Descriptive results for Patient Perception of Patient-Centeredness (PPPC): 14 items (N = 315)

Variables	Range	Mean (Standard Deviation)
PPPC total score	1–2.9	1.5 (0.37)
Patient perception that the illness experience has been explored	1–3.3	1.2 (0.29)
Patient perception that the patient and physician found common ground	1–3.3	1.7 (0.50)

Table 17.4 shows the ranges, means, and standard deviations of the total 14-item PPPC and the two subscores for Components 1 and 3 as found in the study of 39 family physicians and 315 patients (Stewart *et al.*, 2000).

TABLE 17.5 Proportion of one physician's patients who reported high ratings, with the explanation to the physician

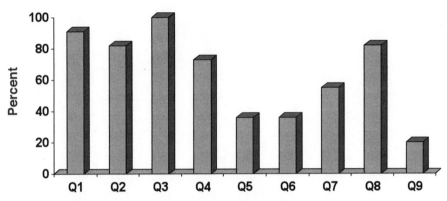

Percentage of Highest Ratings

Q1 To what extent was your main problem(s) discussed today?

Q2 How satisfied were you with the discussion of your problem?

Q3 To what extent did the doctor listen to what you had to say?

Q4 To what extent did the doctor explain this problem to you?

Q5 To what extent did you and the doctor discuss your respective roles? (Who is responsible for making decisions and who is responsible for what aspects of your care?)

Q6 To what extent did the doctor explain treatment?

Q7 To what extent did the doctor explore how manageable this (treatment) would be for you?

Q8 How well do you think your doctor understood you today?

Q9 To what extent did the doctor discuss personal or family issues that might affect your health?

Summary: The vast majority of your patients were completely satisfied with the communication during the visit for Q1, Q2, Q4, and Q8. All eleven patients were completely satisfied regarding you listening to them during the visit – Congratulations! For the remaining questions, the minority were completely satisfied. The lowest percentage occurs for question 9 (20%). Although there may be legitimate reasons for not discussing personal or family issues that may affect health, this is an area that was not covered completely. Less than half of your patients were not completely satisfied with the extent of the discussion regarding respective roles (Q5) and the extent you explained treatment (Q6). This may have been due to something you and the patient either could not cover or only had time to discuss superficially. Also, 46% of patients did not feel that a complete discussion of how manageable treatment would be for them occurred.

Table 17.5 shows the feedback on the proportion of patients giving the most positive rating for each item for one doctor. Physicians can see for which aspects of patient-centered care their patients perceive them positively.

TABLE 17.6 Level of agreement between the physician and that physician's patients, with the explanation to the physician*

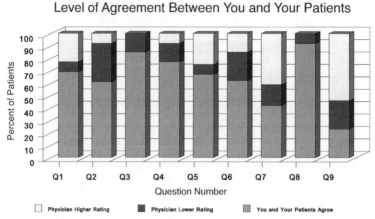

The GREY (bottom) bar represents the percentage of patients for which physician and patient rating agreed. On average, you agreed with 64% of your patients. In general your level of agreement is fairly inconsistent. The highest level of agreement, 92%, occurred on Q8 (How well do you think your doctor understood you today?) with Q3 (To what extent did the doctor listen to what you had to say?) a close second. The lowest level of agreement, 23% occurred on Q9 (To what extent did the doctor discuss personal/family issues that may affect your health?).

Now looking at the BLACK (middle) bar, on average, you rated your communication *lower* than 18% of your patients. The main source of disagreement occurred on Q2 (How satisfied were you with the discussion of your problem?), for which you rated yourself lower than 31% of your patients. There could be many reasons for this: you and your patients may have interpreted the question in different ways, you may have underestimated the impact of what you did discuss, and/or you are not as confident in yourself regarding this area of communication during patient visits. There were no other notable disagreements in this direction.

Now looking at the WHITE (top) bar, on average, you rated your communication higher than 18% of your patients. Q7 (To what extent did the doctor explore how manageable this (treatment) would be for you?) and Q9 (To what extent did the doctor discuss personal or family issues that might affect your health?) both show fairly substantial disagreement in this direction (42% and 54%, respectively).

Note: *These percentages are based on the responses of 13 patients.

Table 17.6 shows the level of agreement between one doctor and his or her patients, along with the written feedback provided to that physician.

CONCLUSION

This chapter shows the versatility of the patient perception measures as both research and education tools. The chapter has presented an overview of two questionnaire measures, showing their items, reliability and validity assessments, and their results. The two measures were the 14-item PPPC and the nine-item questionnaire, which has a patient version and a clinician version.

18 Measuring Patient-Centeredness

Judith Belle Brown, Moira Stewart, and Bridget L Ryan

Concurrent with the development of the concepts of the patient-centered clinical method and subsequent educational programs, was a research initiative to support the empirical basis of the method. Central to the research program was the creation of tools to measure patient-centered care. The patients' perception measures are covered in Chapter 17 of this book. In this chapter, we cover the objective measures based on observation of the clinical encounter. Many methods of measuring communication have been developed since Bales (1950) first introduced the Bales Interaction Analysis (Kaplan *et al.*, 1989a; Roter, 1977; Roter *et al.*, 1990; Stewart, 1984; Shields *et al.*, 2005).

Advances in assessing the patient-physician interaction have led several authors to provide comparisons of various coding schemes. In a special issue of *Health Communication* in 2001, six research teams coded the same data-set using their respective measures (McNeilis, 2001; Meredith *et al.*, 2001; Roter & Larson, 2001; Shaikh *et al.*, 2001; Street & Millay, 2001; von Friederichs-Fitzwater & Gilgun, 2001). Commentaries on the results highlight what certain coding schemes can and cannot measure (Rimal, 2001; Frankel, 2001). In addition, Mead and Bower (2000) have assessed the reliability and validity of various observation-based measures of patient-centered behaviors including an earlier version of the Measure of Patient-Centered Communication (MPCC) described in this chapter.

Many of these measures, while effective in assessing patient-clinician interaction, are not specific to the patient-centered clinical method as we envision it. Thus, rather than import parts of measures relevant to patient-centered care, a new research measure was created and subsequently modified – the MPCC. This chapter describes this measure.

THE MEASURE OF PATIENT-CENTERED COMMUNICATION

Development

Based on the patient-centered clinical method developed in the 1980s, 1990s, and 2000s, a method of assessing and scoring patient-clinician encounters, either audiotaped or videotaped, was developed. The MPCC has evolved significantly since its inception in the early 1980s. The development of the

MPCC is detailed shortly. The MPCC has a couple of advantages over other methods (Bales, 1950; Kaplan *et al.*, 1989a; Roter, 1977; Roter *et al.*, 1990; Stewart, 1984; Shields *et al.*, 2005): (a) it does not require that the recorded interview between the patient and the clinician be transcribed; and (b) it is theory based – that is, it is derived from the conceptual framework described in Chapters 1 and 3–7 of this book.

The initial version of the coding and scoring of the MPCC was published in 1986 and used in a study of family practice residents (Brown *et al.*, 1986). At that time the measure only captured Component 1, Exploring Both the Disease and the Illness Experience. As a result the measure underwent significant expansion, including Component 2, Understanding the Whole Person, and Component 3, Finding Common Ground, and it provided more detailed process categories as well as coding and scoring instructions (Brown *et al.*, 1995). This 1995 version of the measure was used in subsequent studies in family practice (Kinnersley *et al.*, 1999). The 2001 version arose in response to patients' expressed needs regarding communication (McWilliam *et al.*, 2000) and is detailed in the MPCC working paper (Brown *et al.*, 2001). This latest version has been used in a number of funded studies with family physicians, surgeons, and oncologists (Stewart *et al.*, 2007b); family physicians (Epstein *et al.*, 2006; Shields *et al.*, 2005; Cegala & Post, 2009); and oncologists (Clayton *et al.*, 2008). These US and Canadian projects have obtained adequate reliability after 2-day workshops and follow-up telephone advice.

The current measure incorporates coding and scoring of Component 1, Exploring Both the Disease and the Illness Experience; Component 2, Understanding the Whole Person; and Component 3, Finding Common Ground. Component 4, the enhancement of the patient-clinician relationship, is not included. This component evolves over many visits between a clinician and patient; may not be measured in each encounter or may not be verbalized by the clinician or patient. While always an important part of the patient-centered method, this component was not measured explicitly in our previous studies.

It should be noted that the revision of the patient-centered clinical method, as described in this book, from six components to four, and the reframing of the first component to include not only disease and illness but also health is very recent. As such, there has not been the opportunity to develop the necessary revisions and conduct the assessment of psychometric properties, required to capture these changes. This speaks to the need for future research and development of the MPCC.

Application of the Measure of Patient-Centered Communication: Who and Where

The MPCC can be used in a variety of patient-clinician settings. In previous studies, it has been successfully used during office visits when patients are presenting with acute and/or chronic illnesses, routine physical examinations or check-ups, office procedures, and follow-up visits for previous problems. It has also been used in the emergency department where real time coding was conducted. As well as being used with actual patients, the MPCC has been employed in office visits with standardized patients.

This latter application offers the advantage of standardization but presents specific challenges because coders may work with a preset template of patient statements and expected behaviors (i.e., specific feelings, ideas, effects on function, and expectations) on the part of the standardized patient. In reality, these behaviors may not be elicited by the clinician or the encounter may proceed in a manner that does not provide the standardized patient with an opportunity to articulate programmed statements, either at all or at an appropriate time. For example, a standardized patient may be directed to provide the clinician with a statement about the effect of a sore back on his or her ability to work. If the clinician moves quickly to the treatment of the problem, and it is only then that the standardized patient has an opportunity to raise this issue, the coder would normally place the statement in Component 3, coding it as part of the mutual discussion surrounding the treatment. With standardized patients, coders must decide how to handle these situations, balancing the goal of consistency afforded by standardized patients with the goal of accurately capturing the interaction. In the case of the effect of the sore back on work, the coders might decide to move back to Component 1 so as to ensure that this statement was captured in a consistent way for all standardized patient visits.

Occasionally, an additional person such as another health care practitioner will be present during an interview. If the health care practitioner is not an integral part of the visit, this person should not be considered as part of the interview to be coded. However, if the visit does involve two health care practitioners, such as a medical student and a staff physician, who are taking equal part in the interview, these two people, depending on the research question, may be seen as one physician and the interview will be coded as if these two people speak as one physician.

The other situation where an additional person may be present is when another person accompanies a patient. In this case, the coder must decide with whom the interview is being conducted. If, for example, a mother accompanies her child who does not speak for herself, then the interview will be coded between the mother and the clinician. If, however, the child is older and is an active participant in the discussion, the interview will be coded between the child and the clinician. In the case of an adult patient, the interview will usually be coded between the patient and the clinician unless the adult patient is unable to speak independently. This can happen, for example, in the case of a patient who is severely mentally challenged or is cognitively impaired.

Researchers from around the world have requested the working paper that describes the MPCC (Brown *et al.*, 2001). Since publication of the second edition of this book in 2003, over 120 requests have been received from Australia, Austria, Belgium, Brazil, Denmark, Germany, Italy, Japan, Korea, the Netherlands, New Zealand, Nigeria, Norway, Puerto Rico, Spain, Sweden, Switzerland, Taiwan, the United Kingdom, and the United States.

Reliability and Validity of the Measure of Patient-Centered Communication

Interrater reliability of the scoring of the initial version of the MPCC was established among three raters at r = 0.69, 0.84, and 0.80 (Brown *et al.*, 1986). Using the 1995 version (Brown *et al.*, 1995), Stewart *et al.* (2000) established an interrater reliability of 0.83 and an intrarater reliability of 0.73. Three studies using the current version (Brown *et al.*, 2001) report interrater reliabilities of 0.79 (Epstein *et al.*, 2006); 0.77–0.98 (Clayton *et al.*, 2008); and 0.80 (Cegala & Post, 2009).

The validity of the scoring procedure of the 1995 version was established by a high correlation (0.85) with global scores of experienced communication researchers (Stewart *et al.*, 2000).

CODING THE MEASURE OF PATIENT-CENTERED COMMUNICATION

Coding takes place while listening to a recording (either in segments or in full) of a patient's visit to the clinician. It is often necessary to listen to all or parts of the recording a second time in order to fill in gaps in coding that were not captured on the first pass.

Coders listen for statements from the patient and the clinician that are pertinent to the patient-centered clinical method and list only those pertinent statements. Not every statement the patient or clinician makes will be coded. Coders must place statements under the most appropriate component. Components 1, 2, and 3 of the patient-centered clinical method are coded. *See* Figure 18.1 for the coding template of the MPCC.

COMPONENT 1. EXPLORING BOTH THE DISEASE AND THE ILLNESS EXPERIENCE

	Preliminary Exploration	Further Exploration	Validation	Cut-off	SCORE
Symptoms and/or Reason for Visit					
1 _____	Y N	Y N	Y N	Y N	_____
2 _____	Y N	Y N	Y N	Y N	_____
3 _____	Y N	Y N	Y N	Y N	_____
4 _____	Y N	Y N	Y N	Y N	_____
5 _____	Y N	Y N	Y N	Y N	_____
				ST**	
Prompts					
1 _____	Y N	Y N	Y N	Y N	_____
2 _____	Y N	Y N	Y N	Y N	_____
3 _____	Y N	Y N	Y N	Y N	_____
4 _____	Y N	Y N	Y N	Y N	_____
5 _____	Y N	Y N	Y N	Y N	_____
				ST**	
Feelings					
1 _____	Y N	Y N	Y N	Y N	_____
2 _____	Y N	Y N	Y N	Y N	_____
3 _____	Y N	Y N	Y N	Y N	_____
4 _____	Y N	Y N	Y N	Y N	_____
5 _____	Y N	Y N	Y N	Y N	_____
				ST**	
Ideas					
1 _____	Y N	Y N	Y N	Y N	_____
2 _____	Y N	Y N	Y N	Y N	_____
3 _____	Y N	Y N	Y N	Y N	_____
4 _____	Y N	Y N	Y N	Y N	_____
5 _____	Y N	Y N	Y N	Y N	_____
				ST**	

(continued)

FIGURE 18.1 Coding template of the Measure of Patient-Centered Communication*

---

*   As already noted, Component 1 has undergone a change to include health as well as disease and illness. The current measure does not yet reflect this change.

	Preliminary Exploration	Further Exploration	Validation	Cut-off	SCORE
Effect on Function					
1 _____	Y N	Y N	Y N	Y N	_____
2 _____	Y N	Y N	Y N	Y N	_____
3 _____	Y N	Y N	Y N	Y N	_____
4 _____	Y N	Y N	Y N	Y N	_____
5 _____	Y N	Y N	Y N	Y N	_____
				ST**	[ ]
Expectations					
1 _____	Y N	Y N	Y N	Y N	_____
2 _____	Y N	Y N	Y N	Y N	_____
3 _____	Y N	Y N	Y N	Y N	_____
4 _____	Y N	Y N	Y N	Y N	_____
5 _____	Y N	Y N	Y N	Y N	_____
				ST**	[ ]

** Subtotal
*** Grand total

GT*** _____ ÷ = [ ]

COMPONENT 2. UNDERSTANDING OF THE WHOLE PERSON

Any statements relevant to FAMILY, LIFE CYCLE, SOCIAL SUPPORT, PERSONALITY, and CONTEXT are to be listed below:

	Preliminary Exploration	Further Exploration	Validation	Cut-off	SCORE
1 _____	Y N	Y N	Y N	Y N	_____
2 _____	Y N	Y N	Y N	Y N	_____
3 _____	Y N	Y N	Y N	Y N	_____
4 _____	Y N	Y N	Y N	Y N	_____
5 _____	Y N	Y N	Y N	Y N	_____
6 _____	Y N	Y N	Y N	Y N	_____
7 _____	Y N	Y N	Y N	Y N	_____
8 _____	Y N	Y N	Y N	Y N	_____
9 _____	Y N	Y N	Y N	Y N	_____
10 _____	Y N	Y N	Y N	Y N	_____
				ST*	[ ]

* Subtotal
**Grand total

GT** _____ ÷ 5 = [ ]

FIGURE 18.1 Coding template (*cont.*)

COMPONENT 3. FINDING COMMON GROUND

	Clearly Expressed	Opportunity to Ask Questions	Mutual Discussion	Clarification of Agreement	SCORE

Problem Definition:

1 _____	Y N	Y N	Y N	Y N	_____
2 _____	Y N	Y N	Y N	Y N	_____
3 _____	Y N	Y N	Y N	Y N	_____
4 _____	Y N	Y N	Y N	Y N	_____
5 _____	Y N	Y N	Y N	Y N	_____
6 _____	Y N	Y N	Y N	Y N	_____
7 _____	Y N	Y N	Y N	Y N	_____
8 _____	Y N	Y N	Y N	Y N	_____
9 _____	Y N	Y N	Y N	Y N	_____
10 _____	Y N	Y N	Y N	Y N	

ST** [ ]

Goals of Treatment/Management

1 _____	Y N	Y N	Y N	Y N	_____
2 _____	Y N	Y N	Y N	Y N	_____
3 _____	Y N	Y N	Y N	Y N	_____
4 _____	Y N	Y N	Y N	Y N	_____
5 _____	Y N	Y N	Y N	Y N	_____
6 _____	Y N	Y N	Y N	Y N	_____
7 _____	Y N	Y N	Y N	Y N	_____
8 _____	Y N	Y N	Y N	Y N	_____
9 _____	Y N	Y N	Y N	Y N	_____
10 _____	Y N	Y N	Y N	Y N	

ST** [ ]

Responded Appropriately to Disagreement with Flexibility and Understanding

1 _____	Y N	N/A	_____
2 _____	Y N	N/A	

ST** [ ]

** Subtotal
*** Grand total

GT*** _____ ÷ _____ = [ ]

FIGURE 18.1 Coding template (*cont.*)

Coding under Appropriate Headings

Once the appropriate component is identified, the coder will list the patient or clinician statement under the most appropriate heading. In Components 1 and 3, there is a choice of headings. In Component 2, there is only one heading. The headings for each of these components are described here.

Component 1: Exploring Both the Disease and the Illness Experience

Symptoms and/or Reason for Visit

Patients' symptoms are listed using the patients' words in the upper left portion of the Component 1 coding form (*see* Figure 18.1). Patients' symptoms are the stated conscious expression of their physical, emotional, or social problem, usually representing their reason for the visit. While a statement of symptoms normally initiates an office visit, it may occur at any stage of the interaction. For example, a patient may say at the end of the visit, "By the way, doctor, I've also got a pain in my knee."

Symptoms and/or Reasons for Visit fall generally into six categories as follows:

1. The patient initiates the description. ("I've been having a lot of chest pain.")
2. The patient responds positively to a clinician inquiry about a sign or symptom. (The clinician asks: "Have you been having any allergy problems this spring?" The patient responds, "No, they seem to be under control.")
3. The patient responds either positively or negatively to a clinician inquiry regarding a known problem that the patient has not presented at the current visit. (The clinician asks, "So how has it been since your bowel surgery?" The patient responds, "It's been going well, actually.")
4. The patient raises a problem or treatment issue from a previous visit. ("That medication you gave me last time didn't help at all.")
5. The clinician elicits the patient's personal and/or family history or conducts a check-up as part of the visit. (The physician asks, "Any history of heart disease in your family?" Or "Do you smoke?" or "Any hospitalizations?")
6. The patient is present to have a procedure. In this case, there may be very little conversation but it is appropriate to code the clinician's conversation with the patient both before and during the procedure. This is where the clinician would be scored on how he/she handles the issue of informing the patient about the procedure and the issue of patient consent. (The patient begins, "I'm here to have this mole removed." The clinician responds, "OK, now did I explain to you what is going to happen?" The patient indicates, "Yes, we discussed that last time.")

Prompts

Prompts are listed in the patients' words in the second left-hand section of the Component 1 coding form. Prompts are signals from patients that their feelings, ideas or expectations have not yet been explored. Prompts may be verbal, behavioral or arise from the context of the consultation. Prompts are defined as either statements that are out of context or restatements of a problem that has already been mentioned.

Feelings

Feelings are listed in the patients' words in the third left-hand section of the Component 1 coding form. Feelings reflect the emotional content of the patient's illness. They may be the predominant aspect of the illness, as in a grief reaction, or be a contributory factor, as in the anxiety of a discovery about a breast lump. They may arise directly out of the stated Symptoms and/ or Reason for Visit, Prompts, Ideas, Effect on Function, or Expectations, as when a patient who has requested a check-up discloses during the course of the interview that she is anxious (Feeling) about the effects of dyspareunia (Symptom and/or Reason for Visit) on her sexual function. Words commonly used by patients to express their feelings are troublesome, concerned, preoccupied, afraid, fearful, worried, sad, depressed, anxious.

Ideas

Ideas are listed in the patients' words, in the fourth left-hand section of the Component 1 coding form. Patients form ideas about their illness in their attempts to make some meaning or sense of their experience – that is, they develop an explanatory model of their illness. Patients' health beliefs, values, and life experiences can inform this explanatory model. These ideas may be based on prior experiences or influenced by present events such as a recent death of a friend.

Effect on Function

Effects on Function are listed in the patients' words in the fifth left-hand section of the Component 1 coding form. The illness may have an effect on the patient's daily function, including the patient's capacity to fulfil certain roles and responsibilities such as a worker, spouse, or parent. Questions by the clinician may include how the illness limits daily activities, how it impairs family roles, and how it requires a change in lifestyle. Specific activities relevant to the heading Effect on Function include physical mobility, eating, dressing, sleeping, toileting, working, socializing, and leisure activities.

Expectations

Expectations are listed in the patients' words in the last left-hand section of the Component 1 coding form. Every patient who visits a clinician has some expectations of the visit. Patients' expectations often relate to a symptom or a concern about which patients anticipate exploration or response from the clinician. The presentation of the patients' expectations may take many forms, including a question, a request for service, or a statement of the purpose of the visit. Expectations are also reasons for the visit other than symptoms (i.e., annual health visit, request for service, request for completion of a disability form, request for a prescription refill).

Component 2: Understanding the Whole Person

There are five topics specific to component 2 and patient statements relevant to these five topics are to be listed (*see* Figure 18.1, second section, for the Component 2 coding form). The five are Family, Life Cycle, Social Support, Personality, and Context (e.g., employment/schooling, culture, environment, health care system). Often, statements relevant to one topic may also be relevant to another. However, we do not consider it important for these topics to be mutually exclusive and, consequently, we have not separated them by subheadings. This is a difference from the coding for Component 1 with its subheadings.

Component 3: Finding Common Ground

There are two areas specific to Component 3, Finding Common Ground: Problem Definition and Goals of Treatment – which represent (1) establishing the nature of the problems and priorities and (2) the goals of the treatment (*see* Figure 18.1, third section, for the Component 3 coding form).

Problem Definition

Problem Definition is the clinician's statement of the nature of the problem(s). This statement is listed in the top left-hand section of the Component 3 coding form. It is not necessarily a restatement of the patient's initial presentation but is the clinician's formulation after the patient's presentation has been explored. It may be that on certain occasions the clinician does not know what the problem is but may offer a number of possible definitions of the problem. In this instance, each separate hypothesis/problem definition is to be documented under Problem Definition.

Goals of Treatment

Goals of Treatment are the present treatment plan. These are listed in the second left-hand section of the Component 3 coding form. These goals are sometimes future oriented but are reasonable and attainable. Both the clinician's stated goals for treatment and any patient expressions of goals or patient comments on the clinician goals are listed. Goals of Treatment include such things as ordering a test, suggesting an examination, prescribing a medication, or suggesting a treatment. Typically, these are instrumental suggestions on the part of the clinician.

Coding of Appropriate Process Categories

After writing the statement in the appropriate place, the coder must assign process categories to each statement. These process categories describe the clinician's response or lack of response to the patient's statements. The following two sections describe (1) the process categories for Components 1 and 2 (which are identical) and (2) for Component 3, respectively.

Component 1 and Component 2 Process Categories

The process categories include Preliminary Exploration (yes/no); Further Exploration (yes/no); Validation (yes/no); Cut-off (yes/no); and Return (R).

Preliminary Exploration

Preliminary Exploration is the immediate response of the clinician to the patient's expression of Symptoms and/or Reason for Visit, Prompts, Feelings, Ideas, Effect on Function, and Expectations. A code of "Yes" is any acknowledgment that the clinician heard and accepts the patient's Symptoms and/or Reason for Visit, Prompts, Feelings, Ideas, Effect on Function, Expectations. Alternatively, when the clinician cuts off the patient, the categorization would be "No" to Preliminary Exploration and "Yes" to Cut-off. Premature reassurance by the clinician does not count as Preliminary Exploration.

Further Exploration

Further Exploration is the second and subsequent responses of the clinician. Further exploration means that the clinician's response facilitated the patient's further expression either with verbal facilitation or by silence allowing the patient to amplify and/or redirect the conversation.

Validation

Validation is an empathetic response by the clinician to the patient's expression. A code of "Yes" means that the clinician has acknowledged the patient's expression in an empathetic way. Validation would include phrases such as, "I understand that . . .;" "This must be a difficult time . . .;" "These are difficult decisions to make . . .."

Cut-Off

A Cut-off is defined as the clinician blocking the patient's further expression of Symptoms and/or Reason for Visit, Prompts, Feelings, Ideas, Effect on Function, or Expectations – for example, by changing the subject, excessive focus on disease, jargon, or premature reassurance.

Return

The final process category is a specific clinician behavior called a Return. The Return will be indicated by an R in the margin. This occurs where a clinician has cut-off a patient but subsequently in the interview returns to the patient's Symptoms and/or Reason for Visit, Prompts, Feelings, Ideas, Effect on Function, or Expectations. With a Return, the clinician is considered to have initiated Preliminary Exploration of the patient's problem and this nullifies the Cut-off.

Component 3 Process Categories

The process categories include Clearly Expressed (yes/no); Opportunity to Ask Questions (yes/no); Mutual Discussion (yes/no); and Clarification of Agreement (yes/no).

Clearly Expressed

Clearly Expressed requires that the clinician clearly states in language the patient can understand what he/she believes is the problem or what the treatment should be. Statements are not clearly expressed if (1) the statement is garbled, incomplete, or contradictory, or (2) the statement is not comprehensive enough for the patient to understand the reasoning behind the statement.

Providing an Opportunity to Ask Questions

Providing an Opportunity to Ask Questions includes the explicit request from the clinician, "Do you have any questions about this?" It can also be the patient asking a question or the patient making a comment on the problem definition or goal.

Mutual Discussion

Mutual Discussion is not achieved when the clinician describes the problem definition or goal without any evidence of the patient participating in a discussion either by asking questions or stating opinions. The patient also has to provide verbal content for there to be a discussion.

Clarification of Agreement

Clarification of Agreement can take two forms. The first form is where the clinician explicitly asks "Do you agree with this?" and the patient responds to the question. The second form is where the clinician encourages, through silence or the implicit tone of the interaction, the patient to express agreement or disagreement.

Responded Appropriately to Disagreement with Flexibility and Understanding

The final part of scoring the interaction concerns the clinicians' response to disagreement by the patient. In our experience, such disagreements rarely occur. However, although rare, we consider the clinician's response to such disagreement to be important in Finding Common Ground.

SCORING

After the entire interview is coded, coders assign scores on the right side of the coding sheets and calculate the scores for Components 1, 2 and 3. On the last coding sheet, an overall Patient-Centered Score is calculated. Each of the three component scores can range theoretically from 0 to 100. The total Patient-Centered Score score is an average of the three component scores and it too can range theoretically from 0 (not at all patient-centered) to 100 (very patient-centered). A detailed description of the scoring procedure is provided in the MPCC working paper (Brown *et al.*, 2001).

DESCRIPTIVE RESULTS

Table 18.1 shows the means, ranges, and standard deviations of the total MPCC and the three components as found in an observational cohort study of 39 family physicians and 315 of their patients (Stewart *et al.*, 2000).

TABLE 18.1 Measure of Patient-Centered Communication (MPCC) Scores for a Sample of Family Physicians (N = 39) and Patient (N = 315) Encounters*

MPCC	Mean	Standard Deviation	Actual Range
Total score	50.77	17.86	8.13–92.52
Component 1	50.85	19.00	0.00–97.50
Component 2	39.70	42.76	0.00–100.00
Component 3	56.26	22.97	0.00–100.00

Source: *Stewart et al.*, 2000.

CONCLUSION

In this chapter, we have described the development, evolution, and application of the MPCC. The most recent coding and scoring of the MPCC have been outlined in some detail.

19 Conclusions

Moira Stewart

This book makes the point that the patient should be at the center of health care, research, and education. Most medical disciplines and health professions can adapt the patient-centered principles espoused herein to their work with patients. A clinical approach, agreed to by all health care professionals, will not only benefit patients but also enhance the seamlessness of health services by providing a glue to hold all participants together. The four components of the patient-centered clinical method become the shared goals for care, and they are (1) exploring health, disease, and the illness experience; (2) understanding the whole person; (3) finding common ground; and (4) enhancing the patient-clinician relationship.

One strength of the body of material contained in this book is that it represents 3 decades of work on four fronts simultaneously: (1) conceptual/theoretical development; (2) development of practical clinical approaches; (3) educational development; and (4) research. The first decade (1982–1992) saw great strides in the theoretical development of the patient-centered clinical method and patient-centered teaching. The second decade (1992–2002) saw the implementation of undergraduate medical education programs and residency programs based on patient- and learner-centered principles. As well, the second decade saw research programs come to fruition. The third decade (2002–2012) witnessed significant threats to patient-centered clinical care while, at the same time, producing positive research results, telling us of the major benefits of patient-centeredness.

Another strength of the patient-centered method is that it seeks to transcend some of the distinctions and limitations inherent in the conventional medical model – specifically, the dichotomy between mind and body, art and science, feeling and thinking, subjective and objective, and tacit and explicit knowledge. Also, we challenge another false distinction, the notion that patient-centered medicine and evidence-based medicine are incompatible dichotomies; rather, they are synergistic in creating improved clinical practice.

One of the abiding strengths of this book and its previous editions is the presentation of the patient-centered framework in concise diagrams. Clinicians tell us that these pictures guide them even in the thick of an intense patient encounter. Educators have found them to be invaluable. However, these diagrams, even though helpful, are a double-edged sword: there are limitations. We have attempted to overcome the rather linear format of previous diagrams by creating a more circular appearance. Still, none of these representations adequately depicts the complex interactive process that circles around and around, always in motion. Although extremely helpful for clinical practice, for teaching, and for clarity in research, diagrams can never fully capture the mysterious reality of a relationship between a clinician and a patient.

What are the key messages of this book? One message is that patient-centered concepts are evolving while still resting on the bedrock of the original principles from 30 years ago. The clinical method is streamlined with four components replacing six; it is also more integrated, with all clinical activities (acute care, chronic care, and prevention/health promotion) subsumed by the four components. A new conceptual leap clarifies that health promotion, as an exploration of meanings, aspirations, and illness experiences, falls into Component 1, Exploring Health, Disease, and the Illness Experience; while health education and prevention, as activities the clinician can prioritize with the patient, fall into Component 3, Finding Common Ground.

A second key message is the plethora of education approaches and experiences that are available to support learning patient-centered care. Educational scholarship has advanced over the past decade and this book covers the most up-to-date literature.

A third key message is to keep an eye on the context. In the fast pace of change in health care, we may lose more than we gain in terms of models of care that support a patient-centered clinical method. Decreasing continuity of care, the advent of information technology in the clinical setting, and the increasing number of guidelines are examples of contexts that pose substantial threats to patient-centeredness. In this book, we chose to address two potential threats in some detail: (1) teamwork in health care and (2) cost of health care. With regard to teamwork, Chapter 13 espouses a parallel process of four components of building a team matching the four components of the patient-centered clinical method. The case is made that enhanced teamwork promotes patient-centeredness. Regarding the context of cost constraints and accountability, it is crucial that we trumpet far and wide the result indicating cost savings of patient-centered health care, as Chapter 14 reveals.

Finally, the research part of the book provides the most optimistic message, one that can be used for strong advocacy in favor of patient-centered innovations: they work! Patient-centered interventions with practicing clinicians succeed in improving clinicians' behaviors and patient-clinician interactions. The systematic review asks and answers the question: Do the results justify all the effort being placed on patient-centered training? Yes, they do! Furthermore, the majority of studies indicate positive effects of patient-centered care on patient health outcomes.

An important next step in the development and evolution of the patient-centered clinical method will be the application of the principles to a wide variety of problems, thereby evolving the concepts and making them tangibly relevant to concrete clinical situations. An exciting series of books continues this task. They deal with challenges and solutions (Brown *et al.*, 2011); mental illness (Rudnick & Roe, 2011); pregnancy and childbirth (Shields & Candib, 2010); palliative care (Mitchell, 2008); prescribing (Dowell *et al.*, 2007); substance abuse (Floyd & Seale, 2002); chronic fatigue (Murdoch & Denz-Penhey, 2002); eating disorders (Berg *et al.*, 2002); and chronic myofascial pain (Malterud & Hunskaar, 2002).

With encouraging findings on the positive effects that can be enjoyed and using the resources provided in the patient-centered book series, let us move forward with energy and optimism.

References

Aagard E, Teherani A, Irby DM. Effectiveness of the One-Minute Preceptor model for diagnosing the patient and the learner: proof of concept. *Acad Med.* 2004; **79**(1): 42–9.

Abendroth M, Flannery J. Predicting the risk of compassion fatigue. *J Hosp Palliat Nurs.* 2006; **8**(6): 346–56.

Ablesohn A, Stieb D, Sanborn MD, *et al.* Identifying and managing adverse environmental health effects: 2. Outdoor air pollution. *CMAJ.* 2002a; **166**(9): 1161–7.

Ablesohn A, Gibson BL, Sanborn MD, *et al.* Identifying and managing adverse environmental health effects: 5. Persistent organic pollutants. *CMAJ.* 2002b; **166**(12): 1549–54.

Abramson NS, Wald KS, Grenvik AN, *et al.* Adverse occurrences in intensive care units. *JAMA.* 1980; **244**(14): 1582–4.

Adams F. *The Genuine Works of Hippocrates.* Birmingham, AL: The Classics of Medicine Library; 1985.

Adams WG, Mann AM, Bauchner H. Use of an electronic medical record improves the quality of urban paediatric primary care. *Paediatrics.* 2003; **111**(3): 626–32.

Alexander M, Lenahan P, Pavlov A (eds). *Cinemeducation: Using Film and Other Visual Media in Graduate and Medical Education.* Vol. 2. London: Radcliffe Publishing; 2012.

Alguire PC, DeWitt DE, Pinsky LE, *et al. Teaching in Your Office: A Guide to Instructing Medical Students and Residents.* 2nd ed. Philadelphia, PA: ACP Press; 2008.

Alonso A. *The Quiet Profession: Supervisors of Psychotherapy.* Toronto, Canada: Collier Macmillan; 1985.

Alonzo AA. The experience of chronic illness and post-traumatic stress disorder: the consequences of cumulative adversity. *Soc Sci Med.* 2000; **50**(10): 1475–84.

Ambrose SA, Bridges MW, DiPietro M, *et al. How Learning Works: Seven Research-Based Principles for Smart Teaching.* San Francisco, CA: Jossey-Bass; 2010.

Anda RF, Croft JB, Felitti VJ, *et al.* Adverse childhood experiences and smoking during adolescence and adulthood. *JAMA.* 1999; **282**(17): 1652–8.

Anderson ES, Winett RA, Wojcik JR, *et al.* A computerized social cognitive intervention for nutrition behavior: direct and mediated effects on fat, fiber, fruits, and vegetables, self-efficacy, and outcome expectations among food shoppers. *Ann Behav Med.* 2001; **23**(2): 88–100.

Anspach RR. Notes on the sociology of medical discourse: the language of case presentation. *J Health Soc Behav.* 1988; **29**(4): 357–75.

Apker J, Propp KM, Zabava Ford WS, *et al.* Collaboration, credibility, compassion, and coordination: professional nurse communication skill sets in health care team interactions. *J Prof Nurs.* 2006; **22**(3): 180–9.

Archer JC. State of the science in health professional education: effective feedback. *Med Educ.* 2010; **44**: 101–8.

Arman M, Rehnsfeldt A, Lindholm L, *et al.* Suffering related to health care: a study of breast cancer patients' experiences. *Int J Nurs Pract.* 2004; **10**(6): 248–56.

Arnold L, Willoughby TL, Caulkins EV. Self-evaluation in undergraduate medical education: a longitudinal perspective. *J Med Educ.* 1985; **60**(1): 21–8.

Arnold LM, Crofford LJ, Mease PJ, *et al.* Patient perspectives on the impact of fibromyalgia. *Patient Educ Couns.* 2008; **73**(1): 114–20.

Aronoff DM. And then there were none: the consequences of academia losing clinically excellent physicians. *Clin Med Res.* 2009; **7**(4): 125–6.

Aronowitz RA. *Making Sense of Illness: Science, Society, and Disease.* Cambridge: Cambridge University Press; 1998.

Ashley P, Rhodes N, Sari-Kouzel H, *et al.* 'They've all got to learn': Medical students' learning from patients in ambulatory (outpatient and general practice) consultations. *Med Teach.* 2008; **31**(2): e24–31.

Atkins CGK. *My Imaginary Illness: A Journey into Uncertainty and Prejudice in Medical Diagnosis.* Ithica, NY: Cornell University Press; 2010.

Aujoulat I, Luminet O, Deccache A. The perspective of patients on their experience of powerlessness. *Qual Health Res.* 2007; **17**(6): 772–85.

Back AL, Bauer-Wu SM, Rushton CH, *et al.* Compassionate silence in the patient-clinician encounter: a contemplative approach. *J Palliat Med.* 2009; **12**(12): 1113–17.

Bacon F. *The Advancement of Learning* [1605]. New York: PF Collier and Son; 1901.

Bailey P, Jones L, Way D. Family physician/nurse practitioner: stories of collaboration. *J Adv Nurs.* 2006; **53**(4): 381–91.

Bain K. *What the Best College Teachers Do.* Cambridge, MA: Harvard University Press; 2004.

Bainbridge L, Nasmith L, Orchard C, *et al.* Competencies for Interprofessional Collaboration. *Journal of Physical Therapy.* 2010; **24**(1): 6–11.

Baker SS. *Information, Decision-Making and the Relationship between Client and Health Care Professional in Published Personal Narratives.* Ann Arbor, MI: University Microfilms International; 1985.

Baldwin DC Jr, Daugherty SR, Eckenfels EJ. Student perceptions of mistreatment and harassment during medical school: a survey of ten United States schools. *West J Med.* 1991; **155**(2): 140–5.

Bales RF. *Interactive process analysis: a method for the study of small groups.* Reading, MA: Addison-Wesley; 1950.

Balint E, Courtenay AE, Hull S, *et al.* *The Doctor, the Patient, and the Group.* London: Routledge; 1993.

Balint M. *The Doctor, His Patient, and the Illness.* New York, NY: International Universities Press; 1957.

Balint M. *The Doctor, His Patient, and the Illness.* 2nd ed. New York, NY: International Universities Press; 1964.

Balint M. *The Doctor, His Patient and the Illness.* 3rd ed. Philadelphia, PA: Churchill Livingstone; 2000.

Balint M, Hunt J, Joyce D, *et al.* *Treatment or Diagnosis: A Study of Repeat Prescriptions in General Practice.* Philadelphia, PA: JB Lippincott; 1970.

Bandura A. *Social Learning Theory.* Englewood Cliffs, NJ: Prentice-Hall; 1977.

Bandura A. *Social Foundations of Thought and Action: A Social Cognitive Theory.* Englewood Cliffs, NJ: Prentice-Hall; 1986.

Bannister SL, Hanson JL, Maloney CG, *et al.* Using the student case presentation to enhance diagnostic reasoning. *Pediatrics.* 2011; **128**(2): 211–13.

Barbee RA, Feldman SE. A three-year longitudinal study of the medical interview and its relationship to student performance in clinical medicine. *J Med Educ.* 1970; **45**(10): 770–6.

Barilan YM. The Doctor by Luke Fildes: an icon in context. *J Med Humanit.* 2007; **28**(2): 59–80.

Barlow JH, Turner AP, Wright CC. A randomized controlled study of the arthritis self-management programme in the UK. *Health Educ Res.* 2000; **15**(6): 665–80.

Barnett K, Mercer SW, Norbury M, *et al.* Epidemiology of multimorbidity and implications for health care, research, and medical education: a cross-sectional study. *Lancet.* 2012; **380**(9836): 37–43.

Baron RA. Negative effects of destructive criticism: impact on conflict, self-efficacy, and task performance. *J Appl Psychol.* 1988; **73**(2): 199–207.

Barry CA, Bradley CP, Britten N, *et al.* Patients' unvoiced agendas in general practice consultations: qualitative study. *BMJ.* 2000; **320**(7244): 1246–50.

Barry CA, Stevenson FA, Britten N, *et al.* Giving voice to the lifeworld: more humane, more effective medical care? *Soc Sci Med.* 2001; **53**(4): 487–505.

Barry MA. A framework for understanding the conflicting role of clinical instructors. Presented at the International Nursing Research Congress, Toronto, Canada, 2006. Available at : www.nursinglibrary.org/vhl/handle/10755/151354 (accessed September 15, 2013).

Bartz R. *Interpretive Dialogue: a multi-method qualitative approach for studying doctor-patient interactions.*

Paper presented at the Annual Meeting of the North American Primary Care Research Group, San Diego, CA; 1993.

Bartz R. Beyond the biopsychosocial model: new approaches to doctor-patient interactions. *J Fam Pract.* 1999; **48**(8): 601–7.

Bass MJ, Buck C, Turner L, *et al.* The physician's actions and the outcome of illness in family practice. *J Fam Pract.* 1986; **23**(1): 43–7.

Battista RN, Lawrence RS (eds). Implementing preventive services. *Am J Prev Med.* 1988; **4**(Supp 8).

Bayoumi AM, Kopplin PA. The storied case history. *CMAJ.* 2004; **171**(6): 569–70.

Beaudoin C, Maheux B, Côté L, *et al.* Clinical teachers as humanistic caregivers and educators: percep-tions of senior clerks and second-year residents. *CMAJ.* 1998; **159**(7): 765–9.

Beckman HB, Frankel RM. The effect of physician behavior on the collection of data. *Ann Int Med.* 1984; **101**(5): 692–6.

Bellini LM, Shea JA. Mood change and empathy decline persist during three years of internal medicine training. *Acad Med.* 2005; **80**(2): 164–7.

Benjamin WW. Healing by the fundamentals. *N Engl J Med.* 1984; **311**(9): 595–7.

Bentham J, Burke J, Clark J, *et al.* Students conducting consultations in general practice and the accept-ability to patients. *Med Educ.* 1999; **33**(9): 686–7.

Berg KM, Hurley DJ, McSherry JA, *et al. Eating Disorders: A Patient-Centered Approach.* Oxford: Radcliffe Medical Press; 2002.

Berger AS. Arrogance among physicians. *Acad Med.* 2002; **77**(2): 145–7.

Berger J, Mohr J. *A Fortunate Man: The Story of a Country Doctor.* New York, NY: Pantheon Books; 1967.

Berkman LF, Syme SL. Social networks, host resistance, and mortality: a nine-year follow-up of Alameda County residents. *Am J Epidemiol.* 1979; **109**(2): 186–204.

Berman CW, Bezkor MF. Transference in patients and caregivers. *Am J Psychother.* 2010; **64**(1): 107–14.

Berzoff J, Flanagan LM, Hertz P. *Inside Out and Outside In: Psychodynamic Clinical Theory and Practice in Contemporary Multicultural Contexts.* Northvale, N.J.: Jason Aronson; 1996.

Betancourt J, Quinlan J. Personal responsibility versus responsible options: health care, community health promotion, and the battle against chronic disease. *Prev Chronic Dis.* 2007; **4**(3): A41

Bevis O, Watson J. *Towards a Caring Curriculum: A New Pedagogy for Nursing.* Sudbury, MA: Jones & Bartlett; 2000.

Billings ME, Lazarus ME, Wenrich M, *et al.* The effect of the hidden curriculum on resident burnout and cynicism. *J Grad Med Educ.* 2011; **3**(4): 503–10.

Bing-You RG, Trowbridge RL. Why medical educators may be failing at feedback. *JAMA.* 2009; **302**(112): 1330–1.

Blane D, Hart CL, Smith GD, *et al.* Association of cardiovascular disease risk factors with socioeconomic position during childhood and during adulthood. *BMJ.* 1997; **313**(7070): 1434–8.

Blane D, Mercer SW. Compassionate health care: is empathy the key? *J Holist Healthc.* 2011; **8**(3): 18–21.

Bleakley A. Broadening conceptions of learning in medical education: the message from teamworking. *Med Educ.* 2006; **40**(2): 150–7.

Bleakley A, Bligh J, Browne J. *Medical Education for the Future: Identity Power and Location.* New York, NY: Springer; 2011.

Blickem C, Priyadharshini E. Patient narratives: the potential for "patient-centred" interprofessional learning? *J Interprof Care.* 2007; **21**(6): 619–32.

Bodenheimer T, Lorig K, Holman H, *et al.* Patient self-management of chronic disease in primary care. *JAMA.* 2002; **288**(19): 2469–75.

Bombeke K, Symons L, Debaene L, *et al.* Help, I'm losing patient-centredness! Experiences of medical students and their teachers. *Med Educ.* 2010; **44**(7): 662–73.

Bond M. Empirical studies of defense style: relationships with psychopathology and change. *Harv Rev Psychiatry.* 2004; **12**(15): 263–78.

Boon H, Brown JB, Gavin A, *et al.* Breast cancer survivors' perceptions of complementary/alternative medicine (CAM): making the decision to use or not to use. *Qual Health Res.* 1999; **9**(5): 639–53.

Bosma H, Schrijvers C, Mackenbach JP. Socioeconomic inequalities in mortality and importance of perceived control: cohort study. *BMJ.* 1999; **319**(7223): 1469–70.

Boss P, Couden BA. Ambiguous loss from chronic physical illness: clinical interventions with individuals, couples, and families. *J Clin Psychol.* 2002; **58**(11): 1351–60.

Botelho R. *Beyond Advice: Becoming a Motivational Practitioner.* Rochester, NY: Motivative Healthy Habits Press; 2002.

Botha E. Why metaphors matter in education. *S Afr J Educ.* 2009; **29**: 431–44.

Boud A. Avoiding the traps: seeking good practice in the use of self-assessment and reflection in professional courses. *Soc Work Educ.* 1999; **18**(2): 121–32.

Boudreau JD, Cassell EJ, Fuks A. A healing curriculum. *Med Educ.* 2007; **41**(12): 1193–201.

Bowie P, Pope L, Lough M. A review of the current evidence base for significant event analysis. *J Eval Clin Pract.* 2008; **14**(4): 520–36.

Bowie P, Pringle M. *Significant Event Audit: Guidance for Primary Care Teams.* National Health Service for Scotland and the National Patient Safety Agency, 2008. Available at: www.nrls.npsa.nhs.uk/resources/?entryid45=61500 (accessed February 8, 2013).

Bowlby J. *Attachment and Loss: Vol. 1, Attachment.* 2nd ed. New York, NY: Basic Books; 1982.

Bowlby J. *Attachment and Loss: Vol. 2, Separation: Anxiety and Anger.* New York, NY: Basic Books; 1973.

Braddock CH, Edwards KA, Hasenberg NM, *et al.* Informed decision making in outpatient practice: time to get back to basics. *JAMA.* 1999; **282**(4): 2313–20.

Brancati FL. The art of pimping. *JAMA.* 1989; **262**(1): 89–90.

Bransford JD, Brown AL, Cocking RR. *How People Learn: Brain, Mind, Experience, and School.* Washington, DC: National Academy Press; 1999.

Braveman PA, Cubbin C, Egerter S, *et al.* Socioeconomic disparities in health in the United States: what the patterns tell us. *Am J Pub Health.* 2010; **100**(Suppl. 1): S186–96.

Brennan N, Corrigan O, Allard J, *et al.* The transition from medical student to junior doctor: today's experiences of Tomorrow's Doctors. *Med Educ.* 2010; **44**(5): 449–58.

Brennen TA, Leape LL, Laird NM *et al.* Incidence of adverse events and negligence in hospitalized patients: results of the Harvard Medical Practice Study I. *N Engl J Med.* 1991; **324**(6): 370–6.

Brent DA. The residency as a developmental process. *J Med Educ.* 1981; **56**(5): 417–22.

Brett J, Bankhead C, Henderson B, *et al.* The psychological impact of mammographic screening: a systematic review. *Psychooncology.* 2005; **14**(11): 917–38.

Brezis M, Israel S, Weinstein-Birenshtock A, *et al.* Quality of informed consent for invasive procedures. *Int J Qual Health Care.* 2008; **20**(5): 352–7.

Brindle P, Fahey T. Primary prevention of coronary heart disease. *BMJ.* 2002; **325**(7355): 56–7.

Britten N. Understanding medicine taking in context. In: Dowell J, Williams B, Snadden D (eds). *Patient-Centered Prescribing: Seeking Concordance in Practice.* Oxford: Radcliffe Publishing; 2007.

Britten N, Stevenson FA, Barry CA, *et al.* Misunderstandings in prescribing decisions in general practice: qualitative study. *BMJ.* 2000; **320**(7233): 484–8.

Broderick P, Blewitt P. *The Life Span: Human Development for Helping Professionals.* 3rd ed. Upper Saddle River, NJ: Merrill-Prentice Hall; 2010.

Brody H. "My story is broken; can you help me fix it?" Medical ethics and the joint construction of narrative. *Lit Med.* 1994; **13**(1): 79–92.

Brookfield S. *The Skillful Teacher: On Technique, Trust, and Responsiveness in the Classroom.* 2nd ed. San Francisco, CA: Jossey-Bass; 2006.

Brookfield SD, Preskill S. *Discussion as a Way of Teaching: Tools and Techniques for the Democratic Classroom.* 2nd ed. San Francisco, CA: Jossey-Bass; 2005.

Broom B. *Somatic Illness and the Patient's Other Story. A Practical Integrative Mind/Body Approach to Disease for Doctors and Psychotherapists.* New York: Free Association Books Ltd.; 1997.

Broom BC. Medicine and story: a novel clinical panorama arising from a unitary mind/body approach to physical illness. *Adv Mind Body Med.* 2000; **16**(3): 161–77.

Broom B. *Meaning-full Disease: How Personal Experience and Meanings Cause and Maintain Physical Illness.* London: Karnac; 2007.

Brown JB, Carroll J, Boon H, *et al.* Women's decision-making about their health care: views over the life cycle. *Patient Educ Couns.* 2002; **48**(3): 225–31

Brown JB, Handfield-Jones R, Rainsberry P, *et al.* The certification examination of the College of Family Physicians of Canada: IV. Simulated office orals. *Can Fam Physician.* 1996; **42**: 1539–48.

Brown JB, Harris SB, Webster-Bogaert S, *et al.* Point-of-care testing in diabetes management: what role does it play? *Diabetes Spectr.* 2004; **17**(4): 244–8.

Brown JB, Karley ML, Boudville N, *et al.* The experience of living kidney donors. *Health Soc Work.* 2008; **33**(2): 93–100.

Brown JB, Lewis L, Ellis K, *et al.* Mechanisms for communicating on primary health care teams. *Can Fam Physician.* 2009; **55**(12): 1216–22.

Brown JB, Lewis L, Ellis K, *et al.* Research report: sustaining primary health care teams: what is needed? *J Interprof Care.* 2010; **24**(4): 463–5.

Brown JB, Lewis L, Ellis K, *et al.* Conflict on interprofessional primary health care teams: can it be resolved? *J Interprof Care.* 2011; **25**(1): 4–10.

Brown JB, Sangster M, Swift J. Factors influencing palliative care. Qualitative study of family physicians' practices. *Canadian Family Physician.* 1998; **43**: 901–6.

Brown JB, Stewart M, Ryan B. *Assessing Communication between Patients and Physicians: The Measure of Patient-Centered Communication (MPCC).* Paper #95-2 (2e). Working Paper Series. London, ON: Centre for Studies in Family Medicine, The University of Western Ontario; 2001.

Brown JB, Stewart MA, McCracken EC, *et al.* Patient-centered clinical method II. Definition and application. *Fam Pract.* 1986; **3**(2): 75–9.

Brown JB, Stewart MA, Tessier S. *Assessing Communication between Patient and Doctors: A Manual for Scoring Patient-Centred Communication.* CSFM Working Paper Series #95-2. London, ON: Centre for Studies in Family Medicine, The University of Western Ontario; 1995.

Brown JB, Thornton T, Stewart M. *Challenges and Solutions: Narratives of Patient-Centered Care.* London: Radcliffe Publishing; 2012a.

Brown JB, Thorpe C, Paquette-Warren J, *et al.* The mentoring needs of trainees in family practice. *Educ Prim Care.* 2012b; **23**(3): 196–203.

Brown JB, Weston WW, Stewart MA. Patient-centered interviewing Part II: Finding common ground. *Can Fam Physician.* 1989; **35**: 153–7.

Broyard A. *Intoxicated By My Illness: And Other Writings on Life and Death.* New York, NY: Clarkson Potter Publishers; 1992.

Buddeberg-Fischer, Herta K-D. Formal mentoring programmes for medical students and doctors: a review of the Medline literature. *Med Teach.* 2006; **28**(3): 248–57.

Burke V, Giangiulio N, Gillam HF, *et al.* Health promotion in couples adapting to a shared lifestyle. *Health Educ Res.* 1999; **14**(2): 269–88.

Burtt EA. *The Metaphysical Foundations of Modern Science*, 2nd ed. Garden City, NY: Doubleday; 1954.

Byrne PS, Long BEL. *Doctors Talking To Patients.* London: Her Majesty's Stationery Office; 1984.

Cairney J. Socio-economic status and self-rated health among older Canadians. *Can J Aging.* 2000; **19**(4): 456–78.

Campbell C, Lockyer J, Laidlaw T, *et al.* Assessment of a matched-pair instrument to examine doctor-patient communication skills in practising doctors. *Med Educ.* 2007; **41**(2): 123–9.

Canadian Communication Working Group: *Canadian Communication Competency Framework.* Ottawa: Royal College of Physicians and Surgeons of Canada. 2013, In preparation. Personal communication.

Canadian Task Force on Preventive Health Care. *The Canadian Guide to Clinical Preventive Health Care.* Edmonton, AB: Canadian Task Force on Preventive Health Care, University of Alberta; 1994.

Candib LM. *Medicine and the Family: A Feminist Perspective.* New York, NY: Basic Books; 1995.

Candib L. Obesity and diabetes in vulnerable populations: reflection on proximal and distal causes. *Ann Fam Med.* 2007; **5**(6): 547–55.

Cannon WB. The case method of teaching systematic medicine. *Boston Med Surg J.* 1990; **142**: 31–6.

Cantillon P, Macdermott M. Does responsibility drive learning? Lessons from intern rotations in general practice. *Med Teach.* 2008; **30**(3): 254–9.

Cantillon P, Sargeant J. Giving feedback in clinical settings. *BMJ.* 2008; **337**: a1961.

Carel, H. *Illness: the Cry of the Flesh.* Stocksfield, UK: Acumen Publishing; 2008.

Carroll JC, Brown JB, Reid AJ, *et al.* Women's experience of maternal serum screening. *Can Fam Physician.* 2000; **46**: 614–20.

Carroll JG, Lipkin M Jr, Nachtigall L, *et al.* A developmental awareness for teaching doctor/patient communication skills. In: Lipkin M Jr, Putnam SM, Lazare A (eds). *The Medical Interview: Clinical Care, Education, and Research.* New York, NY: Springer; 1995.

Carter AH. Metaphors in the physician-patient relationship. *Soundings.* 1989; **72**(1): 153–64.

Cassell EJ. The nature of suffering and the goals of medicine. *N Engl J Med.* 1982; **306**(11): 639–45.

Cassell EJ. *Talking with Patients: II. Clinical Technique.* Cambridge, MA: MIT Press; 1985.

Cassell EJ. *The Nature of Suffering and the Goals of Medicine.* New York, NY: Oxford University Press; 1991.

Cassell EJ. *The Nature of Suffering and the Goals of Medicine.* 2nd ed. Oxford: Oxford University Press; 2004.

Cassell EJ. *The Nature of Healing: The Modern Practice of Medicine.* New York, NY: Oxford University Press; 2013.

Cavalcanti RB, Detsky AS. The education and training of future physicians: why coaches can't be judges. *JAMA.* 2011; **306**(9): 993–4.

Cavanaugh SH. Professional caring in the curriculum. In: Norman GR, van der Vleuten CPM, Newble DI (eds). *International Handbook of Research in Medical Education.* Dordrecht: Kluwer Academic Publishers; 2002.

Cegala DJ, Coleman MT, Turner JW. The development and partial assessment of the medical communication competence scale. *Health Commun.* 1998; **10**(3): 261–88.

Cegala DJ, Post DM. The impact of patients' participation on physicians' patient-centered communication. *Patient Educ Couns.* 2009; **77**(2): 202–8.

Chakraborti C, Boonyasai RT, Wright SM, *et al.* A systematic review of teamwork training interventions in medical student and resident education. *J Gen Intern Med.* 2008; **23**(6): 846–53.

Chambers D. *A Sociology of Family Life: Change and Diversity in Intimate Relations.* Cambridge: Polity Press; 2012.

Champion VL, Skinner CS. The health belief model. In: Glanz K, Rimer BK, Viswanath K (eds). *Health Behavior and Health Education: Theory, Research, and Practice.* 4th ed. San Francisco, CA: Jossey-Bass; 2008.

Charles C, Gafni A, Whelan T. Decision-making in the physician-patient encounter: revisiting the shared treatment decision-making model. *Soc Sci Med.* 1999; **49**(5): 651–61.

Charon R. To render the lives of patients. *Lit Med.* 1986; **5**: 58–74.

Charon R. Doctor-patient/reader-writer: learning to find the text. *Soundings.* 1989; **72**(1): 137–52.

Charon R. The patient-physician relationship. Narrative medicine: a model for empathy, reflection, profession, and trust. *JAMA.* 2001; **286**(15): 1897–1902.

Charon R. Narrative and medicine. *N Engl J Med.* 2004; **350**(9): 862–4.

Charon R. *Narrative Medicine: Honoring the Stories of Illness.* New York, NY: Oxford University Press; 2006.

Charon R. What to do with stories: the sciences of narrative medicine. *Can Fam Physician.* 2007; **53**(8): 1265–7.

Charon R, Montello M (eds). *Stories Matter: The Role of Narrative in Medical Ethics.* New York, NY: Routledge; 2002.

Cheren M. Helping learners achieve greater self-direction. In: Smith RM (ed). *Helping Adults Learn How to Learn.* San Francisco, CA: Jossey-Bass; 1983.

Cherry JD. The epidemiology of pertussis and pertussis immunization in the United Kingdom and the United States: a comparative study. *Curr Probl Pediatr.* 1984; **14**(2): 1–78.

Chew-Graham CA, Rogers A, Yassin N. 'I wouldn't want it on my CV or their records': medical students' experiences of help-seeking for mental health problems. *Med Educ.* 2003; **37**(10): 873–80.

Chi RC, Neuzil KM. The association of sociodemographic factors and patient attitudes on influenza vaccination in older persons. *American Journal of Medical Sciences.* 2004; **327**(3): 113–17.

Chin JJ. Doctor-patient relationship: from medical paternalism to enhanced autonomy. *Singapore Med J.* 2002; **43**(3): 152–5.

Chipp E, Stoneley S, Cooper K. Clinical placements for medical students: factors affecting patients' involvement in medical education. *Med Teach.* 2004; **26**(2): 114–19.

Churchill LR, Schenck D. Healing skills for medical practice. *Ann Intern Med.* 2008; **149**(10): 720–24.

Claridge M-T, Lewis T. *Coaching for Effective Learning: A Practical Guide for Teachers in Health and Social Care.* Oxford: Radcliffe Publishing; 2005.

Clark MC, Rossiter M. Narrative learning in adulthood. *New Dir Adult Cont Learn.* 2008; **2008**(119): 61–70.

Clarke LE, Nisker J. *In Our Hands: On Becoming a Doctor.* Lawrencetown Beach, NS: Pottersfield Press; 2007.

Clayton MF, Dudley WN, Musters A. Communication with breast cancer survivors. *Health Commun.* 2008; **23**(3): 207–21.

Clayton MF, Dudley WN. Patient-centered communication during oncology follow-up visits for breast cancer survivors: content and temporal structure. *Oncol Nurs Forum.* 2009; **36**(2): E68–79.

Cohen SJ. An educational psychologist goes to medical school. In: Eisner EW (ed). *The Educational Imagination: On the Design and Evaluation of School Programs.* 2nd ed. New York, NY: Macmillan; 1985.

Cole SA, Bird J. *The Medical Interview: The Three-Function Approach.* 3rd ed. Philadelphia, PA: Mosby; 2009.

Collins JL, Giles HW, Holmes-Chavez A. Old dilemmas, new commitments: toward a 21st century strategy for community health promotion. *Prev Chronic Dis.* 2007; **4**(3): A42.

Collins RE, Lopez LM, Marteau TM. Emotional impact of screening: a systematic review and meta-analysis. *BMC Public Health.* 2011; **11**: 603.

Cooke M, Irby DM, O'Brien BC. *Educating Physicians: A Call for Reform of Medical School and Residency.* San Francisco, CA: Jossey-Bass; 2010.

Coombs RH. *Surviving Medical School.* Thousand Oaks, CA: Sage Publications; 1998.

Coombs RH, May DS, Small GW (eds). *Inside Doctoring: Stages and Outcomes in the Professional Development of Physicians.* New York, NY: Praeger; 1986.

Cooper AF. Whose illness is it anyway? Why patient perceptions matter. *Int J Clin Pract.* 1998; **52**(8): 551–6.

Corbin J. Introduction and overview: chronic illness and nursing. In: Hyman R, Corbin J (eds). *Chronic Illness: Research and Theory for Nursing Practice.* New York, NY: Springer; 2001.

Corbin J, Strauss A. A nursing model for chronic illness management based upon the trajectory framework. In: Woog P (ed). *The Chronic Illness Trajectory Framework: The Corbin and Strauss Nursing Model.* New York, NY: Springer; 1992.

Corin E. The social and cultural matrix of health and disease. In: De Gruyter A (ed). *Why Are Some People Healthy and Others Not? The Determinants of Health of Populations.* New York, NY: Hawthorne; 1994.

Cortese L, Malla AK, McLean T, *et al.* Exploring the longitudinal course of psychotic illness: a case study approach. *Can J Psychiatr.* 1999; **44**(9): 881–6.

Coulehan J. You say self-interest, I say altruism. In: Wear D, Aultman JM (eds). *Professionalism in Medicine: Critical Perspectives.* New York, NY: Springer; 2006.

Coulehan J, Williams PC. Vanquishing virtue: the impact of medical education. *Acad Med.* 2001; **76**(6): 598–605.

Coulter A. *The Autonomous Patient: Ending Paternalism in Medical Care.* London: Nuffield Trust; 2002.

Coulter A. What's happening around the world? In: Edwards A, Elwyn G (eds). *Shared Decision-Making in Health Care: Achieving Evidence-Based Patient Choice.* Oxford: Oxford University Press; 2009.

Coulter A, Ellins J. Effectiveness of strategies for informing, educating and involving patients. *BMJ.* 2007; **335**(7609): 24–7.

Cousins N. *Anatomy of an Illness as Perceived by the Patient.* New York, NY: Norton; 1979.

Craigie FC Jr, Hobbs RF 3rd. Spiritual perspectives and practices of family physicians with an expressed interest in spirituality. *Fam Med.* 1999; **31**(8): 578–85.

Craigie FC Jr, Hobbs RF 3rd. Exploring the organizational culture of exemplary community health centre practices. *Fam Med.* 2004; **36**(10): 733–8.

Cramer P. Defense mechanisms in psychology today: further processes for adaptation. *Am Psychol.* 2000; **55**(6): 637–46.

Cramer P. *Protecting the Self: Defense Mechanisms in Action.* New York, NY: Guilford Press; 2006.

Cranton P. *Understanding and Promoting Transformative Learning: A Guide for Educators of Adults.* 2nd ed. San Francisco, CA: Jossey-Bass; 2006.

Crookshank FG. The theory of diagnosis. *Lancet.* 1926; **2**: 934–42, 995–9.

Cruess RL, Cruess SR, Steinert Y (eds). *Teaching Medical Professionalism.* Cambridge: Cambridge University Press; 2009.

Cruess SR, Cruess RL, Steinert Y. Role modelling making the most of a powerful teaching strategy. *BMJ.* 2008; **336**(7646): 718–21.

Crutcher RA, Szafran O, Woloschuk W, *et al.* Family medicine graduates' perceptions of intimidation, harassment, and discrimination during residency training. *BMC Med Educ.* 2011; **11**: 88.

Culhane-Pera KA, Rothenberg D. The larger context: culture, community, and beyond. In: Shields SG, Candib LM (eds). *Woman-Centered Care in Pregnancy and Childbirth.* Oxford: Radcliffe Publishing; 2010.

Curlin FA, Hall DE. Strangers or friends? A proposal for a new spirituality-in-medicine ethic. *J Gen Intern Med.* 2005; **20**(4): 370–4.

Curry L. Individual differences in cognitive style, learning style and instructional preference in medical education. In: Norman GR, van der Vleuten CPM, Newbie DI (eds). *Handbook of Research in Medical Education.* Dordrecht: Kluwer Academic; 2002.

Cushing H. *The Life of Sir William Osler.* Oxford: Clarendon Press; 1925.

Dahan R, Borkan J, Brown JB, *et al.* The challenge of using the low back pain guidelines: a qualitative research. *J Eval Clin Pract.* 2007; **13**(4): 616–20.

Dakubo CY. *Ecosystems and Human Health: A Critical Approach to Ecohealth Research and Practice.* New York, NY: Springer Science+Business Media; 2010.

Dall'Alba G. *Learning to be Professionals.* New York, NY: Springer; 2009.

Daloz LA. *Mentor: Guiding the Journey of Adult Learners.* 2nd ed. San Francisco, CA: Jossey-Bass; 2012.

Daniels N, Kennedy B, Kawachi I. *Is Inequality Bad for Our Health?* Boston, MA: Beacon Press; 2000.

Davidson JE, Jones C, Bienvenu OJ. Family response to critical illness: postintensive care syndrome-family. *Crit Care Med.* 2012; **40**(2): 618–24.

Davis DA, Mazmanian PE, Fordis M, *et al.* Accuracy of physician self-assessment compared with observed measures of competence: a systematic review. *JAMA.* 2006; **296**(9): 1094–102.

Day SC, Grosso LG, Norcini JJ, *et al.* Residents' perception of evaluation procedures used by their training program. *J Gen Intern Med.* 1990; **5**(5): 421–6.

De Bourdeaudhuij I, Van Oost P. Family members' influence on decision making about food: differences in perception and relationship with healthy eating. *Am J Health Promot.* 1998; **13**(2): 73–81.

De Leeuw E. Concepts in health promotion: the notion of relativism. *Soc Sci Med.* 1989; **29**(11): 1281–8.

Denomme LB, Terry AL, Brown JB, *et al.* Primary health care teams' experience of electronic medical record use after adoption. *Fam Med.* 2011; **43**(9): 638–42.

Derose KP, Escarce JJ, Lurie N. Immigrants and health care: sources of vulnerability. *Health Aff (Millwood).* 2007; **26**(5): 1258–68.

Desjardins N, Gritke J, Hill B. Trans-cultural issues in person-centered care for people with serious mental illness. In: Rudnick A, Roe D (eds). *Serious Mental Illness Person-Centered Approaches.* London: Radcliffe Publishing; 2011.

Detsky AS. The art of pimping. *JAMA*. 2009; **301**(13): 1379–81.

Deveugele M, Derese A, De Maesschalck S, *et al.* Teaching communication skills to medical students, a challenge in the curriculum? *Patient Educ Couns.* 2005; **58**(3): 265–70.

Disclosure Working Group. *Canadian Disclosure Guidelines: Being Open and Honest with Patients and Families.* Edmonton, AB: Canadian Patient Safety Institute; 2011.

Doherty WJ, Baird MA. *Family-Centered Medical Care: A Clinical Casebook.* New York, NY: Guildford Press; 1987.

Doherty WJ, McDaniel SH. *Family Therapy.* Washington, DC: American Psychological Association; 2010.

Dombeck MB, Evinger JS. Spiritual care: the partnership covenant. In: Suchman AL, Botelho RJ, Hinton-Walker P (eds). *Partnerships in Healthcare: Transforming Relational Process.* Rochester, NY: University of Rochester Press; 1998.

Donnelly WJ. Medical language as symptom: doctor talk in teaching hospitals. *Perspect Biol Med.* 1986; **30**(1): 81–94.

Donnelly WJ. Righting the medical record: transforming chronicle into story. *Soundings.* 1989; **72**(1): 127–36.

Dowell J, Jones A, Snadden D. Exploring medication use to seek concordance with 'non-adherent' patients: a qualitative study. *Br J Gen Pract.* 2002; **52**(474): 24–32.

Dowell J, Williams B, Snadden D. *Patient-Centered Care Series, Patient-Centered Prescribing: Seeking Concordance in Practice.* Oxford: Radcliffe Publishing; 2007.

Downing R. *Biohealth: Beyond Medicalization: Imposing Health.* Eugene, OR: Pickwick Publications; 2011.

Doxiadis S (ed). *Ethical Dilemmas in Health Promotion.* New York, NY: John Wiley &VA Sons; 1987.

Doyle T. *Learner-Centered Teaching: Putting the Research on Learning into Practice.* Sterling, VA: Stylus Publishing; 2011.

Drewnowski A, Specter SE. Poverty and obesity: the role of energy density and energy costs. *Am J Clin Nutr.* 2004; **79**(1): 6–16.

Dubos R. *Man Adapting.* New Haven, CT: Yale University Press; 1980.

Duffy FD, Holmboe ES. Self-assessment in lifelong learning and improving performance in practice: physician know thyself. *JAMA.* 2006; **296**(9): 1137–9.

Dunning D, Heath C, Suls JM. Flawed self-assessment: implications for health, education, and the workplace. *Psychol Sci Public Interest.* 2004; **5**(3): 69–106.

Dunning D, Johnson K, Ehrlinger J, *et al.* Why people fail to recognize their own incompetence. *Curr Dir Psychol Sci.* 2003; **12**: 83–6.

Dwamena F, Holmes-Rovner M, Gaulden CM, *et al.* Interventions for providers to promote a patient-centred approach in clinical consultations. *Cochrane Database Syst Rev.* 2012; (12): CD003267.

Dyrbye LN, Massie FS Jr, Eacker A, *et al.* Relationship between burnout and professional conduct and attitudes among US medical students. *JAMA.* 2010; **304**(11): 1173–80.

Edwards A. Risk communication: making evidence part of patient choice. In: Edwards A, Elwyn G (eds). *Shared Decision-Making in Health Care: Achieving Evidence-Based Patient Choice.* Oxford: Oxford University Press; 2009.

Edwards A, Elwyn G. *Shared Decision-Making in Health Care: Achieving Evidence-Based Patient Choice.* Oxford: Oxford University Press; 2009.

Egan M, Tannahill C, Petticrew M, *et al.* Psychosocial risk factors in home and community settings and their associations with population health and health inequalities: a systematic meta-review. *BMC Public Health.* 2008; **8**: 239.

Egnew TR. The meaning of healing: transcending suffering. *Ann Fam Med.* 2005; **3**(3): 255–62.

Egnew TR. Suffering, meaning and healing: challenges of contemporary medicine. *Ann Fam Med.* 2009; **7**(2): 170–5.

Egnew TR, Wilson HF. Role modeling the doctor-patient relationship in the clinical curriculum. *Fam Med.* 2011; **43**(2): 99–105.

Eichna L. Medical-school education, 1975–1979: a student's perspective. *N Engl J Med.* 1980; **303**(13): 727–34.

Eisner EW. *The Educational Imagination: On the Design and Evaluation of School Programs (2e).* New York: Macmillan; 1985.

Ellingson LL. Interdisciplinary health care teamwork in the clinic backstage. *J Appl Commun Res.* 2003; **31**(2): 93–117.

Elwyn G, Charles C. Shared decision making: the principles and the competences. In: Edwards GEA (ed). *Evidence-Based Patient Choice: Inevitable or Impossible?* New York, NY: Oxford University Press; 2001.

Elwyn G, Edwards A, Gwyn R, *et al.* Towards a feasible model for shared decision making: focus group study with general practiced registrars. *BMJ.* 1999; **319**(7212): 753–6.

Elwyn G, Edwards A, Kinnersley P, *et al.* Shared decision making and the concept of equipoise: the competences of involving patients in healthcare choices. *Br J Gen Pract.* 2000; **50**(460): 892–7.

Elwyn G, Edwards A, Mowle S, *et al.* Measuring the involvement of patients in shared decision-making: a systematic review of instruments. *Patient Educ Couns.* 2001; **43**(1): 5–22.

Elwyn G, Frosch D, Thomson R, *et al.* Shared decision making: a model for clinical practice. *J Gen Intern Med.* 2012; **27**(10): 1361–7.

Engel GL. The need for a new medical model: a challenge for biomedicine. *Science.* 1977; **196**(4286): 129–36.

Engel GL. The clinical application of the biopsychosocial model. *Am J Psychiatry.* 1980; **137**(5): 535–44.

Entralgo PL. *Mind and Body.* New York, NY: PJ Kennedy; 1956.

Entralgo PL. *The Therapy of the Word in Classical Antiquity.* New Haven, CT: Yale University Press; 1961.

Epp J. *Achieving Health for All: A Framework for Health Promotion.* Ottawa, ON: Health and Welfare Canada; 1986.

Epstein PR. Emerging diseases and ecosystem instability: new threats to public health. *Am J Public Health.* 1995; **85**(2): 168–72.

Epstein RM. Mindful practice. *JAMA.* 1999; **282**(9): 833–9.

Epstein RM. Whole mind and shared mind in clinical decision-making. *Patient Educ Couns.* 2013; **90**(2): 200–6.

Epstein RM, Campbell TL, Cohen-Cole SA, *et al.* Perspectives on patient-doctor communication. *J Fam Pract.* 1993; **37**(4): 377–88.

Epstein RM, Franks P, Fiscella K, *et al.* Measuring patient-centered communication in patient-physician consultations: theoretical and practical issues. *Soc Sci Med.* 2005a; **61**(7): 1516–28.

Epstein RM, Franks P, Shields CG, *et al.* Patient-centered communication and diagnostic testing. *Ann Fam Med.* 2005b; **3**(5): 415–21.

Epstein RM, Shields CG, Meldrum SC, *et al.* Physicians' responses to patients' medically unexplained symptoms. *Psychosom Med.* 2006; **68**(2): 269–76.

Epstein RM, Siegel DJ, Silberman J. Self-monitoring in clinical practice: a challenge for medical educators. *J Contin Educ Health Prof.* 2008; **28**(1): 5–13.

Erikson EH. *Childhood and Society.* New York: Norton; 1950.

Erikson EH. *The Life Cycle Completed: a review.* New York: Norton; 1982.

Ericsson KA. Deliberate practice and acquisition of expert performance: a general overview. *Acad Emerg Med.* 2008; **15**(11): 988–94.

Ericsson KA, Krampe RT, Tesch-Romer C. The role of deliberate practice in the acquisition of expert performance. *Psychol Rev.* 1993; **100**(3): 363–406.

Eva KW, Cunnington JPW, Reiter HI, *et al.* How can I know what I don't know? Poor self-assessment in a well-defined domain. *Adv Health Sci Educ Theory Pract.* 2004; **9**(3): 211–24.

Eva KW, Regehr G. "I'll never play professional football" and other fallacies of self-assessment. *J Contin Educ Health Prof.* 2008; **28**(1): 14–19.

Eva KW, Regehr G, Gruppen LD. Blinded by "insight": self-assessment and its role in performance improvement. In: Hodges BD, Lingard L (eds). *The Question of Competence: Reconsidering Medical Education in the Twenty-First Century.* Ithaca, NY: Cornell University Press; 2012.

Evans JM, Newton RW, Ruta DA, *et al.* Socio-economic status, obesity and prevalence of type 1 and type 2 diabetes mellitus. *Diabet Med.* 2000; **17**(6): 478–80.

Evans RG, Edwards A, Evans S, *et al.* Assessing the practicing physician using patient surveys: a systematic review of instruments and feedback methods. *Fam Pract.* 2007; **24**(2): 117–27.

Faber K. *Nosography in Modern Internal Medicine.* Martin J, trans. New York, NY: Paul B Hoeber; 1923.

Falvo D. *Effective Patient Education: A Guide to Increased Adherence.* 4th ed. Mississauga, ON: Jones & Bartlett; 2011.

Farnan JM, Johnson JK, Meltzer DO, *et al.* Strategies for effective on-call supervision for internal medicine residents: the superb/safety model. *J Grad Med Educ.* 2010; **2**(1): 46–52.

Farrell K, Wicks MN, Martin JC. Chronic disease self-management improved with enhanced self-efficacy. *Clin Nurs Res.* 2004; **13**(4): 289–308.

Fava GA, Sonino N. The biopsychosocial model thirty years later. *Psychother Psychosom.* 2008; **77**(1): 1–2.

Feinstein AR. *Clinical Judgement.* Baltimore, MD: Williams & Wilkins; 1967.

Feinstein JS. The relationship between socioecomonic status and health: a review of the literature. *Milbank Q.* 1993; **71**(2): 279–322.

Feldman RH, Damron D, Anliker J, *et al.* The effect of the Maryland WIC 5-A-Day promotion program on participants' stages of change for fruit and vegetable consumption. *Health Educ Behav.* 2000; **27**(5): 649–63.

Ferenchick G, Simpson D, Blackman J, *et al.* Strategies for efficient and effective teaching in the ambulatory care setting. *Acad Med.* 1997; **72**(4): 277–80.

Festinger L. A theory of cognitive dissonance. 1957. Quoted in: Daloz LA. *Mentor: Guiding the Journey of Adult Learners.* 2nd ed. San Francisco, CA: Jossey-Bass; 1999.

Fiscella K, Franks P, Srinivasan M, *et al.* Ratings of physician communication by real and standardized patients. *Ann Fam Med.* 2007; **5**(2): 151–8.

Flach SD, McCoy KD, Vaughn TE, *et al.* Does patient-centered care improve provision of preventive services? *J Gen Intern Med.* 2004; **19**(10): 1019–26.

Flachmann M. Teaching in the twenty-first century. *Teaching Professor.* 1994; **8**(3): 1–2.

Fleck L. *The Genesis and Development of a Scientific Fact.* Chicago, IL: University Chicago of Press; 1979.

Flexner A. *Medical Education in the United States and Canada. Bulletin No. 4.* New York, NY: Carnegie Foundation for the Advancement of Teaching; 1910.

Flexner A. *The American College: A Criticism.* New York, NY: Century, 1908. Reprinted by Arno Press and the New York Times; 1969.

Flocke SA. Measuring attributes of primary care: development of a new instrument. *J Fam Pract.* 1997; **45**(1): 64–74.

Floyd MR, Seale JP (eds). *Substance Abuse: A Patient-Centered Approach.* Oxford: Radcliffe Medical Press; 2002.

Fogarty CT, Schultz S. Team huddles: the role of the primary care educator. *Clin Teach.* 2010; **7**(3): 157–60.

Fong J, Longnecker N. Doctor-patient communication: a review. *Ochsner J.* 2010; **10**: 38–43.

Ford S, Schofield T, Hope T. Are patients' decision-making preferences being met? *Health Expect.* 2003; **6**(1): 72–80.

Ford-Gilboe M. Family strengths, motivation, and resources as predictors of health promotion behavior in single-parent and two-parent families. *Res Nurs Health.* 1997; **20**(3): 205–17.

Forsythe GB. Identity development in professional education. *Acad Med.* 2005; **80**(10): S112–17.

Foss L. *The End of Modern Medicine: Biomedical Science Under a Microscope.* Albany: State University of New York; 2002.

Fossum B, Arborelius E. Patient-centred communication: videotaped consultations. *Patient Educ Couns.* 2004; **54**(2): 163–9.

Foster CR, Dahill LE, Golemon LA, *et al. Educating Clergy: Teaching Practices and Pastoral Imagination.* San Francisco, CA: Jossey-Bass; 2006.

Foster K. Becoming a professional doctor. In: Scanlon L (ed). *"Becoming" a Professional: An Interdisciplinary Analysis of Professional Learning.* New York, NY: Springer; 2011.

Fowler JW. *Stages of Faith: The Psychology of Human Development and the Quest for Meaning.* San Francisco, CA: Harper & Row; 1981.

Fraiberg S, Adelson E, Shapiro V. Ghosts in the nursery: a psychoanalytic approach to the problems of impaired infant-mother relationships. *J Am Acad Child Psychiatry.* 1975; **14**(3): 387–421.

Frank A. *At the Will of the Body: Reflections on Illness.* Boston, MA: Houghton, Mifflin; 1991.

Frank AW. *The Wounded Storyteller: Body, Illness, and Ethics.* Chicago, IL: University of Chicago Press; 1995.

Frank AW. *The Renewal of Generosity: Illness, Medicine and How to Live.* Chicago, IL: University of Chicago Press; 2004.

Frank AW. Reflective healthcare practice: claims, phonesis and dialogue. In: Kinsella EA, Pitman A (eds). *Phronesis as Professional Knowledge: Practical Wisdom in the Professions.* Rotterdam: Sense Publishers; 2012.

Frank E, Carrera JS, Stratton T, *et al.* Experiences of belittlement and harassment and their correlates among medical students in the United States: longitudinal survey. *BMJ.* 2006; **333**(7570): 682.

Frank E, Elon L, Naimi T, *et al.* Alcohol consumption and alcohol counselling behaviour among US medical students: a cohort study. *BMJ.* 2008; **337**: a2155.

Frankel RM. Cracking the code: theory and method in clinical communication analysis. *Health Commun.* 2001; **13**(1): 101–10.

Frankel RM, Quill TE, McDaniel SH. *The Biopsychosocial Approach: Past, Present, Future.* Rochester: University of Rochester Press; 2003.

Freeman GK. Progress with relationship continuity 2012, a British perspective. *Int J Integr Care.* 2012; **12**(29): 1–6.

Freeman R. *Mentoring in General Practice.* Oxford: Butterworth–Heinemann; 1998.

Freeth D. Sustaining interprofessional collaboration. *J Interprof Care.* 2001; **15**(1): 37–46.

Fried JM, Vermillion M, Parker NH, *et al.* Eradicating medical student mistreatment: a longitudinal study of one institution's efforts. *Acad Med.* 2012; **87**(9): 1191–8.

Friedman M, Prywes M, Benbassat J. Hypothesis: Cognitive development of medical students is relevant for medical education. *Med Teach.* 1987; **9**(1): 91–6.

Friere P. *Pedagogy of the Oppressed.* 30th anniversary ed. New York, NY: Continuum; 2006.

Frostholm L, Fink P, Christensen KS, *et al.* The patients' illness perceptions and the use of primary health care. *Psychosom Med.* 2005; **67**(6): 997–1005.

Fugelli P. Trust in general practice. *Br J Gen Pract.* 2001; **51**(468): 575–9.

Furney SL, Orsini AN, Orsetti KE, *et al.* Teaching the One-Minute Preceptor: a randomized controlled trial. *J Gen Intern Med.* 2001; **16**(9): 620–4.

Gaissmaier W, Gigerenzer G. Statistical illiteracy undermines informed shared decision making. *Zeitschrift für Evidenz, Fortbildung und Qualität im Gesundheitswesen.* 2008; **102**(7): 411–13.

Galassi JP, Ware W, Schanberg R. The Patient Reactions Assessment: a brief measure of the quality of the patient-provider medical relationship. *Psychol Assess.* 1992; **4**(3): 346–51.

Galazka SS, Eckert JK. Clinically applied anthropology: concept for the family physician. *J Fam Pract.* 1986; **22**(2): 159–65.

Galbraith MW (ed). *Adult Learning Methods: A Guide for Effective Instruction.* 3rd ed. Malabar, FL: Krieger Publishing; 2004.

Gamble J. Modelling the invisible: the pedagogy of craft apprenticeship. *Stud Cont Educ.* 2001; **23**(2): 185–200.

Garrett L. *The Coming Plague: Newly Emerging Diseases in a World Out Of Balance.* New York, NY: Penguin Books; 1994.

Gawande A. *The Checklist Manifesto.* London: Profile Books; 2010.

Gerhardt U. Qualitative research on chronic illness: the issue and the story. *Soc Sci Med.* 1990; **30**(11): 1149–59.

Gieger JH. Community oriented primary care: the legacy of Sidney Kark. *Am J Public Health.* 1993; **83**(7): 946–7.

Gill VT, Maynard DW. Explaining illness; patients' proposals and physicians' responses. In: Heritage J,

Maynard DW (eds). *Communication in Medical Care: Interactions Between Primary Care Physicians and Patients.* Cambridge: Cambridge University Press; 2006.

Gilligan C. *In a Different Voice: psychological theory and women's development.* Cambridge, MA: Harvard University Press; 1982.

Gilligan C, Pollack S. The vulnerable and invulnerable physician. In: Gilligan C, Ward JV, Taylor JM (eds). *Mapping the Moral Domain: A Contribution of Women's Thinking to Psychological Theory and Education.* Cambridge, MA: Harvard University Press; 1988.

Gillis AJ. Determinants of a health-promoting lifestyle: an integrative review. *J Adv Nurs.* 1993; **18**(3): 345–53.

Gilman S. *Disease and Representation: Images of Illness from Madness to AIDS.* Ithaca, NY: Cornell University Press; 1988.

Glaser B, Strauss A. *Time for Dying.* Chicago, IL: Aldine; 1968.

Glass TA, de Leon CM, Marottoli RA, *et al.* Population base study of social and productive activities as predictors of survival among elderly Americans. *BMJ.* 1999; **319**(7208): 478–83.

Glasser M, Pelto GH. *The Medical Merry-Go-Round: A Plea for Reasonable Medicine.* Pleasantville, NY: Redgrave Publishing; 1980.

Godolphin W, Towle A, McKendry R. Challenges in family practice related to informed and shared decision-making: a survey of preceptors of medical students. *JAMA.* 2001; **165**(4): 434–5.

Godolphin W. Shared decision-making. *Healthcare Q.* 2009; **12**: e186–90.

Goldberg PE. The physician-patient relationship: three psychodynamic concepts that can be applied to primary care. *Arch Fam Med.* 2000; **9**(10): 116–48.

Goldstein K. *The Organism.* New York, NY: Zone Books; 1995.

Golin CE, DiMatteo MR, Gelberg L. The role of patient participation in the doctor visit. implications for adherence to diabetes care. *Diabetes Care.* 1996; **19**(10): 1153–64.

Good BJ, Good M. Meaning of symptoms: a cultural-hermeneutic model for clinical practice. In: Eisenberg L, Kleinman A (eds). *Relevance of Social Science for Medicine.* Boston, MA: D Reidel; 1981.

Goodyear-Smith F, Buetow S. Power issues in the doctor-patient relationship. *Health Care Anal.* 2001; **9**(4): 449–62.

Gordon J. Fostering students' personal and professional development in medicine: a new framework for PPD. *Med Educ.* 2003; **37**(4): 341–9.

Gordon MJ. A review of the validity and accuracy of self-assessments in health professions training. *Acad Med.* 1991; **66**(12): 762–9.

Gordon T, Edwards WS. *Making the Patient Your Partner: Communication Skills for Doctors and Other Caregivers.* New York, NY: Auburn House; 1997.

Gorman E. Chronic degenerative conditions, disability and loss. In: Harris DL (ed). *Counting Our Losses: Reflecting on Change, Loss and Transition in Everyday Life.* New York, NY: Routledge; 2011.

Graham H, Power C. Childhood disadvantage and health inequalities: a framework for policy based on lifecourse. *Child Care Health Dev.* 2007; **30**(6): 671–8.

Grant J. Learning needs assessment: assessing the need. *BMJ.* 2002; **324**(7330): 156–9.

Greco M, Brownlea A, McGovern J. Impact of patient feedback on the interpersonal skills of general practice registrars: results of a longitudinal study. *Med Educ.* 2001; **35**(8): 748–56.

Green AR, Carrillo JE, Betancourt JR. Why the disease-based model of medicine fails our patients. *West J Med.* 2002; **176**(2): 141–3.

Green EH, Durning AJ, DeCherrie L, *et al.* Expectations for oral case presentations for clinical clerks: opinions of internal medicine clerkship directors. *Journal of General Internal Medicine.* 2009; **24**(3): 370–3.

Green EH, DeCherrie L, Fagan MJ, *et al.* The oral case presentation: what internal medicine clinician-teachers expect from clinical clerks. 2011; **23**(1): 58–61.

Green LA, Fryer GE Jr, Yawn BP, *et al.* The ecology of medical care revisited. *N Engl J Med.* 2001; **344**(26): 2021–5.

Greenberg CC, Regenbogen SE, Studdert DM, *et al.* Patterns of communication breakdowns resulting in injury to surgical patients. *J Am Coll Surg.* 2007; **204**(4): 533–40.

Greenfield S, Kaplan SH, Ware JE Jr, *et al.* Patients' participation in medical care: effects on blood sugar control and quality of life in diabetes. *J Gen Intern Med.* 1988; **3**(5): 448–57.

Greenhalgh T, Hurwitz B. *Narrative Based Medicine: Dialogue and Discourse in Clinical Practice.* London: BMJ Books; 1998.

Greenhalgh T. Narrative based medicine: narrative base medicine in an evidence based world. *BMJ.* 1999; **318**(7179): 323–5.

Greenhalgh T. *What Seems to be the Trouble? Stories in Illness and Healthcare.* Oxford: Radcliffe Publishing; 2006.

Greveson GC, Spencer JA. Self-directed learning: the importance of concepts and contexts. *Med Educ.* 2005; **39**(4): 348–9.

Griffin SJ, Kinmonth AL, Veltman MWM, *et al.* Effect on health-related outcomes of interventions to alter the interaction between patients and practitioners: a systematic review of trials. *Ann Fam Med.* 2004; **2**(6): 595–608.

Groopman J. God at the bedside. *N Engl J Med.* 2004; **350**(12): 1176–8.

Grow G. Teaching learners to be self-directed. *Adult Educ Q.* 1991; **41**: 125–49.

Grunfeld E, Whelan TJ, Zitzelsberger L, *et al.* Cancer care workers in Ontario: prevalence of burnout, job stress and job satisfaction. *CMAJ.* 2000; **163**(7): 166–9.

Guest A. *Taking Sides: Clashing Views on Lifespan Development.* Dubuque, IA: McGraw-Hill; 2007.

Gupta RP, de Wit ML, Margaret L, *et al.* The impact of poverty on the current and future health status of children. *Paediatr Child Health.* 2007; **12**(8): 667–72.

Gutkind L (ed). *Becoming a Doctor: From Student to Specialist, Doctor-Writers Share Their Experiences.* New York, NY: WW Norton; 2010.

Guttman N, Salmon CT. Guilt, fear, stigma and knowledge gaps: ethical issues in public health communication interventions. *Bioethics.* 2004; **18**(6): 531–2.

Guy K. *Our Promise to Children.* Ottawa, ON: Canadian Institute of Child Health; 1997.

Haber RJ, Lingard La. Learning oral presentation skills: A rhetorical analysis with pedagogical and professional implications. *Journal of General Internal Medicine.* 2001; **16**(5): 308–14.

Hadas R. *Strange Relation-A Memoire of Marriage, Dementia and Poetry.* Philadelphia, PA: Paul Dry Books; 2011.

Haddad S, Potvin L, Roberge D, *et al.* Patient perception of quality following a visit to a doctor in a primary care unit. *Fam Pract.* 2000; **17**(1): 21–9.

Hadler NM. *Worried Sick: A Prescription for Health in an Overtreated America.* Chapel Hill: University of North Carolina Press; 2008.

Hafferty FW. Beyond curriculum reform: confronting medicine's hidden curriculum. *Acad Med.* 1998; **73**(4): 403–7.

Hafferty FW. Professionalism and the socialization of medical students. In: Cruess RL, Cruess SR, Steinert Y (eds). *Teaching Medical Professionalism.* Cambridge: Cambridge University Press; 2009.

Hafferty FW, Levinson D. Moving beyond nostalgia and motives: towards a complexity science view of medical professionalism. *Perspect Biol Med.* 2008; **51**(4): 599–615.

Haidet P. Patient-centredness and its challenge of prevailing professional norms. *Med Educ.* 2010; **44**(7): 643–4.

Haidet P, Kroll TL, Sharf BF. The complexity of patient participation: lessons learned from patients' illness narratives. *Patient Educ Couns.* 2006; **62**(3): 323–9.

Haidet P, Morgan RO, O'Malley K, *et al.* A controlled trial of active versus passive learning strategies in a large group setting. *Adv Health Sci Educ Theory Pract.* 2004; **9**(1): 15–27.

Hajek P, Najberg E, Cushing A. Medical students' concerns about communicating with patients. *Med Educ.* 2000; **34**(8): 656–8.

Hall P. Interprofessional teamwork: professional cultures as barriers. *J Interprof Care.* 2005; **19**(2): 188–96.

Halpern H, Morrison S. Narrative-based supervision. In: Owen D, Shohet R (eds). *Clinical Supervision in the Medical Profession: Structured Reflective Practice.* New York, NY: Open University Press; 2012.

Hanckel FS. The problem of induction in clinical decision making. *Med Decis Making.* 1984; **4**(1): 59–68.

Handzo G, Koenig HG. Spiritual care: whose job is it anyway? *South Med J.* 2004; **97**(12): 1242–4.

Hani MA, Keller H, Vandenesch J, *et al.* Different from what the textbooks say: how GPs diagnose coronary heart disease. *Fam Pract.* 2007; **24**(6): 622–7.

Hanson JL. Shared decision making: have we missed the obvious? *Arch Intern Med.* 2008; **168**(13): 1368–70.

Harden RM, Crosby J. The good teacher is more than a lecturer: the twelve roles of a teacher. AMEE Medical Education Guide No 20. *Med Teach.* 2000; **22**(4): 334–47.

Harris DL. *Counting Our Losses: Reflecting on Change, Loss and Transition in Everyday Life.* New York, NY: Routledge; 2011.

Hart JT. The inverse care law. *Lancet.* 1971; **297**(7676): 405–12.

Hatcher S, Arroll B. Assessment and management of medically unexplained symptoms. *BMJ.* 2008; **336**(7653): 1124–8.

Hattie J. *Visible Learning for Teachers: Maximizing Impact on Learning.* New York, NY: Routledge; 2012.

Hattie J, Timperley H. The power of feedback. *Rev Educ Res.* 2007; **77**: 81–112.

Hawk J, Scott CD. A case of family medicine: sources of stress in residents and physicians in practice. In: Scott CD, Hawk J (eds). *Heal Thyself: The Health of Health Care Professionals.* New York, NY: Brunner/Mazel; 1986.

Hawkins AH. A. R. Luria and the art of clinical biography. *Lit Med.* 1986; **5**: 1–15.

Hawkins AH. *Reconstructing Illness: Studies in Pathology.* West Lafayette, IN: Purdue University Press; 1993.

Hawkins SC, Osborne A, Schofield SJ, *et al.* Improving the accuracy of self-assessment of practical clinical skills using video feedback: the importance of including benchmarks. *Med Teach.* 2012; **34**(4): 279–84.

Hayes JA, Gelso CJ, Hummel AM. Managing countertransference. *Psychotherapy.* 2011; **48**(1): 88–97.

Haynes RB, Devereaux PJ, Guyatt GH. Physicians' and patients' choices in evidence based practice. *BMJ.* 2002; **324**(7350): 1350.

Headache Study Group of the University of Western Ontario. Predictors of outcome in headache patients presenting to family physicians: a one year prospective study. *Headache.* 1986; **26**(6): 285–94.

Health Council of Canada. *Decisions, Decisions: Family Doctors as Gatekeepers to Prescription Drugs and Diagnostic Imaging in Canada.* Toronto, ON: Author; 2010. Available at: http://healthcouncilcanada.ca/en/index.php?page=shop.product_details&flypage=shop.flypage&product_id=116&category_id=16&manufacturer_id=0&option=com_virtuemart&Itemid=170 (accessed April 1, 2011).

Heidenreich C, Lye P, Simpson D, *et al.* The search for effective and efficient ambulatory teaching methods through the literature. *Pediatrics.* 2000; **105**(1): 231–7.

Helfer RE. An objective comparison of pediatric interviewing skills on freshman and senior medical students. *Pediatrics.* 1970; **45**(4): 623–7.

Helman C. *Suburban Shaman: Tales from Medicine's Front Line.* London: Hammersmith Press; 2006.

Helman CG. *Culture, Health and Illness.* 5th ed. London: Hodder Arnold; 2007.

Henbest RJ, Stewart M. Patient-centredness in the consultation 2: Does it really make a difference? *Fam Pract.* 1990; **7**(1): 28–33.

Hendley B. Martin Buber on the teacher-student relationship: a critical appraisal. *J Philos Educ.* 1978; **12**(1): 141–8.

Hendry GD, Schrieber L, Bryce D. Patients teach students: partners in arthritis education. *Med Educ.* 1999; **33**(9): 674–7.

Herbert CP. Stories in family medicine commentary: the power of stories. *Can Fam Physician.* 2013; **59**(1): 62–5.

Herwaldt LA. Treating the patient, not the disease. In: Herwaldt LA. *The Stories: Experiences of Relationship-Centered Care.* Kalamazoo, MI: Fetzer Institute; 2001.

Heshusius L. *Inside Chronic Pain-An Intimate and Critical Account.* Ithica, NY: Cornell University Press; 2009.

Hewa S, Hetherington RW. Specialists without spirit: limitations of the mechanistic biomedical model. *Theor Med.* 1995; **16**(2): 129–39.

Higgins SE, Routhieaux RL. A multiple-level analysis of hospital team effectiveness. *Health Care Superv.* 1999; **17**(4): 1–13.

Hilnan J. Physician use of patient-centered weblogs and online journals. *Clin Med Res.* 2003; **1**(4): 333–5.

Hinds PS, Chaves DE, Cypress SM. Context as a source of meaning and understanding. In: Morse JM (ed). *Qualitative Health Research.* Newbury Park, CA: Sage Publications; 1992.

Hippocrates. *Hippocrates; Airs, Waters, Places: an Essay on the Influence of Climate, Water Supply and Situation on Health. Hippocratic Writings.* Hammondsworth: Penguin Books; 1986.

Hodges BD. Clinical commentary. In: Atkins CGK. *My Imaginary Illness.* Ithaca, NY: Cornell University Press; 2010.

Hodges B, Regehr G, Martin D. Difficulties in recognizing one's own incompetence: novice physicians who are unskilled and unaware of it. *Acad Med.* 2001; **76**(10 Suppl.): S87–9.

Hodson R. Work life and social fulfillment: does social affiliation at work reflect a carrot or a stick. *Soc Sci Q.* 2004; **85**(2): 221–39.

Hoffmaster B. Values: the hidden agenda in prevention medicine. *Can Fam Physician.* 1992; **38**: 321–7.

Hojat M, Mangione S, Nasca TJ, *et al.* An empirical study of decline in empathy in medical school. *Med Educ.* 2004; **38**(9): 934–41.

Hojat M, Vergare Mj, Maxwell K, *et al.* The devil is in the third year: a longitudinal study of erosion of empathy in medical school. *Acad Med.* 2009; **84**(9): 1182–91.

Hollander MJ, Kadlec H, Hamdi R, *et al.* Increasing value for money in the Canadian healthcare system: new findings on the contribution of primary care services. *Healthc Q.* 2009; **12**(4): 32–44.

Holman H, Lorig K. Patient self-management: a key to effectiveness and efficiency in care of chronic disease. *Public Health Rep.* 2004; **119**(3): 239–43.

Holmes SM, Ponte M. En-case-ing the Patient: Disciplining Uncertainty in Medical Student Patient Presentations. *Cult Med Psychiatry.* 2011; 35: 163–82.

Hopkins P, Balint Society. Patient-centred medicine: based on the First International Conference of the Balint Society in Great Britain on "The doctor, his patient, and the illness," held March 23–25, 1972 at the Royal College of Physicians, London. Regional Doctor Publications Ltd.

House JS, Landis KR, Umberson D. Social relationships and health. *Science.* 1988; **241**(4865): 540–5.

Hudon C, Fortin M, Haggerty JL, *et al.* Measuring patients' perceptions of patient-centered care: a systematic review of tools for family medicine. *Ann Fam Med.* 2011; **9**(2): 155–64.

Humphrey HJ. *Mentoring in Academic Medicine.* Philadelphia, PA: ACP Press; 2010.

Humphrey-Murto S, Smith CD, Touchie C, *et al.* Teaching the musculoskeletal examination: are patient educators as effective as rheumatology faculty? *Teach Learn Med.* 2004; **16**(2): 175–80.

Hunter KM. *Doctors' Stories – The Narrative Structure of Medical Knowledge.* Princeton, NJ: Princeton University Press; 1991.

Hurowitz JC. Toward a social policy for health. *N Engl J Med.* 1993; **329**(2): 130–3.

Ingelfinger FJ. On arrogance. *N Engl J Med.* 1980; **33**(206): 507–11.

Institute for Healthcare Communication. *Choices and Changes: Clinician Influence and Patient Action. Workshop Syllabus.* New Haven, CT: Institute for Healthcare Communication; 2010.

Institute of Medicine. *Resident Duty Hours: Enhancing Sleep, Supervision, and Safety.* Washington, DC: National Academies Press; 2009.

Inui TS. *A Flag in the Wind: Educating for Professionalism in Medicine.* Washington, DC: Association of American Medical Colleges; 2003.

Irby DM. How attending physicians make instructional decision when conducting teaching rounds. *Acad Med.* 1992; **67**(10): 630–8.

Irby DM, Bowen JL. Time-efficient strategies for learning and performance. *Clin Teach.* 2004; **1**(1): 23–8.

Ishikawa H, Hashimoto H, Roter DL, *et al.* Patient contribution to the medical dialogue and perceived patient-centeredness: an observational study in Japanese geriatric consultations. *J Gen Intern Med.* 2005; **20**(10): 906–10.

Jacobson RM, Targonski PV, Poland GA. A taxonomy of reasoning flaws in the anti-vaccine movement. *Vaccine.* 2007; **25**: 3146–52.

Jamal MH, Rosseau MC, Hanna WC, *et al.* Effect of the ACGME duty hours restrictions on surgical residents and faculty: a systematic review. *Acad Med.* 2011; **86**(1): 34–42.

James W. *The Varieties of Religious Experience: A Study in Human Nature.* New York, NY: New American Library; 1958.

Jani B, Bikker AP, Higgins M, *et al.* Patient centredness and the outcome of primary care consultations with patients with depression in areas of high and low socioeconomic deprivation. *Br J Gen Pract.* 2012; **62**(601): e576–81.

Janicik R, Kalet AL, Schwartz MD, *et al.* Using bedside rounds to teach communication skills in the internal medicine clerkship. *Med Educ Online.* 2007; **12**: 1.

Janz NK, Becker MH. The Health Belief Model: A Decade Later. *Health Educ Behav.* 1984; **11**: 1–48.

Jarvis-Selinger S, Halwani Y, Joughin K, *et al.* Supporting the Development of Residents as Teachers: Current Practices and Emerging Trends. *Members of the FMED PG Consortium.* 2011.

Jauhar S. *Intern: A Doctor's Initiation.* New York, NY: Farrar, Straus & Giroux; 2008.

Jiménez X, Thorkelson G. Medical countertransference and the trainee: identifying a training gap. *J Psychiatr Pract.* 2012; **18**(2): 109–17.

Jones I, Morrell D. General practitioners' background knowledge of their patients. *Fam Pract.* 1995; **12**(1): 49–53.

Jones S, Oswald N, Date J, *et al.* Attitudes of patients to medical student participation: general practice consultations on the Cambridge Community-Based Clinical Course. *Med Educ.* 1996; **30**(1): 14–17.

Juckett G. Cross-cultural medicine. *Am Fam Physician.* 2005; **72**(11): 2267–74.

Kalén S, Ponzer S, Silén C. The core of mentorship: medical students' experiences of one-to-one mentoring in a clinical environment. *Adv Health Sci Educ Theory Pract.* 2012; **17**(3): 389–401.

Kalet A, Pugnaire MP, Cole-Kelly K, *et al.* Teaching communication in clinical clerkships: models from the Macy Initiative in Health Communications. *Acad Med.* 2004; **79**(6): 511–20.

Kant AK. Dietary patterns and health outcomes. *J Am Diet Assoc.* 2004; **104**(4): 615–35.

Kaplan GA, Neil JE. Socioecomonic factors and cardiovascular disease: a review of the literature. *Circulation.* 1993; **88**(4): 1973–98.

Kaplan SH, Greenfield S, Ware JE. Impact of the doctor-patient relationship on outcomes of chronic disease. In: Stewart M, Roter D (eds). *Communicating with Medical Patients.* Beverly Hills, CA: Sage Publications; 1989a. pp.228–245

Kaplan SH, Greenfield S, Ware JE Jr. Assessing the effects of physician-patient interactions on the outcomes of chronic disease. *Med Care.* 1989b; **27**: S110–27.

Karr-Morse R, Wiley MS. *Scared Sick: The Role of Childhood Trauma in Adult Disease.* New York, NY: Basic Books; 2012.

Kasman DL. Socialization in medical training: exploring "lifelong curiosity" and a "community of support". *Am J Bioethics.* 2004; **4**(2): 52–5.

Kata A. Anti-vaccine activists, Web 2.0, and the postmodern paradigm: an overview of tactics and tropes used online by the anti-vaccination movement. *Vaccine.* 2012; **30**(25): 3778–89.

Katon W, Kleinman A. Doctor-patient negotiation and other social science strategies in patient care. In: Eisenberg L, Kleinman A (eds). *Relevance of Social Science for Medicine.* Boston, MA: D Reidel; 1981.

Kaufman DM, Mann KV, Jennett PA. *Teaching and Learning in Medical Education: How Theory Can Inform Practice.* Edinburgh: Association for the Study of Medical Education; 2000.

Kawachi I, Kennedy BP, Wilkinson RG. Crime: social disorganization and relative deprivation. *Soc Sci Med.* 1999a; **48**(6): 719–31.

Kawachi I, Kennedy B, Wilkinson R. *The Society and Population Health Reader: Income Inequality and Health*. New York, NY: The New Press; 1999b.

Keller VF, White MK. Choices and changes: a new model for influencing patient health behavior. *J Clin Outcomes Manag*. 1997; **4**(6): 33–6.

Kelly L. *Community-Based Medical Education: A Teacher's Handbook*. London: Radcliffe Publishing; 2012.

Kelly L, Brown JB. Listening to native patients. *Can Fam Physician*. 2002; **48**: 1645–52.

Kelman EG, Straker KC. *Study without Stress: Mastering Medical Sciences*. Thousand Oaks, CA: Sage; 2000.

Kennedy TJT, Regehr G, Baker GR, *et al.* Point-of-care assessment of medical trainee competence for independent clinical work. *Acad Med*. 2008; **83**(10 Suppl.): 589–92.

Kenny N, Shelton W (eds). *Lost Virtue: Character Development in Medical Education*. Amsterdam: Elsevier; 2006.

Kern DE, Thomas PA, Hughes MT. *Curriculum Development for Medical Education: A Six-Step Approach*. 2nd ed. Baltimore, MD: Johns Hopkins University Press; 2009.

Kern DE, Wright SM, Carrese JA, *et al.* Personal growth in medical faculty: a qualitative study. *West J Med*. 2001; **175**(2): 92–8.

Kestenbaum V. *Humanity of the Ill: Phenomenological Perspectives*. Knoxville: University of Tennessee Press; 1982.

Kilminster S, Cottrell D, Grant J, *et al.* AMEE Guide No. 27: Effective educational and clinical supervision. *Med Teach*. 2007b; **29**(1): 2–19.

Kilminster S, Downes J, Gough B, *et al.* Women in medicine: is there a problem? A literature review of the changing gender composition, structures and occupational cultures in medicine. *Med Educ*. 2007a; **41**(1): 39–49.

Kim S. Content analysis of cancer blog posts. *J Med Libr Assoc*. 2009; **97**(4): 260–6.

King J. Giving feedback. *BMJ*. 1999; **318**: S2–7200.

Kinnersley P, Stott N, Peters TJ, *et al.* The patient-centredness of consultations and outcome in primary care. *Br J Gen Pract*. 1999; **49**(446): 771–6.

Kinra S, Nelder RP, Lewendon GJ. Deprivation and childhood obesity: a cross sectional study of 20,973 children in Plymouth, United Kingdom. *J Epidemiol Commun Health*. 2000; **54**(6): 456–60.

Kinsella EA. Practitioner reflection and judgement as phonesis. In: Kinsella EA, Pitman A (eds). *Phronesis as Professional Knowledge: Practical Wisdom in the Professions*. Rotterdam: Sense Publishers; 2012.

Kinsella EA, Pitman A (eds). *Phronesis as Professional Knowledge: Practical Wisdom in the Professions*. Rotterdam: Sense Publishers; 2012.

Kitagawa EM, Hauser PM. *Differential Mortality in the United States: A Study in Socio-Economic Epidemiology*. Cambridge, MA: Harvard University Press; 1973.

Kjeldmand D, Holmström I, Rosenqvist U. Balint training makes GPs thrive in their job. *Patient Educ Couns*. 2004; **55**(2): 230–5.

Klass P. *A Not Entirely Benign Procedure: Four Years as a Medical Student*. New York, NY: GP Putman; 1987.

Klass P. *Baby Doctor*. New York, NY: Random House; 1992.

Klaus MH, Kennell JH, Klaus PH. *Bonding: Building the Foundation of Secure Attachment and Independence*. Cambridge, MA: De Capo Press; 1996.

Kleinman A. *The Illness Narratives: Suffering, Healing and the Human Condition*. New York, NY: Basic Books; 1988.

Kleinman A. Prologue. In: Borkan J, Reis S, Steinmetz D, *et al.* (eds). *Patients and Doctors: Life-Changing Stories for Primary Care*. Madison: University of Wisconsin Press; 1999.

Kleinman AM, Eisenberg L, Good B. Culture, illness, and care: clinical lessons from anthropologic and cross-cultural research. *Ann Intern Med*. 1978; **88**(2): 251–8.

Klitzman R. *A Year-Long Night*. New York, NY: Penguin Books; 1989.

Knight JK, Wood WB. Teaching more by lecturing less. *Cell Biol Educ*. 2005; **4**(4): 298–310.

Knowles M. *Self-Directed Learning: A Guide for Learners and Teachers.* Chicago, IL: Follett Publishing; 1975.

Knowles MS, Holton EF 3rd, Swanson RA. *The Adult Learner: The Definitive Classic in Adult Education and Human Resource Development.* 5th ed. Houston, TX: Gulf Publishing; 1998.

Knowles MS, Holton EF 3rd, Swanson RA. *The Adult Learner: The Definitive Classic in Adult Education and Human Resource Development.* 7th ed. Oxford: Butterworth–Heinemann; 2011.

Koenig HG. Religion, spirituality, and medicine: research findings and implications for clinical practice. *South Med J.* 2004; **97**(12): 1194–200.

Koenig HG, King DE, Larson VB. *Handbook of Religion and Health.* 2nd ed. Oxford: Oxford University Press; 2012.

Koenig HG, McCullough ME, Larson DB. *Handbook of Religion and Health.* Oxford: Oxford University Press; 2001.

Kohlhammer Y, Schnoor M, Schwartz M. *et al.* Determinants of influenza and pneumococal vaccination in elderly people: a systematic review. *Public Health.* 2007; **121**(10): 742–51.

Kohn KT, Corrigan JM, Donaldson MS. *To Err is Human: Building a Safer Health System.* Washington, DC: National Academy Press; 2000.

Kohut H. *the Analysis of the Self.* New York: International Universities Press; 1971.

Kohut H. *The Restoration of the Self.* New York: International Universities Press; 1977.

Konner M. *Becoming a Doctor: A Journey of Initiation in Medical School.* New York, NY: Viking-Penguin; 1987.

Korsch B, Negrete V. Doctor-patient communication. *Sci Am.* 1972; **227**(2): 66–74.

Korzybski A. *Science and Sanity: An Introduction to Non-Aristotelian Systems and General Semantics.* 4th ed. Lake Bille, CT: International Non-Aristotelian Library Publishing; 1958.

Krasner MS, Epstein RM, Beckman H, *et al.* Association of an educational program in mindful communication with burnout, empathy, and attitudes among primary care physicians. *JAMA.* 2009; **302**(12): 1284–93.

Kruger J. Lake Wobegon be gone! The "below-average effect" and the egocentric nature of comparative ability judgments. *J Pers Soc Psychol.* 1999; **77**(2): 221–32.

Kruger J, Dunning D. Unskilled and unaware of it: how difficulties in recognizing one's own incompetence lead to inflated self-assessments. *J Pers Soc Psychol.* 1999; **77**(6): 1121–34.

Krupat E, Rosenkranz SL, Yeager CM, *et al.* The practice orientations of physicians and patients: the effect of doctor-patient congruence on satisfaction. *Patient Educ Couns.* 2000; **39**(1): 49–59.

Kumagai AK Forks in the road: disruption and transformation in professional development. *Acad Med.* 2010; **85**(12): 1819–20.

Kumar P, Basu D. Substance abuse by medical students and doctors. *J Indian Med Assoc.* 2000; **98**(8): 447–52.

Kurth RJ, Irigoyen M, Schmidt HJ. A model to structure student learning in ambulatory care settings. *Acad Med.* 1997; **72**(7): 601–6.

Kurtz S, Silverman J, Benson J, *et al.* Marrying content and process in clinical method teaching: enhancing the Calgary-Cambridge Guides. *Acad Med.* 2003; **78**(8): 802–9.

Kurtz S, Silverman J, Draper J. *Teaching and Learning Communication Skills in Medicine.* 2nd ed. Oxford: Radcliffe Publishing; 2005.

Lacasse M. *Educational Diagnosis and Management of Challenging Learning Situations in Medical Education.* Quebec City, QC: University of Laval; 2009.

Lacasse M, Théorêt J, Skalenda P, *et al.* Challenging learning situations in medical education: innovative and structured tools for assessment, educational diagnosis, and intervention. Part 1: history and data gathering. *Can Fam Physician.* 2012a; **58**(4): 481–4.

Lacasse M, Théorêt J, Skalenda P, *et al.* Challenging learning situations in medical education: innovative and structured tools for assessment, educational diagnosis, and intervention. Part 2: objective examination, assessment, and plan. *Can Fam Physician.* 2012b; **58**(7): 802–3.

Lai DW, Tsang KT, Chappell N, *et al.* Relationships between culture and health status: a multi-site study of the older Chinese in Canada. *Can J Aging.* 2007; **26**(3): 171–83.

Laing RD. *The Divided Self.* London: Tavistock Publications; 1960.

Lake FR, Vickery AW, Ryan G. Teaching in the run tips 7: effective use of questions. *Med J Aust.* 2005; **182**(3): 126–7.

Lakoff G, Johnson M. *Metaphors We Live By.* Chicago, IL: University of Chicago Press; 1980.

Lam V. *Bloodletting and Miraculous Cures.* Toronto, ON: Doubleday Canada; 2006.

Lane JL, Gottlieb RP. Improving the interviewing and self-assessment skills of medical students: is it time to readopt videotaping as an educational tool. *Ambul Pediatr.* 2004; **4**(3): 244–8.

Lang F, Floyd MR, Beine KL. Clues to patients' explanations and concerns about their illness: a call for active listening. *Arch Fam Med.* 2000; **65**(7): 1351–4.

Lang F, Marvel K, Sanders D, *et al.* Interviewing when family members are present. *Am Fam Physician.* 2002; **65**(7): 1351–4.

Lantz PM, House JS, Lepkowski JM, *et al.* Socioeconomic factors, health behaviors, and mortality: results from a nationally representative prospective study of US adults. *JAMA.* 1998; **279**(21): 1703–8.

Larsen A, Boggild H, Mortensen JT, *et al.* Psychology, defense mechanisms, and the psychosocial work environment. *Int J Soc Psychiatry.* 2010; **56**(6): 563–77.

Laschinger HKS, Shamian J, Thomson D. Impact of magnet hospital characteristics on nurses' perceptions of trust, burnout, quality of care, and work satisfaction. *Nurs Econ.* 2001; **19**(Pt. 5): 209–20.

Launer J. *Narrative-Based Primary Care: A Practical Guide.* Oxford: Radcliffe Medical Press; 2002.

Launer J, Lindsey C. Training for systemic general practice: a new approach from the Tavistock Clinic. *Br J Gen Pract.*1997; **47**(420): 453–6.

Lave J, Wenger E. *Situated Learning: Legitimate Peripheral Participation.* Cambridge: Cambridge University Press; 1991.

LeBaron C. *Gentle Vengeance.* New York, NY: Richard Marek Publishers; 1981.

Leder D. Clinical interpretation: the hermeneutics of medicine. *Theor Med.* 1990; **11**(1): 9–24.

Lee FJ, Stewart M, Brown JB. Stress, burnout, and strategies for reducing them. *Can Fam Physician.* 2008; **54**(2): 234–5.

Lee JM. Screening and informed consent. *N Engl J Med.* 1993; **328**(6): 438–40.

Lee-Poy M. *The Role of Religion and Spirituality in the Care of Patients in Family Medicine* [master's thesis], Western University; 2012a.

Lee-Poy M, Brown JB, Stewart M, *et al.* Let's get spiritual: talking to patients about their religion and spirituality. Paper presented at 2012 Family Medicine Forum, Toronto, Ontario, Canada, November 14, 2012b.

Légaré F, Ratté S, Gravel K, *et al.* Barriers and facilitators to implementing shared decision-making in clinical practice: update of a systematic review of health professionals' perceptions. *Patient Educ Couns.* 2003; **73**(3): 526–35.

Légaré F, Ratté S, Stacey D, *et al.* Interventions for improving the adoption of shared decision making by healthcare professionals. *Cochrane Database Syst Rev.* 2010; (5): CD006732.

Légaré F, Stacey D, Pouliot S, *et al.* Interprofessionalism and shared decision-making in primary care: a stepwise approach towards a new model. *J Interprof Care.* 2011; **25**(1): 18–25.

Légaré F, Turcotte S, Stacey D, *et al.* Patients' perceptions of sharing in decisions: a systematic review of interventions to enhance shared decision making in routine clinical practice. *Patient.* 2012; **5**(1): 1–19.

Lemieux-Charles L, McGuire WL. What do we know about health care team effectiveness? A review of the literature. *Med Care Res Rev.* 2006; **63**(3): 263–300.

Leonard M, Graham S, Bonacum D. The human factor: the critical importance of effective teamwork and communication in providing safe care. *Qual Saf Health Care.* 2004; **13**(Suppl. 1): i85–90.

Lerman CE, Brody DS, Caputo GC, *et al.* Patients' perceived involvement in care scale: relationship to attitudes about illness and medical care. *J Gen Intern Med.* 1990; **5**(1): 29–33.

Leung ASO, Epstein RM, Moulton CAE. The competent mind: beyond cognition. In: Hodges BD, Lingard L (eds). *The Question of Competence.* Ithaca, NY: Cornell University Press; 2012.

Leung L. Whose difficulty is it? *Can Fam Physician.* 2012; **58**(9): 987–8.

Levenstein JH, McCracken EC, McWhinney IR, *et al.* The patient-centred clinical method: 1. A model for the doctor-patient interaction in family medicine. *Fam Pract.* 1986; **3**(1): 24–30.

Levine RB, Haidet P, Kern DE, *et al.* Personal growth during internship: a qualitative analysis of interns' responses to key questions. *J Gen Intern Med.* 2006; **21**(6): 564–9.

Levinson DJ. *Seasons of a Man's Life.* New York, NY: Knopf; 1978.

Levinson W, Gorawara-Bhat R, Lamb J. A study of patient clues and physician responses in primary care and surgical settings. *JAMA.* 2000; **284**(8): 1021–7.

Levinson W, Kao A, Kuby A, *et al.* Not all patients want to participate in decision making: a national study of public preferences. *J Gen Intern Med.* 2005; **20**(6): 531–5.

Levinson W, Lurie N. When most doctors are women: what lies ahead? *Ann Intern Med.* 2004; **141**(6): 471–4.

Lewin SA, Skea ZC, Entwistle V, *et al.* Interventions for providers to promote a patient-centred approach in clinical consultations. *Cochrane Database Syst Rev.* 2001; (4): CD003267.

Liben S, Chin K, Bourdreau JD, *et al.* Assessing a faculty development workshop in narrative medicine. *Med Teac.* 2012; **34**(12): e813–19.

Liberante L. The importance of teacher-student relationships, as explored through the lens of the NSW Quality Teaching Model. *Journal of Student Engagement: Education Matters.* 2012; **2**(1): 2–9.

Lillich DW, Mace K, Goodell M, *et al.* Active precepting in the residency clinic: a pilot study of a new model. *Fam Med.* 2005; **37**(3): 205–10.

Lindeman EC. *The Meaning of Adult Education.* New York, NY: New Republic; 1926.

Lingard L. Rethinking competence in the context of teamwork. In: Hodges BD, Lingard L (eds). *The Question of Competence.* Ithaca, NY: Cornell University Press; 2012.

Lingard L, Schryer C, Garwood K, *et al.* 'Talking the talk': school and workplace genre tension in clerkship case presentations. *Med Educ.* 2003; **37**(7): 612–20.

Little M, Midtling JE. *Becoming a Family Physician.* New York, NY: Springer-Verlag; 1989.

Little P, Everitt H, Williamson I, *et al.* Observational study of effect of patient centredness and positive approach on outcomes of general practice consultations. *BMJ.* 2001b; **323**(7318): 908–11.

Little P, Everitt H, Williamson I, *et al.* Preferences of patients for patient-centred approach to consultation in primary care: observational study. *BMJ.* 2001a; **322**(7284): 468–72.

Livneh H, Antonak RF. Psychosocial adaptation to chronic illness and disability: a primer for counselors. *J Couns Dev.* 2005; **83**(1): 12–20.

Lorig K. Self-management education: more than a nice extra. *Med Care.* 2003; **41**(6): 699–701.

Lorig K and Associates. *Patient Education: A Practical Approach.* 3rd ed. Thousand Oaks, CA: Sage Publications; 2001a.

Lorig KR, Holman HR. Self-management education: history, definition, outcomes, and mechanisms. *Ann Behav Med.* 2003; **26**(1): 1–7.

Lorig K, Sobel D, Ritter P, *et al.* Effects of a self-management program on patients with chronic disease. *Eff Clin Pract.* 2001b; **4**(6): 256–62.

Lowenstein SR, Fernandez G, Crane LA. Medical school discontent: prevalence and predictors of intent to leave academic careers. *BMC Med Educ.* 2007; **7**: 37.

Lown BA, Hanson JL, Clarke WD. Mutual influence in shared decision making: a collaborative study of patients and physicians. *Health Expect.* 2009; **12**(2): 160–74.

Lown BA, Rodriguez D. Lost in translation/How EHRs structure communication, relationships, and meaning. *Academic Medicine.* 2012; **7**(4): 392–4.

Loxterkamp D. The headwaters of family medicine. *BMJ.* 2008; **337**: 2575.

Lubkin IM, Larsen PD. *Chronic Illness: Impact and Intervention.* 8th ed. Nurlington, MA: James & Bartlett Learning; 2013.

Ludmerer KM. Learner-centered education. *N Engl J Med.* 2004; **351**(12): 1163–4.

Lussier MT, Richard C. Because one shoe doesn't fit all: : a repertoire of doctor-patient relationships. *Can Fam Physician.* 2008; **54**(8): 1089–92.

Lynch JW, Kaplan GA, Salonen JT. Why do poor people behave poorly? Variation in adult health behaviours and psychosocial characteristics by stages of socioeconomic lifecourse. *Soc Sci Med.* 1997; **44**(6): 809–19.

Lyn-Cook R, Halm EA Wishivesky JP. Determinants of adherence to influenza vaccination among inner-city adults with persistent asthma. *Primary Care Respiratory Journal.* 2007; **16**(4): 229–35.

Ma GX, Fang CY, Shive SE, *et al.* Risk perceptions and barriers to hepatitis B screening and vaccination among Vietnamese immigrants. *J Immigrant Minority Health.* 2007; **9**: 213–20.

Maguire P, Fairbairn S, Fletcher C. Consultation skills of young doctors: benefits of undergraduate feedback training in interviewing. In: Stewart M, Roter D (eds). *Communicating With Medical Patients.* Thousand Oaks, CA: Sage Publications; 1989.

Makoul G, Krupat E, Chang CH. Measuring patient views of physician communication skills: development and testing of the Communication Assessment Tool. *Patient Educ Couns.* 2007; **67**(3): 333–42.

Malterud K. Key questions: a strategy for modifying clinical communication. Transforming tacit skills into a clinical method. *Scand J Prim Health Care.* 1994; **12**(2): 121–7.

Malterud K. Symptoms as a source of medical knowledge: understanding medically unexplained disorders in women. *Fam Med.* 2000; **32**(9): 603–11.

Malterud K, Hunskaar S (eds). *Chronic Myofascial Pain: A Patient-Centered Approach.* Oxford: Radcliffe Medical Press; 2002.

Mann K, van der Vleuten C, Eva K, *et al.* Tensions in informed self-assessment: how the desire for feedback and reticence to collect and use it can conflict. *Acad Med.* 2011; **86**(9): 1120–7.

Margalit RS, Roter D, Dunevant MA, *et* al. Electronic medical record use and physician-patient communication: an observational study of Israeli primary care encounters. *Patient Educ Couns.* 2006; **61**(1): 134–41.

Margolis E (ed). *The Hidden Curriculum in Higher Education.* New York, NY: Routledge; 2001.

Marini I, Stebnicki M. *The Psychological and Social Impact of Illness and Disability.* New York, NY: Springer; 2012.

Markle GE, McCrea FB. *What If Medicine Disappeared?* New York: State University of New York Press; 2008.

Marmoreo J, Brown JB, Batty HR, *et al.* Hormone replacement therapy: determinants of women's decisions. *Patient Educ Couns.* 1998; **33**(3): 289–98.

Marmot MG, Kogevinas M, Elston MA. Social/economic status and disease. *Annu Rev Public Health.* 1987; **8**: 111–35.

Marra M, Angouri J. Investigating the negotiation of identity: a view from the field of workplace discourse. In: Angouri J, Marra M (eds). *Constructing Identities at Work.* New York, NY: Palgrave Macmillan; 2011.

Marshall KG. Prevention. How much harm? How much benefit? 4: The ethics of informed consent for preventive screening programs. *CMAJ.* 1996; **155**(4): 377–83.

Marshall L, Weir E, Ablesohn A, *et al.* Identifying and managing adverse environmental health effects: 1. Taking an exposure history. *CMAJ.* 2002; **166**(8): 1041–3.

Marteau TM. Reducing the psychological costs. *BMJ.* 1990; **301**(6742): 26–8.

Marteau TM. Screening for cardiovascular risk: public health imperative or matter for individual informed choice? *BMJ.* 2002; **325**(7355): 78–80.

Martin D, Regehr G, Hodges B, *et al.* Using videotape benchmarks to improve the self-assessment ability of family practice residents. *Acad Med.* 1998; **73**(11): 1201–6.

Martinelli AM. An explanatory model of variables influencing health promotion behaviors in smoking and nonsmoking college students. *BMJ.* 1999; **16**(4): 263–9.

Marvel MK, Epstein RM, Flowers K, *et al.* Soliciting the patient's agenda: have we improved? *JAMA.* 1999; **281**(3): 283–7.

Marwan Y, Al-Saddique M, Hassan A, *et al.* Are medical students accepted by patients in teaching hospitals. *Med Educ Online.* 2012; **17**: 171–2.

Mattingly C, Fleming MH. *Clinical Reasoning: Forms of Inquiry in a Therapeutic Practice.* Philadephia, PA: FA Davis; 1994.

Mavis B, Vasilenko P, Schnuth R, *et al.* Medical students' involvement in outpatient clinical encounters: a survey of patients and their obstetricians-gynecologists. *Academic Medicine.* 2006; **81**: 290–6.

Maxfield D, Grenny J, McMillan R, *et al. Silence Kills: The Seven Crucial Conversations for Healthcare.*

Provo, UT: VitalSmarts; 2005. Available at: www.silenttreatmentstudy.com/silencekills/ (accessed January 6, 2013).

May WF. *The Patient's Ordeal.* Bloomington, IN: Indiana University Press; 1991.

Mayer JD. Medical geography: an emerging discipline. *JAMA.* 1984; **251**(20): 2680–3.

McConnell MM, Regehr G, Wood TJ, *et al.* Self-monitoring and its relationship to medical knowledge. *Adv Health Sci Educ.* 2012; **17**: 311–23.

McCord G, Gilchrist VJ, Grossman SD, *et al.* Discussing spirituality with patients: a rational and ethical approach. *Ann Fam Med.* 2004; **2**(4): 356–61.

McCullough LB. The abstract character and transforming power of medical language. *Soundings.* 1989; **72**(1): 111–25.

McDaniel SH, Campbell TL, Hepworth J, *et al. Family-Oriented Primary Care.* 2nd ed. New York, NY: Springer; 2005.

McEwen BS. Stress, adaptation, and disease: allostasis and allostatic load. *Ann N Y Acad Sci.* 1998; **840**: 33–44.

McEwen BS. Allostatis and allostatic load: implications for neuropharmacology. *Neuropharmacology.* 2000; **22**(2): 108–24.

McGeehin MA, Mirabelli M. The potential impacts of climate variability and change on temperature-related morbidity and mortality in the United States. *Environ Health Perspect.* 2001; **109**(Suppl. 2): 185–9.

McGoldrick M, Carter B, Garcia-Preto N. *The Expanded Family Life Cycle: Individual, Family, and Social Perspectives.* 4th ed. Boston, MA: Pearson Allyn & Bacon; 2010.

McKeachie WJ. *Teaching Tips: A Guidebook for the Beginning College Teacher.* 7th ed. Lexington, MA: DC Health; 1978.

McKee A, Eraut M (eds). *Learning Trajectories, Innovation and Identity for Professional Development.* New York, NY: Springer; 2011.

McKinstry B. Do patients wish to be involved in decision making in the consultation? A cross sectional survey with video vignettes. *BMJ.* 2000; **321**(7265): 867–71.

McLeod ME. Doctor-patient relationships: perspectives, needs, and communication. *Am J Gastroenterol.* 1998; **93**(5): 676–80.

McMurray C, Smith R. *Diseases of Globalization: Socioeconomic Transitions and Health.* London and Sterling, VA: Earthscan Publications; 2001.

McNeilis KS. Analyzing communication competence in medical consultations. *Health Commun.* 2001; **13**(1): 5–18.

McQueen DV, Jones CM. *Global Perspectives on Health Promotion Effectiveness.* New York, NY: Springer; 2010.

McWhinney IR. Beyond diagnosis: an approach to the integration of behavioural science and clinical medicine. *N Engl J Med.* 1972; **287**(8): 384–7.

McWhinney I. *Through Clinical Method to a More Humane Medicine in the Task of Medicine: Dialogue at Wickenberg.* Menlo Park, CA: Henry J Kaiser Foundation; 1988.

McWhinney IR. *An Acquaintance with Particulars.* The Curtis Hames Lecture. Society of Teachers of Family Medicine, Annual Spring Conference, Denver, CO; 1989a.

McWhinney IR. *A Textbook of Family Medicine.* New York, NY: Oxford University Press; 1989b.

McWhinney IR. The William Pickles Lecture 1996: the importance of being different. *Br J Gen Pract.* 1996; **46**(408): 433–6.

McWhinney IR. *A Textbook of Family Medicine.* 2nd ed. New York, NY: Oxford University Press; 1997a.

McWhinney IR. Being a general practitioner: what it means. *Eur J Gen Pract.* 2000; **6**: 135–9.

McWhinney IR. The value of case studies. *Eur J Gen Pract.* 2001; **7**: 88–9.

McWhinney IR. *A Call to Heal: Reflections on a Life in Family Medicine.* Saskatoon, SK: Benchmark Press; 2012.

McWhinney IR, Epstein RM, Freeman TR. Rethinking somatization. *Ann Intern Med.* 1997b; **126**(9): 747–50.

McWhinney IR, Freeman T. *Textbook of Family Medicine.* 3rd ed. Oxford: Oxford University Press; 2009.

McWilliam CL, Brown JB, Stewart M. Breast cancer patients' experiences of patient-doctor communication: a working relationship. *Patient Educ Couns.* 2000; **39**(2–3): 191–204.

McWilliam CL, Hoch J, Coyte P, *et al.* Can we afford consumers choice in home care? *Care Manag J.* 2007; **8**(4): 108.

McWilliam CL, Stewart M, Brown JB, *et al.* Creating health with chronic illness. *Adv Nurs Sci.* 1996; **18**(3): 1–15.

McWilliam CL, Stewart M, Brown JB, *et al.* Creating empowering meaning: an interactive process of promoting health with chronically ill older Canadians. *Health Promot Int.* 1997; **12**(2): 111–23.

McWilliam CL, Stewart M, Brown JB, *et al.* A randomized controlled trial of a critical reflection approach to home-based health promotion for chronically ill older persons. *Health Promot Int.* 1999; **14**(1): 27–41.

McWilliam CL, Stewart M, Vingilis E, *et al.* Flexible client-driven case management. *J Case Manag.* 2004; **5**(2): 73–86.

Mead N, Bower P. Patient-centredness: a conceptual framework and review of the empirical literature. *Soc Sci Med.* 2000; **51**(7): 1087–110.

Meade MS. Geographic analysis of disease and care. *Ann Rev Public Health.* 1986; **7**: 313–35.

Meade M, Emch M. *Medical Geography.* 3rd ed. New York, NY: Guildford Press; 2010.

Medalie J, Borkan J, Reis S, *et al. Patients and Doctors: Life Changing Stories from Primary Care.* Madison: University of Wisconsin Press; 1999.

Medalie JH, Cole-Kelly K. The clinical importance of defining family. *Am Fam Physician.* 2002; **65**(7): 1277–9.

Mercer S. Empathy is key. In: *Working Towards People Powered Health: Insights from Practitioners.* London: Nesta; 2012.

Mercer SW, Maxwell M, Heaney D, *et al.* The consultation and relational empathy (CARE) measure: development and preliminary validation and reliability of an empathy-based consultation process measure. *Fam Pract.* 2004; **21**(6): 699–705.

Mercer SW, Reynolds WJ. Empathy and quality of care. *Br J Gen Pract.* 2002; **52**(Suppl.): S9–12.

Meredith L, Stewart M, Brown JB. Patient-centered communication scoring method report on nine coded interviews. *Health Commun.* 2001; **13**(1): 19–31.

Merriam SB. Adult learning theory for the twenty-first century. *New Directions for Adult and Continuing Education.* 2008; **119**: 93–8.

Merriam SB, Caffarella RS, Baumgartner LM. *Learning in Adulthood: A Comprehensive Guide.* 3rd ed. San Francisco, CA: Jossey-Bass; 2007.

Mezirow J and Associates. *Learning as Transformation: Critical Perspectives on a Theory in Progress.* San Francisco, CA: Jossey-Bass; 2000.

Mickan S, Rodger S. Characteristics of effective teams: a literature review. *Aust Health Rev.* 2000; **23**(3): 201–8.

Miflin BM, Price DA, Mitchell MG, *et al.* Briefing students before seeing patients. *Med Teach.* 1997; **19**(2): 143–4.

Miksanek T. On caring for 'difficult' patients. *Health Aff (Millwood).* 2008; **27**(5): 1422–8.

Milan FB, Dyche L, Fletcher J. "How am I doing?" Teaching medical students to elicit feedback during their clerkships. *Med Teach.* 2011; **33**(11): 904–10.

Miller GA. The magical number seven, plus or minus two: some limits on our capacity for processing information. *Psychol Rev.* 1956; **63**(2): 81–97.

Miller GE, Abrahamson S, Cohen IS, *et al. Teaching and Learning in Medical School.* Cambridge, MA: Harvard University Press; 1961.

Miller NP, Garretson HJ. Preserving law school's signature pedagogy and great subjects. *Mich B J.* 2009; **88**(5): 46–7.

Miller WL. Routine, ceremony, or drama: an exploratory field study of the primary care clinical encounter. *J Fam Pract.* 1992; **34**(3): 289–96.

Miller WR, Rollnick S. *Motivational Interviewing: Helping People Change.* 3rd ed. New York, NY: Guilford Press; 2013.

Milstein JM. Introducing spirituality in medical care: transition from hopelessness to wholeness. *JAMA.* 2008; **299**(20): 2440–1.

Ministry of Health and Long-Term Care (MOHLTC). *Externally Informed Annual Health Systems Trends Report.* 2nd ed. Toronto, ON: MOHLTC Health Systems Planning and Research Branch; 2009.

Mishler EG. *Discourse of Medicine: Dialectics of Medical Interviews.* Norwood, NJ: Ablex; 1984.

Mitchell G (ed). *Palliative Care: A Patient-Centered Approach.* Oxford: Radcliffe Publishing; 2008.

Mohanna K, Wall D, Chambers R. *Teaching Made Easy.* Oxford: Radcliffe Publishing; 2004.

Mokdad AH, Marks JS, Stroup DF, *et al.* Actual causes of death in the United States. 2000. *JAMA.* 2004; **291**(10): 1238–45.

Molloy E, Borell-Carrió F, Epstein R. The impact of emotions in feedback. In: Boud D, Molloy E (eds). *Feedback in Higher and Professional Education: Understanding It and Doing It Well.* New York, NY: Routledge; 2013.

Molyneux J. Interprofessional teamworking: what makes teams work well? *J Interprof Care.* 2001; **15**(1): 29–35.

Monrouxe LV. Identity, identification and medical education: why should we care? *Med Educ.* 2010; **44**(1): 40–9.

Moonesinghe SR, Lowery J, Shahi N, *et al.* Impact of reduction in working hours for doctors in training on postgraduate medical education and patients' outcomes: systematic review. *BMJ.* 2011; **342**: d1580.

Mooney CG. *Theories of Attachment: An Introduction to Bowlby, Ainsworth Gerber, Brazelton, Kennell, and Kraus.* St. Paul, MN: Redleaf Press; 2010.

Moore J. What Sir Luke Fildes' 1887 painting The Doctor can teach us about the practice of medicine today. *Br J Gen Pract.* 2008; **58**(548): 210–13.

Moore WS. Student and faculty epistemology in the college classroom: the Perry schema of intellectual and ethical development. In: Prichard KW, Sawyer RM (eds). *Handbook of College Teaching: Theory and Applications.* Westport, CT: Greenwood Press; 1994.

Morris A. *Illness and Culture in the Postmodern Age.* Berkeley: University of California Press; 1998.

Morris BAP. Case reports: Boon or Bane? In: Norton PG *et al.* (eds). *Primary Care Research: Traditional and Innovative Approaches.* Newbury Park, CA: Sage; 1991.

Mosack KE, Abbott M, Singer M, *et al.* If I didn't have HIV, I'd be dead now: illness narratives of drug users living with HIV/AIDS. *Qual Health Res.* 2005; **15**(5): 586–605.

Moss E, Maxfield D. Silence kills: a case manager's guide to communication breakdowns in healthcare: part I of III. *Prof Case Manag.* 2007; **12**(1): 52–4.

Moulton CA, Regehr G, Myopoulos M, *et al.* Slowing down when you should: a new model of expert judgment. *Acad Med.* 2007; **82**(10 Suppl.): S109–116.

Mukand J. Vital lines: contemporary fiction about medicine. New York, NY: St. Martin's Press; 1990.

Mundy GR. Presidential address of the SSCI: can the triple threat survive biotech? *Am J Med Sci.* 1991; **302**(1): 38–41.

Murdin, L. *Understanding Transference: The Power of Patterns in the Therapeutic Relationships.* Hampshire: Palgrave Macmillan; 2010.

Murdoch C, Denz-Penhey H. *Chronic Fatigue Syndrome: A Patient-Centered Approach.* Oxford: Radcliffe Medical Press; 2002.

Murray CJL, Ezzati M, Lopez AD, *et al.* Comparative quantification of health risks: conceptual framework and methodological issues. *Popul Health Metr.* 2003; **1**(1): 1–20.

Murray M. *Beyond the Myths and Magic of Mentoring: How to Facilitate an Effective Mentoring Process.* San Francisco, CA: Jossey-Bass; 2001.

Myers MF. *Intimate Relationships in Medical School: How to Make them Work.* Thousand Oaks, CA: Sage; 2000.

National Research Council, Committee on Risk Perception and Communication. *Improving Risk Communication.* Washington, DC: National Academy Press; 1989.

Navarro AM, Voetsch KP, Liburd LC, *et al.* Charting the future of community health promotion:

recommendations from the National Expert Panel on Community Health Promotion. *Prev Chronic Dis.* 2007; **4**(3): A68.

Neher JO, Stevens NG. The One-Minute Preceptor: shaping the teaching conversation. *Fam Med.* 2003; **35**(6): 391–3.

Neilson S. *Call Me Doctor.* Lawrencetown, NS: Pottersfield Press; 2006.

Nelson WL, Han PKJ, Fagerlin A, *et al.* Rethinking the objectives of decision aids: a call for conceptual clarity. *Med Decis Making.* 2007; **27**(5): 609–18.

Nettleton S, Watt I, O'Malley L, *et al.* Understanding the narratives of people who live with medically unexplained illness. *Patient Educ Couns.* 2005; **56**(2): 205–10.

Neumann M, Edelhäuser F, Tauschel D, *et al.* Empathy decline and its reasons: a systematic review of studies with medical students and residents. *Acad Med.* 2011; **86**(8): 996–1009.

Newman B, Young RJ. A model for teaching total person approach to patient problems. *Nurs Res.* 1972; **21**(3): 264–9.

Newman D. *Families: A Sociological Perspective.* New York, NY: McGraw-Hill; 2008.

Nilsen S, Baerheim A. Feedback on video recorded consultations in medical teaching: why students loathe and love it – a focus-group based qualitative study. *BMC Med Educ.* 2005; **5**: 28.

Noonan WDM. Must an internship be miserable? *The Pharos.* 1995: 19–23. Quoted in Coombs RH. *Surviving Medical School.* London: Sage Publications; 1998.

Noordman J, Verhaak P, van Beljouw I, *et al.* Consulting room computers and their effect on general practitioner-patient communication. *Fam Pract.* 2010; **27**(6): 644–51.

Norcini J. The power of feedback. *Med Educ.* 2010; **44**(1): 16–17.

Norcini J, Burch V. Workplace-based assessment as an educational tool: AMEE Guide No. 31. *Med Teach.* 2007; **29**(9): 855–71.

Norman GR. The adult learner: a mythical species. *Acad Med.* 1999; **74**(8): 886–9.

Norman G. Editorial: what's the active ingredient in active learning? *Adv Health Sci Educ.* 2004; **9**(1): 1–3.

Novack DH, Epstein RM, Paulsen RH. Toward creating physician-healers: fostering medical students' self-awareness, personal growth, and well-being. *Acad Med.* 1999; **74**(5): 516–20.

Novack DH, Suchman AL, Clark W, *et al.* Calibrating the physician: personal awareness and effective patient care. *JAMA.* 1997; **278**(6): 502–9.

Nutting PA (ed). *Community-Oriented Primary Care: From Principle to Practice.* Albuquerque: University of New Mexico Press; 1990.

O'Connell D, White MK, Platt FW. Disclosing unanticipated outcomes of medical errors. *J Clin Outcomes Manag.* 2003; **10**(1): 26–9.

O'Connor AM, Stacey D, Légaré F. Coaching to support patients in making decisions. *BMJ.* 2008; **336**(7638): 228–9.

Ofri D. *Singular Intimacies: Becoming a Doctor at Bellevue.* Boston, MA: Beacon Press; 2003.

Ofri D. *Incidental Findings: Lessons from My Patients in the Art of Medicine.* Boston, MA: Beacon Press; 2005.

Ofri D. *Medicine in Translation: Journeys with My Patients.* Boston, MA: Beacon Press; 2010.

Oldham J. Aspects of countertransference. *J Psychiatr Pract.* 2012; **18**(2): 69.

Olesen J. Understanding the biologic basis of migraine. *N Engl J Med.* 1994; **331**(25): 1713–14.

Osler W. *Aequanimitas With Other Addresses to Medical Students, Nurses and Practitioners of Medicine.* 3rd ed. London: The Blakiston Division, McGraw-Hill Book Company; 1932.

Ottawa Charter for Health Promotion. *Ottawa Charter for Health Promotion.* 1986.

Oxford Textbook of Medicine. The maladies of modernization: sickness in the system itself; Oxford: Oxford University Press; 2002.

Paas F, Renkl A, Sweller J. Cognitive load theory and instructional design: recent developments. *Educational Psychologist.* 2003; **38**(1): 1–4.

Paas F, Renkl A, Sweller J. Cognitive load theory: instructional implications of interaction between information structures and cognitive structure. *Instructional Science.* 2004; **32**: 1–8.

Palaccia T, Tardif J, Triby E, *et al.* An analysis of clinical reasoning through a recent and comprehensive approach: the dual-process theory. *Med Educ Online.* 2011; **16**: 10.3402/meo.v16i0.5890.

Paling J. Strategies to help patients understand risks. *BMJ.* 2003; **327**(7417): 745–8.

Paling J. *Helping Patients Understand Risks.* Gainsville, FL: The Risk Communication Institute; 2006.

Palmer PJ. *The Courage to Teach: Exploring the Inner Landscape of a Teacher's Life.* 10th anniversary ed. San Francisco, CA: Jossey-Bass; 2007.

Pangaro L. A new vocabulary and other innovations for improving descriptive in-training evaluations. *Acad Med.* 1999; **74**(11): 1203–7.

Papadopoulos R, Lay M, Lees S, *et al.* The impact of migration on health beliefs and behaviours: the case of Ethiopian refugees in the UK. *Contemp Nurse.* 2003; **15**(3): 210–21.

Pappas G, Queen S, Hadden W, *et al.* The increasing disparity in mortality between socioeconomic groups in the United States, 1960 and 1986. *N Engl J Med.* 1993; **329**(2): 103–9.

Parchman M, Ferrer R, Blanchard S. Geography and geographic information systems in family medicine research. *Fam Med.* 2002; **34**(2): 132–7.

Paro HBMS, Morales NMO, Silva CHM, *et al.* Health-related quality of life of medical students. *Med Educ.* 2010; **44**(3): 227–35.

Patz JA, Epstein PR, Burke TA, *et al.* Global climate change and emerging infectious diseases. *JAMA.* 1996; **275**(3): 217–23.

Pavis S, Cunningham-Burley S, Amos A. Health related behavioural change in context: young people in transition. *Soc Sci Med.* 1998; **47**(10): 1407–18.

Payne M. *Teamwork in Multiprofessional Care.* Chicago, IL: Lyceum Books; 2000.

Peek ME, Wilson SC, Gorawara-Bhat R, *et al.* Barriers and facilitators to shared decision-making among African-Americans with diabetes. *J Gen Intern Med.* 2009; **24**(10): 1135–9.

Pendleton D, Schofield T, Tate P, *et al. The New Consultation.* Oxford: Oxford University Press; 2003.

Perera J, Nagarajah L, Win K, *et al.* Formative feedback to students: the mismatch between faculty perceptions and student expectations. *Med Teach.* 2008; **30**(4): 395–9.

Perry WG Jr. *Forms of Intellectual and Ethical Development in the College Years.* New York: Holt, Rinehart and Winston; 1970.

Perry WG. Cognitive and ethical growth: the making of meaning. In: Chickering AW and Associates. *The Modern American College.* San Francisco, CA: Jossey-Bass; 1981.

Peterkin AD. *Staying Human during Residency Training: How to Survive and Thrive after Medical School.* 4th ed. Toronto, ON: University of Toronto Press; 2008.

Petrini C, Thomas R. Meetings, stressful meetings. *Training Dev.* 1995; **49**(10): 11.

Piaget J. *The Psychology of Intelligence.* New York: Harcourt Brace; 1950.

Piazza J, Conrad K, Wilbur J. Exercise behavior among female occupational health nurses: influence of self-efficacy, perceived health control, and age. *AAOHN J.* 2001; **49**(2): 79–86.

Pincus H. Alcohol, drug and mental disorders, psychosocial problems, and behavioural intervention in primary care. In: Showstack J, Rothman AA, Hassmiller SB (eds). *The Future of Primary Care.* San Francisco, CA: Jossey-Bass; 2004.

Pincus T, Esther R, DeWalt DA, *et al.* Social conditions and self-management are more powerful determinants of health than access to care. *Ann Intern Med.* 1998; **129**(5): 406–11.

Pink D. *Drive: The Surprising Truth About What Motivates Us.* New York, NY: Riverhead Books; 2011.

Plsek PE, Greenhalgh T. Complexity science: the challenge of complexity in health care. *BMJ.* 2001; **323**(7313): 625–8.

Poirier S. *Doctors in the Making.* Iowa City: University of Iowa Press; 2009.

Polanyi M. *The Tacit Dimension.* London: Routledge & Kegan Paul; 1966.

Polanyi M. *Knowing and Being: Essays by Michael Polanyi.* London: Routledge & Kegan Paul; 1969.

Poole G. The culturally sculpted self in self-directed learning. *Med Educ.* 2012; **46**(8): 728–37.

Porter-O'Grady T. Embracing conflict: building a healthy community. *Health Care Manag Rev.* 2004; **29**(3): 181–7.

Post SG, Puchalski CM, Larson DB. Physicians and patient spirituality: professional boundaries, competency, and ethics. *Ann Intern Med.* 2000; **132**(7): 578–83.

Pottie K, Brown JB, Dunn S. The resettlement of central American men in Canada: from emotional distress to successful integration. *Refugee.* 2005; **22**(2): 101–11.

Power C, Li L, Manor O. A prospective study of limiting longstanding illness in early adulthood. *Int J Epidemiol.* 2000; **29**(1): 131–9.

Pratt DD and Associates. *Five Perspectives on Teaching in Adult and Higher Education.* Malabar, FL: Krieger Publishing; 1998.

Preven DW, Kachur EK, Kupfer RB, *et al.* Interviewing skills of first-year medical students. *J Med Educ.* 1986; **61**(10): 842–4.

Prochaska JO. Decision making in the transtheoretical model of behavior change. *Med Decis Making.* 2008; **28**(6): 845–9.

Prochaska JO, DiClemente CC. *The Transtheoretical Approach: Crossing Traditional Boundaries of Therapy.* Homewood, IL: Dow/Jones Irwin; 1984.

Pronovost PJ, Freischlag JA. Improving teamwork to reduce surgical mortality. *JAMA.* 2010; **304**(15): 1721–2.

Puddester D, Edward S. The future of medical education in Canada: brief literature review physician wellness and work/life balance. In: *The Future of Medical Education in Canada: Environmental Scan Project; National Literature Reviews.* Toronto, ON: Wilson Centre for Research in Education, University of Toronto; 2008. Available at: www.afmc.ca/future-of-medical-education-in-canada/medical-doctor-project/pdf/National%20Literature%20Reviews.pdf (accessed February 1, 2013).

Pullen C, Fiandt K, Walker SN. Determinants of preventive service utilization in rural older women. *Journal of Gerontological Nursing.* 2001; **27**(1): 40–51.

Quill TE, Brody H. Physician recommendations and patient autonomy: finding a balance between physician power and patient choice. *Ann Intern Med.* 1996; **125**(9): 763–9.

Ramsay J, Campbell JL, Schroter S, *et al.* The General Practice Assessment Survey (GPAS): tests of data quality and measurement properties. *Fam Pract.* 2000; **17**(5): 372–9.

Rao JK, Anderson LA, Inui TS, *et al.* Communication interventions make a difference in conversations between physicians and patients: a systematic review of the evidence. *Med Care.* 2007; **45**(4): 340–9.

Reber AS. *Implicit Learning and Tacit Knowledge: An Essay on the Cognitive Unconscious.* Oxford: Oxford University Press; 1993.

Rees CE, Monrouxe LV. "A morning since eight of just pure grill": a multischool qualitative study of student abuse. *Acad Med.* 2011; **86**(11): 1374–82.

Reeves S, Lewin S, Espin S, *et al. Interprofessional Teamwork for Health and Social Care.* Oxford: Wiley-Blackwell; 2010.

Reifman A, Barnes GM, Dintcheff BA, *et al.* Health values buffer social-environmental risks for adolescent alcohol misuse. *Psychol Addict Behav.* 2001; **15**(3): 249–51.

Reilly P. *To Do No Harm: A Journey through Medical School.* Dover, MA: Auburn House Publishing; 1987.

Reinders ME, Blankenstein AH, Knol DL, *et al.* Validity aspects of the patient feedback questionnaire on consultation skills (PFC), a promising learning instrument in medical education. *Patient Educ Couns.* 2009; **76**(2): 202–6.

Reinders ME, Blankenstein AH, van der Horst HE, *et al.* Does patient feedback improve the consultation skills of general practice trainees? a controlled trial. *Med Educ.* 2010; **44**(2): 156–64.

Reiser D, Schroder AK. *Patient Interviewing: The Human Dimension.* Baltimore, MD: Williams & Wilkins; 1980.

Reiser SJ. *Technological Medicine: The Changing World of Doctors and Patients.* Cambridge: Cambridge University Press; 2009.

Remen RN. Educating for the mission, meaning, and compassion. In: Glazier S (ed). *The Heart of Learning: Spirituality in Education.* New York, NY: Penguin Group; 1999.

Rhoades DR, McFarland KF, Finch WH, *et al.* Speaking and interruptions during primary care office visits. *Fam Med.* 2001; **33**(7): 528–32.

Rimal RN. Closing the knowledge-behavior gap in health promotion: the mediating role of self-efficacy. *Health Commun.* 2000; **12**(3): 219–37.

Rimal RN. Analyzing the physician-patient interaction: an overview of six methods and future research directions. *Health Commun.* 2001; **13**(1): 89–99.

Roberts LW, Turner TD, Lyketsos C, *et al.* Perceptions of academic vulnerability associated with personal illness: a study of 1,027 students at nine medical schools. Collaborative Research Group on Medical Student Health. *Compr Psychiatry.* 2001; **42**(1): 1–15.

Roff S, McAleer S. What is educational climate? *Med Teach.* 2001; **23**(4): 333–4.

Rogers C. *Client-Centered Therapy: Its Current Practice Implications and Theory.* Cambridge, MA: Riverside Press; 1951.

Rogers CR. *Freedom to Learn for the 80s.* Columbus, OH: Merrill Publishing; 1982.

Rogers H, Carline JD, Paauw DS. Examination room presentations in general internal medicine clinic: patients' and students' perceptions. *Acad Med.* 2003; **78**(9): 945–9.

Rollnick S, Miller WR, Butler CC. *Motivational Interviewing in Health Care: Helping Patients Change Behavior.* New York, NY: Guilford Press; 2008.

Rose G. Strategy of prevention: lessons from cardiovascular disease. *Br Med J (Clin Res Ed).* 1981; **282**(6279): 1847–51.

Rosenbaum L, Lamas D. Residents' duty hours: toward an empirical narrative. *N Engl J Med.* 2012; **367**(21): 2044–9.

Rosenthal GE, Shannon SE. The use of patient perceptions in the evaluation of health-care delivery systems. *Med Care.* 1997; **35**(11): NS58–68.

Roter DL. Patient participation in the patient-provider interaction: the effects of patient question-asking on the quality of interaction, satisfaction and compliance. *Health Educ Monogr.* 1977; **5**(4): 281–315.

Roter DL, Cole KA, Kern DE, *et al.* An evaluation of residency training in interviewing skills and the psychosocial domain of medical practice. *J Gen Intern Med.* 1990; **5**(4): 347–54.

Roter DL, Hall JA. Physicians' interviewing styles and medical information obtained from patients. *J Gen Intern Med.* 1987; **2**(5): 325–9.

Roter DL, Hall JA. Physician gender and patient-centered communication: a critical review of empirical research. *Annu Rev Public Health.* 2004; **25**: 497–519.

Roter DL, Hall JA, Aoki Y. Physician gender effects in medical communication: a meta-analytic review. *JAMA.* 2002; **288**(6): 756–64.

Roter DL, Larson S. The relationship between residents' and attending physicians' communication during primary care visits: an illustrative use of the Roter Interaction Analysis System. *Health Commun.* 2001; **13**(1): 33–48.

Rourke L, Leduc D, Constantin E, *et al.* Update on well-baby and well-child care from 0 to 5 years: what's new in the Rourke Baby Record? *Can Fam Physician.* 2010; **56**(12): 1285–90.

Roux AVD. Invited commentary: places, people, health. *Am J Epidemiol.* 2002; **155**(6): 516–19.

Rowe MB. Wait time: slowing down may be a way of speeding up. *J Teach Educ.* 1986; **37**(1): 43–50.

Rubenstein W, Talbot Y. *Medical Teaching in Ambulatory Care.* 3rd ed. Toronto, ON: University of Toronto Press; 2013.

Ruddy G, Rhee K. Transdisciplinary teams in primary care for the underserved: a literature review. *J Health Care Poor Underserved.* 2005; **16**(2): 248–56.

Rudebeck CE. Imagination and empathy in the consultation. *Br J Gen Pract.* 2002; **52**(479): 450–3.

Rudland J, Wilkinson T, Wearn A, *et al.* A student-centred feedback model for educators. *Clin Teach.* 2013; **10**(2): 99–102.

Rudnick A, Roe D (eds). *Serious Mental Illness: Person-Centered Approaches.* Oxford: Radcliffe Publishing; 2011.

Russell G, Brown JB, Stewart M. Managing injured workers: family physicians' experiences. *Can Fam Physician.* 2005; **51**: 78–9.

Sackett D, Rosenberg W, Gray JAM, *et al.* Evidence-based medicine: what it is and what it isn't. *BMJ.* 1996; **312**(7023): 71–2.

Sackett DL, Straus SE, Richardson WS, *et al. Evidence-Based Medicine: How to Practice and Teach EBM.* 2nd ed. New York, NY: Churchill Livingstone; 2000.

Sacks O. *Awakenings.* London: Pan Books; 1982.

Sacks O. *One Leg to Stand On.* London: Gerald Duckworth; 1984.

Sacks O. Clinical tales. *Lit Med.* 1986; **5**: 16–23.

Sacks O. *Seeing Voices: A Journey into the World of the Deaf.* Berkeley: University of California Press; 1989.

Safran DG, Kosinski M, Tarlov AR, *et al.* The Primary Care Assessment Survey: tests of data quality and measurement performance. *Med Care.* 1998; **36**(5): 728–39.

Sakalys JA. Restoring the patient's voice: the therapeutics of illness narratives. *J Holist Nurs.* 2003; **21**(3): 228–41.

Salmon DA, Moulton LH, Omer SB, *et al.* Factors associated with refusal of childhood vaccines among parents of school-aged children: a case-control study. *Arch Pediatr Adolesc Med.* 2005; **159**(5): 470–6.

Salmon DA, Pan WK, Omer SB, *et al.* Vaccine knowledge and practices of primary care providers of exempt vs. vaccinated children. *Hum Vaccin.* 2008; **4**(4): 286–91.

Sandhu H, Adams A, Singleton L, *et al.* The impact of gender dyads on doctor-patient communication: a systematic review. *Patient Educ Couns.* 2009; **76**(3): 348–55.

Sands SA, Stanley P, Charon R. Pediatric narrative oncology: interprofessional training to promote empathy, build teams, and prevent burnout. *J Support Oncol.* 2008; **6**(7): 307–12.

Santrock J. *A Topical Approach to Life-Span Development.* New York, NY: McGraw-Hill; 2007.

Sargeant J, Armson H, Chesluk B, *et al.* The processes and dimensions of informed self-assessment: a conceptual model. *Acad Med.* 2010; **85**(7): 1212–20.

Sargeant J, Loney E, Murphy G. Effective interprofessional teams: "Contact is not enough" to build a team. *J Contin Educ Health Prof.* 2008; **28**(4): 228–34.

Saunders JC. Families living with severe mental illness: a literature review. *Issues Ment Health Nurs.* 2003; **24**(2): 175–98.

Sawicki W. We are not like other people: identity loss and reconstruction following migration. In: Harris DL (ed). *Counting Our Losses: Reflecting on Change, Loss and Transition in Everyday Life.* New York, NY: Routledge; 2011.

Scanlon L (ed). *"Becoming" a Professional: An Interdisciplinary Analysis of Professional Learning.* New York, NY: Springer; 2011.

Scarf M. *Intimate Worlds: Life Inside the Family.* New York, NY: Random House; 1995.

Schaeffer JA. *Transference and Countertransference in Non-Analytic Therapy: Double-Edge Swords.* Lanham, MD: University Press of America; 2007.

Schamess G. Ego psychology. In: Berzoff J, Melano Flanzagn I, Hertz P (eds). *Inside Out and Outside In. Psychodynamic clinical theory and practice in contemporary multicultural contexts.* London: Jason Aronson; 1996.

Schechter GP, Blank LL, Godwin HA Jr, *et al.* Refocusing on history-taking skills during internal medicine training. *Am J Med.* 1996; **101**(2): 210–16.

Schleifer R, Vannatta JB. *The Chief Concern of Medicine: The Integration of the Medical Humanities and Narrative Knowledge into Medical Practices.* Ann Arbor: University of Michigan Press; 2013.

Schlesinger EG. *Health Care Social Work Practice: Concepts and Strategies.* St. Louis, MO: Times Mirror/ Mosby College Publishing; 1985.

Schoenbach VJ, Wagner EH, Karon JM. The use of epidemiologic data for personal risk assessment in health hazard/health risk appraisal programs. *J Chronic Dis.* 1983; **36**(9): 625–38.

Schön DA. *Educating the Reflective Practitioner.* San Francisco, CA: Jossey-Bass; 1987.

Schriver J. *Human Behavior and the Social Environment.* 4th ed. New York, NY: Pearson; 2004.

Schulz R, Beach SR. Caregiving as a risk factor for mortality. *JAMA.* 1999; **282**(23): 2215–19.

Schulz R, Mendelsohn AB, Haley WE, *et al.* End-of-life care and the effects of bereavement on family caregivers of persons with dementia. *N Engl J Med.* 2003; **349**(20): 1936–42.

Schunk DH, Zimmerman BJ. *Motivation and Self-Regulated Learning: Theory, Research, and Applications.* London: Routledge; 2008.

Schwartz LM, Woloshin S, Welch HG. Helping consumers to know their chances. In: Edwards A, Elwyn

G (eds). *Shared Decision-Making in Health Care: Achieving Evidence-Based Patient Choice*. Oxford: Oxford University Press; 2009.

Schwartz MA, Wiggins O. Science, humanism and the nature of medical practice: a phenomenological view. *Perspect Biol Med*. 1985; **28**(3): 331–61.

Scott GS, Cohen D, DiCicco-Bloom B, *et al*. Understanding healing relationships in primary care. *Ann Fam Med*. 2008; **6**(4): 315–22.

Scott JG, Cohen D, DiCicco-Bloom B, *et al*. Antibiotic use in acute respiratory infections and the ways patients pressure physicians for a prescription. *J Fam Pract*. 2001; **50**(10): 853–8.

Searight HR, Gafford J. Cultural diversity at the end of life: issues and guidelines for family physicians. *Am Fam Physician*. 2005; **71**(3): 515–22.

Seeman TE. Social ties and health: the benefits of social integration. *Ann Epidemiol*. 1996; **6**(5): 442–51.

Seifert MH Jr. Qualitative designs for assessing interventions in primary care: examples from medical practice. In: Tudiver F, Bass MJ, Dunn EV (eds). *Assessing Interventions: Traditional and Innovative Methods*. Newbury Park, CA: Sage; 1992.

Selwyn PA. The Island. *Ann Fam Med*. 2008; **6**(1): 78–9.

Sfard A. On two metaphors for learning and the dangers of choosing just one. *Educ Res*. 2008; **27**(2): 4–13.

Shachak A, Reis S. The impact of electronic medical records on patient-doctor communication during consultation: a narrative literature review. *J Eval Clin Pract*. 2009; **15**(4): 641–9.

Shaikh A, Knobloch LM, Stiles WB. The use of a verbal response mode coding system in determining patient and physician roles in medical interviews. *Health Commun*. 2001; **13**(1): 49–60.

Shanafelt TD. Enhancing meaning in work: a prescription for preventing physician burnout and promoting patient-centered care. *JAMA*. 2009; **302**(12): 1338–40.

Shanafelt TD, Bradley KA, Wipf JE, *et al*. Burnout and self-reported patient care in an internal medicine residency program. *Ann Intern Med*. 2002; **136**(5): 358–67.

Shann S, Wilson JD. Patients' attitudes to the presence of medical students in a genitourinary medicine clinic: a cross sectional survey. *Sex Transm Infect*. 2006; **82**: 52–4.

Shannon J, Kirkley B, Ammerman A, *et al*. Self-efficacy as a predictor of dietary change in a low-socioeconomic-status southern adult population. *Health Educ Behav*. 1997; **24**(3): 357–68.

Sherwood NE, Jeffery RW. The behavioral determinants of exercise: implications for physical activity interventions. *Annu Rev Nutr*. 2000; **20**: 21–44.

Shi L, Starfield B, Xu J. Validating the adult primary care assessment tool. *J Fam Pract*. 2001; **50**(2): 161–75.

Shields CG, Epstein RM, Fiscella K, *et al*. Influence of accompanied encounters on patient-centeredness with older patients. *J Am Board Fam Pract*. 2005; **18**(5): 344–54.

Shields SG, Candib LM (eds). *Woman-Centered Care in Pregnancy and Childbirth*. Oxford: Radcliffe Publishing; 2010.

Shulman LS. Signature pedagogies in the professions. *Daedalus*. 2005a; **134**(3): 52–9.

Shulman LS. Pedagogies of uncertainty. *Liberal Education*. 2005b; **91**(2): 18–25.

Shute VJ. Focus on formative feedback. *Rev Educ Res*. 2008; **78**(1): 153–89.

Sidell J. Adult adjustment to chronic illness: a review of the literature. *Health Soc Work*. 2001; **22**(1): 5–12.

Silver HK. Medical students and medical school. *JAMA*. 1982; **247**: 309–10.

Silver KH, Glicken AD. Medical student abuse: incidence, severity, and significance. *JAMA*. 1990; **263**(4): 527–32.

Silverman J, Kurtz S, Draper J. *Skills for Communicating with Patients*. 2nd ed. Oxford: Radcliffe Publishing; 2004.

Simpson MA. *Medical Education: A Critical Approach*. London: Butterworths; 1972.

Skeff KM, Mutha S. Role models: guiding the future of medicine. *N Engl J Med*. 1998; **339**(27): 2015–17.

Skeff KM, Stratos GA. *Methods for Teaching Medicine*. Philadelphia, PA: American College of Physicians; 2010.

Smith GD, Hart C, Blane D, *et al.* Lifetime socioeconomic position and mortality: prospective observational study. *BMJ.* 1997; **314**(7080): 547–52.

Smith PJ, Chu SY, Barker LE. Children who have received no vaccines: who are they and where do they live? *Pediatrics.* 2004; **114**(1): 187–95.

Smith RC, Dorsey AM, Lyles JS, *et al.* Teaching self-awareness enhances learning about patient-centered interviewing. *Acad Med.* 1999; **74**(11): 1242–8.

Söderlund LL, Madson MB, Rabak S, *et al.* A systematic review of motivational interviewing training for general health care practitioners. *Patient Educ Couns.* 2011; **84**(1): 16–26.

Sotile WM, Sotile MO. *The Resilient Physician: Effective Emotional Management for Doctors and Their Medical Organizations.* Chicago, IL: American Medical Association; 2002.

Spafford MM, Lingard L, Schryer CF, *et al.* Tensions in the field: teaching standards of practice in optometry case presentations. *Optom Vis Sci.* 2004; **81**(10): 800–6.

Speidel J. Environment and health: 1. Population consumption and human health. *CMAJ.* 2000; **163**(5): 551–6.

Spence JC. *The Purpose and Practice of Medicine: Selections from the Writings of Sir James Spence.* London: Oxford University Press; 1960.

Spencer JA, Jordan RK. Learner centred approaches in medical education. *BMJ.* 1999; **318**(7193): 1280–83.

Squire S, Hill P. The expert patient program. *Clin Govern.* 2006; **11**: 17–23.

Stacey D, Bennett CL, Barry MJ, *et al.* Decision aids for people facing health treatment or screening decisions. *Cochrane Database Syst Rev.* 2011; (10): CD001431.

Stachtchenko S, Jenicek M. Conceptual differences between prevention and health promotion: research implications for community health programs. *Can J Public Health.* 1990; **81**(1): 53–9.

Stagnaro-Green A. Applying adult learning principles to medical education in the United States. *Med Teach.* 2004; **26**(1): 79–85.

Starfield B. *Primary Care: Balancing Health Needs, Services, and Technology.* New York, NY: Oxford University Press; 1998.

Starfield B. New paradigms for quality in primary care. *Br J Gen Pract.* 2001; **51**(465): 303–9.

Starfield B, Gervas J, Mangin D. Clinical care and health disparities. *Annu Rev Public Health.* 2012; **33**: 89–106.

Starfield B, Wray C, Hess K, *et al.* The influence of patient-practitioner agreement on outcome of care. *Am J Public Health.* 1981; **71**(2): 127–31.

Statistics Canada. *The Daily: Canada's Population Estimates.* Ottawa, ON: Author; 2010. Available at: www.statcan.gc.ca/daily-quotidien/100628/dq100628a-eng.htm (accessed April 1, 2011).

Stein HF. What is therapeutic in clinical relationships? *Fam Med.* 1985a; **17**(5): 188–94.

Stein HF. *The Psycho-Dynamics of Medical Practice: Unconscious Factors in Patient Care.* Berkeley: University of California Press; 1985b.

Stein M. *The Lonely Patient: How We Experience Illness.* New York, NY: HarperCollins; 2007.

Steine S, Finset A, Laerum E. A new, brief questionnaire (PEQ) developed in primary health care for measuring patients' experience of interaction, emotion and consultation outcome. *Fam Pract.* 2001; **18**(4): 410–18.

Steinert Y. Educational theory and strategies for teaching and learning professionalism. In: Cruess RL, Cruess SR, Steinert Y (eds). *Teaching Medical Professionalism.* Cambridge: Cambridge University Press; 2009.

Steinhauser KE, Voils CI, Clipp EC, *et al.* "Are You at Peace?" One item to probe spiritual concerns at the end of life. *Arch Intern Med.* 2006; **166**(1): 101–5.

Stensland P, Malterud K. Unravelling empowering internal voices: a case study on the interactive use of illness diaries. *Fam Pract.* 2001; **18**(4): 425–9.

Sterkenburg A, Barach P, Kalkman C, *et al.* When do supervising physicians decide to entrust residents with unsupervised tasks? *Acad Med.* 2010; **85**(9): 1408–17.

Stern DT (ed). *Measuring Medical Professionalism.* Oxford: Oxford University Press; 2006.

Stern DT, Papadakis M. The developing physician: becoming a professional. *N Engl J Med*. 2006; **355**(17): 1794–9.

Stetten D Jr. Coping with blindness. *N Engl J Med*. 1981; **305**(8): 458–60.

Stevens J. Brief encounter. *J R Coll Gen Pract*. 1974; **24**(138): 5–22.

Stevenson FA, Barry CA, Britten N, *et al*. Doctor-patient communication about drugs: The evidence for shared decision making. *Soc Sci Med*. 2000; **50**(6): 829–40.

Stevenson FA, Cox K, Britten N, *et al*. A systematic review of the research on communication between patients and health care professionals about medicines: the consequences for concordance. *Health Expect*. 2004; **7**(3): 235–45.

Steverink N, Lindenberg S, Slaets J. How to understand and improve older people's self-management of well-being. *Eur J Ageing*. 2005; **2**(4): 235–44.

Stewart AL, Nápoles-Springer AM, Gregorich SE, *et al*. Interpersonal processes of care survey: patient-reported measures for diverse groups. *Health Serv Res*. 2007a; **42**(3 Pt. 1): 1235–56.

Stewart EE, Johnson BC. Huddles improve office efficiency in mere minutes. *Fam Pract Manag*. 2007; **14**(6): 27–9.

Stewart MA. What is a successful doctor-patient interview? A study of interactions and outcomes. *Soc Sci Med*. 1984; **19**(2): 167–75.

Stewart M. Towards a global definition of patient centred care. *BMJ*. 2001; **322**(7284): 444–5.

Stewart M. Continuity, care, and commitment: the course of patient-clinician relationships. *Ann Fam Med*. 2004; **2**(5): 388–90.

Stewart M. Reflections on the doctor-patient relationship: from evidence and experience. *Br J Gen Pract*. 2005; **55**: 793–801.

Stewart M, Brown JB, Boon H, *et al*. Evidence on patient-doctor communication. *Cancer Prev Control*. 1999; **3**(1): 25–30.

Stewart M, Brown JB, Donner A, *et al*. The impact of patient-centred care on patient outcome. *J Fam Pract*. 2000; **49**(9): 796–804.

Stewart M, Brown JB, Hammerton J, *et al*. Improving communication between doctors and breast cancer patients. *Ann Fam Med*. 2007b; **5**(5): 387–94.

Stewart MA, Brown JB, Levenstein JH, *et al*. The patient-centred clinical method: III. Changes in resident's performance over two months of training. *Fam Pract*. 1986; **3**: 164–7.

Stewart M, Brown JB, Weston W. Patient-centred interviewing part III: five provocative questions. *Can Fam Physician*. 1989; **35**: 159–61.

Stewart M, Brown JB, Weston WW, *et al*. *Patient-Centered Medicine: Transforming the Clinical Method*. Thousand Oaks, CA: Sage Publications; 1995.

Stewart M, Brown JB, Weston WW, *et al*. *Patient-Centered Medicine: Transforming the Clinical Method*. 2nd ed. Oxford: Radcliffe Medical Press; 2003.

Stewart MA, Buck CW. Physicians' knowledge of and response to patients' problems. *Med Care*. 1977; **15**(7): 578–85.

Stewart M, Maddocks H. Making the case for research on symptoms in family practice. Manuscript in preparation; 2013.

Stewart MA, McWhinney IR, Buck CW. How illness presents: a study of patient behavior. *J Fam Pract*. 1975; **2**(6): 411–14.

Stewart MA, McWhinney IR, Buck CW. The doctor/patient relationship and its effect upon outcome. *J R Coll Gen Pract*. 1979; **29**(199): 77–81.

Stewart M, Meredith L, Ryan BL, *et al*. *The Patient Perception of Patient-Centredness Questionnaire (PPPC)*. Centre for Studies in Family Medicine, editor. Paper #04–1. London, ON: The University of Western Ontario Working Papers; 2004.

Stewart M, Ryan BL. *Catalogue of Curricula for Medical Education in Patient-Centred Care*. Report commissioned and prepared for the Canadian Medical Association; 2012.

Stewart M, Ryan BL, Bodea C. Is patient-centred care associated with lower diagnostic costs? *Healthcare Policy*. 2011; **6**(4): 27–31.

Stiggelbout AM, Van der Weijden T, De Wit MPT, *et al.* Shared decision making: really putting patients at the centre of healthcare. *BMJ.* 2012; **344**: e256.

Strasser T, Jeanneret I, Raymond L. Ethical aspects of prevention trials. In: Doxiadis S (ed). *Ethical Dilemmas in Health Promotion.* Toronto: John Wiley and Sons; 1987.

Strauss A, Glaser B. *Anguish: A Case History of a Dying Trajectory.* Mill Valley, CA: Sociology Press; 1970.

Street RL. Aiding medical decision-making: a communication perspective. *Med Decis Making.* 2007: **27**(5): 550–3.

Street RL, Haidet P. How well do doctors know their patients? Factors affecting patient understanding of patients' health beliefs. *J Gen Intern Med.* 2011; **26**(1): 21–7.

Street RL Jr, Millay B. Analyzing patient participation in medical encounters. *Health Commun.* 2001; **13**(1): 61–73.

Stroebe M, Schut H, Stroebe W. Health outcomes of bereavement. *Lancet.* 2007; **370**(9603): 1960–73.

Stuifbergen AK, Seraphine A, Roberts G. An explanatory model of health promotion and quality of life in chronic disabling conditions. *Nurs Res.* 2000; **49**(3): 122–9.

Styron W. *Darkness Visible.* New York, NY: Random House; 1990.

Susser M. A South Africa Odyssey in community health: a memoir of the impact of the teachings of Sidney Kark. *Am J Public Health.* 1993; **83**(7): 1039–42.

Sutcliffe KM, Lewton E, Rosenthal MM. Communication failures: an insidious contributor to medical mishaps. *Acad Med.* 2004; **79**(2): 186–94.

Sutkin G, Wagner E, Harris I, *et al.* What makes a good clinical teacher in medicine? A review of the literature. *Acad Med.* 2008; **83**(5): 452–66.

Svinicki MD. New directions in learning and motivation. *New Dir Teach Learn.* 1999; **80**: 5–27.

Svinicki M, McKeachie W. *McKeachie's Teaching Tips.* 13th ed. Belmont, CA: Wadsworth; 2011.

Swift TL, Dieppe PA. Using expert patients' narratives as an educational resource. *Patient Educ Couns.* 2004; **57**(1): 115–21.

Tait I. The history and function of clinical records [unpublished MD dissertation thesis]. University of Cambridge; 1979.

Takakua KM, Rubashkin N, Herzig KE (eds). *What I Learned in Medical School: Personal Stories of Young Doctors.* Berkley: University of California Press; 2004.

Takemura Y, Liu J, Atsumi R, Tsuda T. Development of a questionnaire to evaluate patient satisfaction with medical encounters. *Tohoku J Exp Med.* 2006; **210**(4): 373–81.

Tate P, Foulkes J, Neighbour R, *et al.* Assessing physicians' interpersonal skills via videotaped encounters: a new approach for the Royal College of General Practitioners Membership examination. *J Health Commun.* 1999; **4**(2): 143–52.

Tauber AI. *Patient Autonomy and the Ethics of Responsibility.* Cambridge, MA: MIT Press; 2005.

Taylor RB. *Medical Wisdom and Doctoring: The Art of 21st Century Practice.* New York, NY: Springer; 2010.

Teh CF, Karp JF, Kleinman A, *et al.* Older people's experiences of patient-centered treatment for chronic pain: a qualitative study. *Pain Med.* 2009; **10**(3): 521–30.

Ten Cate O. Trust, competence, and the supervisor's role in postgraduate training. *BMJ.* 2006; **333**(7571): 748–51.

Thorsen H, Witt K, Hollnagel H, *et al.* The purpose of the general practice consultation from the patient's perspective: theoretical aspects. *Fam Pract.* 2001; **18**(6): 638–43.

Thurman AR, Litts PL, O'Rourke K, *et al.* Patient acceptance of medical student participation in an outpatient obstetric/gynecologic clinic. *J Reprod Med.* 2006; **51**(2): 109–14.

Tiberius RG. Metaphors underlying the improvement of teaching and learning. *Br J Educ Technol.* 1986; **2**(17): 144–56.

Tiberius RG. The why of teacher/student relationships. *Teaching Excellence: Toward the Best in the Academy.* 1993–94; **5**(8): 1–5.

Tiberius RG, Sinai J, Flak EA. The role of teacher-learner relationships in medical education. In:

Norman GR, van der Vleuten CPM, Newble DI (eds). *International Handbook of Research in Medical Education*. Dordrecht: Kluwer Academic Publishers; 2002.

Tobias S, Duffy TM. *Constructivist Instruction: Success of Failure?* New York, NY: Routledge; 2009.

Tompkins J. Pedagogy of the distressed. *College English.* 1990; **52**(6): 653–60.

Tong A, Biringer A, Ofner-Agnostini M, *et al.* A cross-sectional study of maternity care providers and womens' knowledge, attitudes and behaviours towards influenza vaccination during pregnancy. *JOGC.* 2008; **30**(5): 404–10.

Toombs K. *The Meaning of Illness: A Phenomenological Account of the Different Perspectives of Physician and Patient.* Norwell, MA: Kluwer Academic Publishing; 1992.

Tosteson DC. Learning in medicine. *N Engl J Med.* 1979; **301**(13): 690–4.

Tough A. *The Adult's Learning Projects: A Fresh Approach to Theory and Practice in Adult Learning.* 2nd ed. Toronto: Ontario Institute for Studies in Education; 1979.

Toulmin S. *Return to Reason.* Cambridge, MA: Harvard University Press; 1991.

Toulmin S. *Cosmopolis: The Hidden Agenda of Modernity.* Chicago, IL: University of Chicago Press; 1992.

Towle A, Godolphin W. Framework for teaching and learning informed shared decision making. *BMJ.* 1999; **319**(7212): 766–71.

Tran P, Laurence JM, Weston KM, *et al.* The effect of parallel consulting on the quality of consultations in regional general practice. *Educ Prim Care.* 2012; **23**(3): 153–7.

Trevalon D, Murray-Garcia J. Cultural humility versus cultural competence: a critical distinction in defining physician training outcomes in multicultural education. *J Health Care Poor Underserved.* 1998; **9**(2): 117–25.

Tsimtsiou Z, Kerasidou O, Efstathiou N, *et al.* Medical students' attitudes toward patient-centred care: a longitudinal study. *Med Educ.* 2007; **41**(2): 146–53.

Tuckett D, Boulton M, Olson C, *et al. Meetings Between Experts: An Approach to Sharing Ideas in Medical Consultations.* London: Tavistock Publications; 1985.

Tudiver F, Brown JB, Medved W, *et al.* Making decisions about cancer screening when the guidelines are unclear or conflicting. *J Fam Pract.* 2001; **50**(8): 682–7.

US Preventive Services Task Force. *The Guide to Clinical Preventive Services.* Washington, DC: Department of Health and Human Services, Agency for Healthcare Research and Quality; 2012.

Uygur J, Brown JB, Jordan JM. *Understanding Compassion in Family Medicine: A Qualitative Study.* Paper presented at 40th North American Primary Care Research Group (NAPCRG) Annual Meeting. New Orleans, LA; 2012.

Van den Brink-Muinen A, van Dulmen SM, de Haes HCJM, *et al.* Has patients' involvement in the decision-making process changed over time? *Health Expect.* 2006; **9**(4): 333–42.

van der Heijden AG, Huysmans FT, van Hamersvelt HW. Foot volume increase on nifedipine is not prevented by pretreatment with diuretics. *J Hypertens.* 2004; **22**(2): 425–30.

van Hamersvelt HW, Kloke HJ, de Jong DJ, *et al.* Oedema formation with the vasodilators nifedipine and diazoxide: direct local effect or sodium retention? *J Hypertens.* 1996; **14**(8): 1041–5.

Van Tartwijk J, Driessen EW. Portfolios for assessment and learning: AMEE Guide no. 45. *Med Teach.* 2009; **31**(9): 790–801.

Van Thiel J, Kraan HF, van der Vleuten CPM. Reliability and feasibility of measuring medical inter-viewing skills: the revised Maastricht history-taking and advice checklist. *Med Educ.* 1991; **25**(3): 224–9.

Van Weel-Baumgarten E, Bolhuis S, Rosenbaum M, *et al.* Bridging the gap: how is integrating com-munication skills with medical content throughout the curriculum valued by students? *Patient Educ Couns.* 2013; **90**(2): 177–83.

Värlander S. The role of students' emotions in formal feedback situations. *Teach High Educ.* 2008; **13**(2): 145–56.

Vassilas C, Ho L. Video for teaching purposes. *Adv Psychiatr Treat.* 2000; **6**: 304–11.

Verby JE, Holden P, Davis RH. Peer review of consultations in primary care: the use of audiovisual recordings. *Br Med J.* 1979; **1**(6179): 1686–8.

Verghese A. The Gordon Wilson Lecture: "The Doctor in our own time": Fildes' painting and perceptions of physician attentiveness. *Trans Am Clin Climatol Assoc.* 2008; **119**: 117–26.

Vinson DC, Paden C, Devera-Sales A. Impact of medical student teaching on family physicians' use of time. *J Fam Pract.* 1996; **42**(3): 243–9.

Virshup BB, Oppenberg AA, Coleman MM. Strategic risk management: reducing malpractice claims through more effective patient-doctor communication. *Am J Med Qual.* 1999; **14**(4): 153–9.

Von Friederichs-Fitzwater MM, Gilgun J. Relational control in physician-patient encounters. *Health Commun.* 2001; **13**(1): 75–87.

Wade DT, Halligan PW. Do biomedical models of illness make for good healthcare systems? *BMJ.* 2004; **329**(7479): 1398–401.

Wagner E, Austin B, Hindmarsh M, *et al.* Improving chronic illness care: translating evidence into action. *Health Aff (Millwood).* 2001; **20**(6): 64–78.

Wainwright D (ed). *A Sociology of Health.* Thousand Oaks, CA: Sage; 2008.

Waitzkin H. Doctor-patient communication: clinical implications of social scientific research. *JAMA.* 1984; **252**(17): 2441–6.

Walker EA, Gelfand A, Katon WJ, *et al.* Adult health status of women with histories of childhood abuse and neglect. *Am J Med.* 1999; **107**(4): 332–9.

Walsh F (ed). *Spiritual Resources in Family Therapy.* 2nd ed. New York, NY: Guilford Press; 2009.

Walters L, Worley P, Prideaux D, *et al.* Do consultations in rural general practice take more time when pracitioners are precepting medical students? *Med Educ.* 2008; **42**(1): 69–73.

Walters L. Setting up a teaching practice. In: Kelly L (ed). *Community Medical Education: A Teacher's Handbook.* London: Radcliffe Publishing; 2012.

Wanek V, Born J, Novak P, *et al.* [Attitudes and health status determinants of participation in individually oriented health promotion] [German]. *Gesundheitswsen.* 1999; **61**(7): 346–52.

Ward M, MacRae H, Schlachta C, *et al.* Resident self-assessment of operative performance. *Am J Surg.* 2003; **185**(6): 521–4.

Watson WH, McDaniel SH. Relational therapy in medical settings: working with somatizing patients and their families. *J Clin Psychol.* 2000; **56**(8): 1065–82.

Watts D. *The Orange Wire Problem and Other Tales from the Doctor's Office.* Iowa City: University of Iowa Press; 2009.

Ways P, Engel JD, Finkelstein P. *Clinical Clerkships: The Heart of Professional Development.* Thousand Oaks, CA: Sage; 2000.

Wear D, Aultman JM (eds). *Professionalism in Medicine: Critical Perspectives.* New York, NY: Springer; 2006.

Wear D, Bickel J (eds). *Educating for Professionalism: Creating a Culture of Humanism in Medical Education.* Iowa City: University of Iowa Press; 2000.

Wear D, Kuczewski MG. The professionalism movement: can we pause? *Am J Bioeth.* 2004; **4**(2): 1–10.

Wear D, Zarconi J, Dhillon N. Teaching fearlessness: a manifesto. *Educ Health (Abingdon).* 2011; **24**(3): 668–75.

Weed LL. *Medical Records, Medical Education and Patient Care.* Chicago, IL: Year Book Medical Publishers; 1969.

Weimer M. *Learner-Centered Teaching: Five Key Changes to Practice.* San Francisco, CA: Jossey-Bass; 2002.

Weimer M. Focus on learning, transform teaching. *Change.* 2003; **35**(5): 48–54.

Weimer M. *Learner-Centered Teaching: Five Key Changes to Practice.* 2nd ed. San Francisco, CA: Jossey-Bass; 2013.

Wenger E. *Communities of Practice: Learning, Meaning, and Identity.* Cambridge: Cambridge University Press; 1998.

Wenger E, McDermott R, Snyder WM. *Cultivating Communities of Practice: A Guide to Managing Knowledge.* Boston, MA: Harvard Business School Press; 2002.

Westberg J, Jason H. *Collaborative Clinical Education: The Foundation of Effective Health Care.* New York, NY: Springer Publishing; 1993.

Weston WW. The person: a missing dimension in medical care and medical education. *Can Fam Physician.* 1988; **34**: 1705–803.

Weston WW. The teacher-student-patient relationship in family practice: common dilemmas. *Can Fam Physician.* 1989; **35**: 139–43.

Weston WW. Informed and shared decision-making: the crux of patient-centred care. *CMAJ.* 2001; **165**(4): 438–9.

Weston WW, Brown JB, Stewart MA. Patient-centred interviewing. Part I: Understanding patients' experiences. *Can Fam Physician.* 1989; **35**: 147–51.

Weston WW, Lipkin M Jr. Doctors learning communication skills: developmental issues. In: Stewart M, Roter D (eds). *Communicating With Medical Patients.* Newbury Park, CA: Sage; 1989.

Wheatley RR, Kelley MA, Peacock N, *et al.* Women's narratives on quality in prenatal care: a multicultural perspective. *Qual Health Res.* 2008; **18**(11): 1586–98

White KL. *The Task of Medicine: Dialogue at Wickenburg.* Menlo Park, CA: Henry J Kaiser Family Foundation; 1988.

Whitehead AN. *Science and the Modern World.* San Francisco, CA: Collins, Fontana Books; 1975.

Whitehead C. The doctor dilemma in interprofessional education and care: how and why will physicians collaborate? *Med Educ.* 2007; **41**(10):1010–6.

Whyte A, Burton I. Perception of risks in Canada. In: Burton I, McCullough R (eds). *Living With Risk: Institute for Environmental Studies.* Toronto, ON: University of Toronto; 1982.

Wilkinson JM, Targonski PV. Health promotion in a changing world: preparing for the genomics revolution. *Am J Health Promot.* 2003; **18**(2): 157–61.

Williams GC, Deci EL. The importance of supporting autonomy in medical education. *Ann Intern Med.* 1998; **129**(4): 303–8.

Williams MV, Davis T, Parker RM, *et al.* The role of health literacy in patient-physician communication. *Fam Med.* 2002; **34**(5): 383–9.

Williams SA, Rayman G, Tooke JE. Dependent oedema and attenuation of postural vasoconstriction associated with nifedipine therapy for hypertension in diabetic patients. *Eur J Clin Pharmacol.* 1989; **37**(4): 333–5.

Willis JAR. *The sea monster and the whirlpool.* Keynote address. Birmingham: Royal College of General Practitioners; 2002.

Winkleby MA, Fortmann SP, Barrett DC. Social class disparities in risk factors for disease: eight-year prevalence patterns by level of education. *Prev Med.* 1999; **19**(1): 1–12.

Woloschuk W, Harasym PH, Temple W. Attitude change during medical school: a cohort study. *Med Educ.* 2004; **38**(5): 522–34.

Wolpaw TM, Wolpaw DR, Papp KK. SNAPPS: a learner-centered model for outpatient education. *Acad Med.* 2003; **78**(9): 893–8.

Wood ML. Naming the illness: the power of words. *Fam Med.* 1991; **23**(7): 534–8.

Woodrow SI, Segouin C, Armbruster J, *et al.* Duty hour reforms in the United States, France, and Canada: is it time to refocus our attention on education. *Acad Med.* 2006; **81**(12): 1045–51.

Woolhouse S, Brown JB, Thind A. Meeting people where they're at: the experiences of family physicians engaging women using illicit drugs. *Ann Fam Med.* 2011; **9**(3): 244–9.

Woolhouse S, Brown JB, Thind A. Building through grief: vicarious trauma in a group of inner-city family physicians. *J Am Board Fam Med.* 2012; **25**(6): 840–6.

World Health Organization (WHO). *New Approaches to Health Education in Primary Health Care: Technical Report of a WHO Committee.* Geneva: WHO; 1983.

World Health Organization (WHO). Health promotion: a discussion document on the concept and principles. ICP/HSR 602. In: Health Promotion. Geneva: WHO; 1986a; **1**: 736.

World Health Organization (WHO). *Health Promotion: Concepts and Principles in Action; A Policy Framework.* London: WHO; 1986b.

Wouda JC, van de Wiel HBM. The communication competency of medical students, residents and consultants. *Patient Educ Couns.* 2012; **86**(1): 57–62.

Wouda JC, van de Wiel HBM. Education in patient-physician communication: how to improve effectiveness. *Patient Educ Couns.* 2013; **90**(1): 46–53.

Wright HJ, MacAdam DB. *Clinical Thinking and Practice: Diagnosis and Decision in Patient Care.* Edinburgh: Churchill Livingstone; 1979.

Wright SM, Carrese JA. Excellence in role modelling: insight and perspectives from the pros. *CMAJ.* 2002; **167**(6): 638–43.

Wright SM, Dern DE, Kolodner K, *et al.* Attributes of excellent attending-physician role models. *N Engl J Med.* 1998; **339**(27): 1986–93.

Wulff HR, Andur S, Rosenberg R. Philosophy of medicine: an introduction. Oxford: Blackwell Scientific Publications; 1986.

Wykurz G, Kelly D. Developing the role of patients as teachers: literature review. *BMJ.* 2002; **325**(7368): 818–21.

Xyrichis A, Lowton K. What fosters or prevents interprofessional teamworking in primary and community care? A literature review. *Int J Nurs Stud.* 2008; **45**(1): 140–53.

Yates FE. Self-organizing systems. In: Boyd CAR (ed). *The Logic of Life: The Challenge of Integrative Physiology.* New York, NY: Oxford University Press; 1993.

Yeates PJA, Stewart J, Barton JR. What can we expect of clinical teachers? Establishing consensus on applicable skills, attitudes and practices. *Med Educ.* 2008; **42**(2): 134–42.

You JJ, Alter DA, Iron K, *et al. Diagnostic Services in Ontario: Descriptive Analysis and Jurisdictional Review.* Toronto, ON: Institute for Clinical Evaluative Sciences; 2007.

Young A. *What Patients Taught Me: A Medical Student's Journey.* Seattle, WA: Sasquatch Books; 2004.

Zolnierek KB, DiMatteo MR. Physician communication and patient adherence to treatment: a meta-analysis. *Med Care.* 2009; **47**(8): 826–34.

Zwarenstein M, Reeves S. Working together but apart: Barriers and routes to nurse-physician collaboration. *Jt Comm J Qual Improv.* 2002; **28**(5): 242–7.

Index

Numbers in **bold** refer to figures, tables and boxes.

CPD with Radcliffe

You can now use a selection of our books to achieve CPD (Continuing Professional Development) points through directed reading.

We provide a free online form and downloadable certificate for your appraisal portfolio. Look for the CPD logo and register with us at: www.radcliffehealth.com/cpd

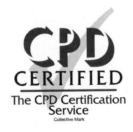